The Praeger Handbook of Chiropractic Health Care

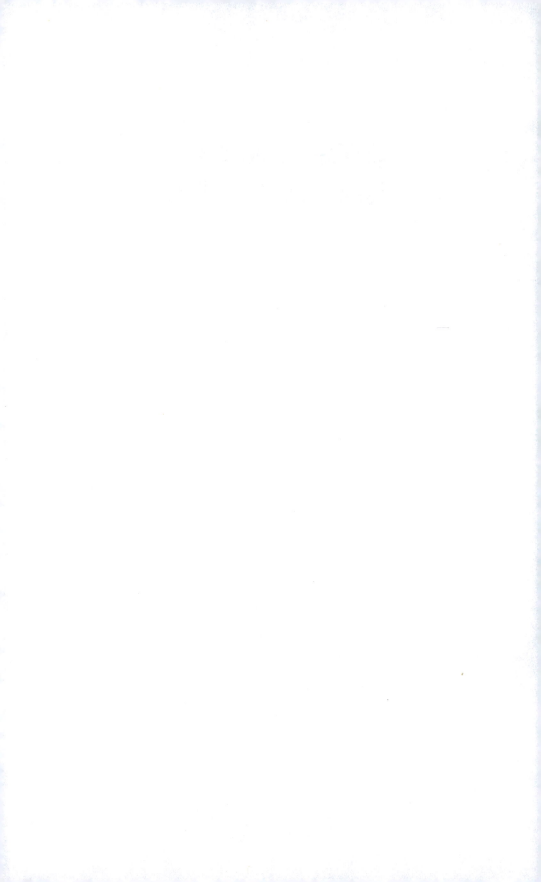

The Praeger Handbook of Chiropractic Health Care

Evidence-Based Practices

Cheryl Hawk, DC, PhD, CHES, Editor

Foreword by John Weeks

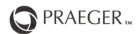

An Imprint of ABC-CLIO, LLC

Santa Barbara, California • Denver, Colorado

Library of Congress Cataloging-in-Publication Data

Names: Hawk, Cheryl, editor.
Title: The Praeger handbook of chiropractic health care : evidence-based
    practices / Cheryl Hawk, editor ; foreword by John Weeks.
Other titles: Handbook of chiropractic health care
Description: Santa Barbara, California : Praeger, An Imprint of ABC-CLIO,
    LLC, [2017] | Includes bibliographical references and index.
Identifiers: LCCN 2017000720 (print) | LCCN 2017001435 (ebook) | ISBN
    9781440837463 (alk. paper) | ISBN 9781440837470 (eISBN)
Subjects: | MESH: Chiropractic | Manipulation, Chiropractic
Classification: LCC RZ241 (print) | LCC RZ241 (ebook) | NLM WB 905.7 | DDC
    615.5/34—dc23
LC record available at https://lccn.loc.gov/2017000720

ISBN: 978-1-4408-3746-3
EISBN: 978-1-4408-3747-0

21 20 19 18 17   1 2 3 4 5

This book is also available as an eBook.

Praeger

An Imprint of ABC-CLIO, LLC

ABC-CLIO, LLC
130 Cremona Drive, P.O. Box 1911
Santa Barbara, California 93116-1911
www.abc-clio.com

This book is printed on acid-free paper ∞

Manufactured in the United States of America

Contents

Foreword

The chiropractic profession has held a series of unique positions in the emergence of what many today call the movement for integrative health and medicine.

By the time the integrative era began in earnest in the early 1990s, chiropractic was already licensed in 50 states and had achieved Medicare inclusion. Limited chiropractic services were included in benefits plans of most large corporations and in state-run disability programs. These thresholds were yet distant horizons for the emerging "complementary and alternative medicine" (CAM) fields, such as acupuncture and Oriental medicine, naturopathic medicine, massage therapy, and direct-entry midwifery. Their then-tenuous existences were a good distance down the food chain from chiropractic on what might be called Maslow's hierarchy of professional needs. These fields struggled with fundamental campaigns for recognition and survival.

Yet the path for chiropractic in the last half century has hardly been smooth. It is strange from our present vantage point to recall that in the 1960s, most medical thinking didn't link nutrition and health. Nor were mind and body considered as a whole. "Healing" was rarely discussed. Chiropractic's patient-centered, hands-on approaches were similarly far removed from the mainstream of medical practice.

All that is changing. Some changes have come through developments internal to the chiropractic field. Chiropractic's research leaders actively responded to new opportunities for funding through the National Center for Complementary and Integrative Health at the National Institutes of Health. Some colleges developed significant research departments. Key chiropractic researchers took positions at major academic health centers at places like the University of Minnesota and the University of Pittsburgh. A chiropractor was appointed to the Board of Governors of the quasi-governmental, influential Patient-Centered Outcomes Research Institute.

On the policy front, through the support of the profession's Congressional allies, chiropractors created paths into providing care through the U.S. Veterans Administration (VA) and the Department of Defense. A chiropractor chaired a key American Medical Association review committee. Chiropractic colleges placed their first residents in VA facilities. The profession developed a powerful media presence through the unifying Foundation for Chiropractic Progress. A chiropractic summit helped frame a shared plan of action across the profession's multiple organizations.

These steps toward engaging leaders of regular medicine came at a convergent time. Over the past 20 years, regular medicine has increasingly shifted its focus from the production of services to what is called "value-based" health care. This movement highlighted outcomes such as patient-centeredness and cost savings through strategies like team care that fostered greater interprofessional understanding and respect. Medicare, for instance, which had only paid chiropractors for spinal manipulation, opened a dialogue with the profession to explore respecting the chiropractor's time and skills in evaluation and management of patients.

The opportunity for chiropractic at the present moment is immense. Crises such as that over opioids cry out for new approaches. The value-based movement is elevating a focus on prevention and on health outcomes. These two principles are foundational to chiropractic's favored self-image. The developments all align well with chiropractic's promotion of conservative care—of a new therapeutic order in care delivery.

As the most politically powerful and institutionally strong of the natural health-oriented fields, chiropractic has a terrific opening here. The profession's leaders are making connections with other professions—wherever they may be on Maslow's hierarchy of professional development—to lead this movement toward optimal, timely use of integrative approaches. Such leadership toward a more balanced, patient-centered approach to health and medicine is the future for chiropractic.

John Weeks
Publisher-Editor, *The Integrator Blog News & Reports*
Editor-in-Chief, *Journal of Alternative and Complementary Medicine*

CHAPTER ONE

Overview of Chiropractic Health Care

Claire Johnson, DC, MSEd, PhD; and
Bart Green, DC, MSEd, PhD

A Brief History of Chiropractic

The chiropractic profession has a long history of serving the public by healing people through the use of natural methods. Chiropractic has been seen as both an alternative and a complementary health care profession and is currently one of the largest primary health care professions and the largest complementary and alternative medicine (CAM) licensed primary health care profession in the United States.[1]

Knowing how chiropractic developed will assist in the understanding and appreciation of this remarkable profession. Chiropractic's unique philosophical approach to health care was born out of social and cultural factors present in the United States during the late 1800s.

Development of American Medicine and the Rise of Alternative Health

Before chiropractic existed, medical care in the United States in the 1800s was limited to a small number of procedures and medicines. None of the scientific advancements that we are familiar with today, such as antibiotics and sterile surgery techniques, were available since they had not yet been discovered. The germ theory of disease, which was only introduced in the 1860s, was still unknown. When the concept of sterile surgery (e.g., doctors washing their hands prior to performing surgery) was introduced, it was met with opposition in the medical profession. Medical science was still crude, and there was no research infrastructure to test which were the most safe and effective methods of care. Formal medical education in the United States developed slowly. Early medical schools were proprietary and had short curricula (e.g., six months). Apprenticeship or self-training was the typical path to becoming a medical doctor. It was not until the mid-1800s that the American Medical Association (AMA) advocated for states to introduce licensing laws for the practice of medicine.[2]

For infectious and systemic diseases, little was available for orthodox medical doctors to use except for heroic medicine.[3] The practice of heroic medicine included bloodletting and purging to attempt to rid the body of "impurities." Most drugs were proprietary, with strong doses of alcohol or opiates and poisons such as mercury or arsenic. Those who used heroic medicine were taught that the strongest doses should be given to the sickest patients. Thus, medical treatment was often more harmful to the patient than the disease for which it was given.[4]

Due to the harsh nature of the medical treatments, people often sought alternatives to medical care of that time. Whether legitimate or not, due to a lack of licensing laws and professional controls, alternative health care practitioners were abundant in the 1800s. Because alternative practitioners offered conservative, and often less potentially damaging, healing treatments, they might have seen positive results where orthodox heroic medicine practitioners did not. Alternative providers used natural healing agents, such as diet changes, herbs and plants, exercise, bonesetting, manipulation, religious healing, magnetic healing, sunshine therapy, and baths. The most commonly known professions that arose toward the end of the century included homeopathy, osteopathy, naturopathy, and chiropractic.[3]

With the rise in alternative healers, orthodox medicine was threatened. To maintain better control over the business of health care, medical doctors gathered together, and the AMA was founded in 1847. This organization began on the path that would eventually establish orthodox medicine as the dominant health profession in the United States. To protect its members and promote its existence, the AMA developed a code of ethics and educational standards and established an agenda to attempt to control and eliminate competing health professions.[2,3]

One of the AMA's goals was to standardize medical practice and eliminate alternate forms of medicine. In doing so, health care practitioners who used alternative practices were labeled by the AMA as "irregular practitioners." Since the alternative health professions—such as osteopathy, chiropractic, naturopathy, and homeopathy—were external to orthodox medicine at the time, they were not allowed to be included in the AMA or under AMA's protection. Since no laws governed the practice of health care at that time, battles for survival ensued in each of the states. Many alternative health care providers, including chiropractors, were prosecuted and jailed for practicing medicine without a license. Over the decades, organized medicine developed cultural dominance, especially when new scientific discoveries began to influence medical practice.[3] It would be many years later that each of the U.S. states would develop its own unique licensing laws that allow chiropractic to be practiced legally. This tension between the professions largely explains why chiropractic has always been distinct and separate from orthodox medicine.

Emergence of Chiropractic

It was into this environment that chiropractic was born in the late 1800s. Chiropractic was founded by Daniel David Palmer, who was born in the small Canadian town of Pickering, Ontario, in 1845.[5] At the age of 20, he moved to the United States. He engaged in several occupations, including grocer, beekeeper, horticulturist, and grade-school teacher, and during this time, he became interested in health care.[3] In the early 1800s, anyone in the United States who provided health care could be called a "doctor" and provide this care using the "practice of medicine." Many doctors did not obtain formal medical education, and of those who did, the education was limited. D. D. Palmer was one of these early American healers.

Palmer was influenced by many of the alternative practices of the period, including "magnetic healing." Derived from the work of Anton Mesmer, magnetic healing involved the "laying on of hands" in order to transfer "vital magnetic energy" from the doctor to the patient. The practice of magnetic healing and metaphysics influenced Palmer,[6] and he opened an office as a magnetic healer around 1885.[3]

D. D. Palmer practiced in Iowa and helped hundreds of patients as a magnetic healer. He developed an infirmary where patients stayed for an extended time while they received his magnetic healing treatments. Palmer provided his patients with clean accommodations and healthy food to eat. Although he had started with only an eighth-grade education, which was the same as the traditional medical doctors at that time, he was a voracious reader and kept a personal library of advanced medical texts.[6]

In the 1890s, his practice of magnetic healing transformed into the practice of chiropractic. Palmer began to practice when the state of Iowa began to license medical doctors. As a strong-minded individual, he was critical of the medical practices of his day. He believed that many common drugs and heroic therapies were harmful to patients who were already weakened by illness and proposed that resistance to disease was related to a person's vital energy and overall health. He supported the Hippocratic philosophy, including the idea that the cause of disease is not due to agents external to the body but that illness is "dis-ease," a natural response to imbalance. These concepts influenced his teachings and were included in the formation of the chiropractic profession.

D. D. Palmer continually sought to improve his practice and began to add quick hand thrusts to his patients' spines during his magnetic sessions. Patients reported that they healed faster with his new method. It was during this time, in 1895, while Palmer was practicing magnetic healing, that he made a clinical observation that launched the new chiropractic profession. Palmer reported that the critical moment when magnetic healing transformed into chiropractic came after a patient's response to a healing session. The patient was Harvey Lillard, a building superintendent where Palmer practiced. Palmer reported that Lillard complained of hearing loss that began several years earlier when he felt something give way in his spine while straining himself during work. He said that immediately after the injury, he lost his hearing.[3] Palmer reported that when examining Lillard's spine, he found a prominent vertebra in the midthoracic area. Palmer used the spinous process of the vertebra as a lever and provided a quick thrust to Lillard's spine. Palmer reported that the patient said his hearing improved greatly after the treatment. Following this, Palmer worked to understand the relationship between his newly discovered form of hands-on healing and its influence on health and disease.[3] His new idea of delivering a quick, isolated thrust to the spinous process of the vertebra later came to be called a "chiropractic adjustment."

As more of his patients received the new style of treatment, Palmer noted that other types of disorders improved with the "hand thrust" treatments. In search of a name for this new treatment, Palmer asked one of his patients, Reverend Samuel Weed, to offer a name for something that is "done by hand." Weed offered *cheiro* (hand) and *practikos* (practice). Thus, from these roots the term "chiropractic" was created.[3,5]

Over the years, Palmer incorporated revisions as technology and science evolved, and he continued to revise his theories of chiropractic many times up to his death in 1913. Palmer's theories of chiropractic primarily focused on the relationship between the nervous system and health and how the chiropractic adjustment could influence the nervous system.

Early Chiropractic Growth

D. D. Palmer taught magnetic healing to others before the discovery of chiropractic. He opened his first school, Palmer's School of Magnetic Cure, in 1896 in Davenport, Iowa, and after the discovery, he taught chiropractic there. He changed the name to Palmer School and Cure the next year.[7] The first classes were small, but they continued to grow over the years. In 1904, it was estimated that there were only 50 chiropractors in the United States.[3]

Palmer encouraged his graduates to start teaching by noting on their diplomas that they were competent to "teach and practice" chiropractic. Following this, new chiropractic institutions started in several locations. However, Palmer may not have been prepared for his graduates to teach new chiropractic theories and methods that varied from his own. New graduates that diverged from his strict teachings were shunned by the founder. He demanded that if it was to be called "chiropractic," the method must be done by hand, as defined by the word "chiropractic" itself. When graduates incorporated other forms of care, including the use of naturopathy or mechanical devices, Palmer was outraged. However, these early efforts at improvement may have assisted the profession by offering other mechanisms for how chiropractic worked.

Only a few years after graduating from the Palmer School of Magnetic Cure, Solon Langworthy, a doctor of chiropractic (DC), opened the American School of Chiropractic and Nature Cure in Cedar Rapids, Iowa. This was the first school to rival Palmer's. Langworthy contributed substantially to the early years of the chiropractic profession's development. He started the first chiropractic journal, called *Backbone*, is credited as the first to use the term "subluxation" in the chiropractic literature, and was instrumental in early investigations into the anatomy of the spine. His school was one of the earliest institutions to use therapeutic agents in addition to spinal adjustments to help patients heal.

Oakley Smith, DC, and Minora Paxson, DC, two other early Palmer graduates, joined Langworthy's school, and the trio was very productive. In 1906, they published the first chiropractic textbook, *Modernized Chiropractic*.[8] At the American School of Chiropractic, they offered the first structured chiropractic curriculum, consisting of four five-month terms.[7] This was a tremendous accomplishment, since at that time chiropractors were trained in the same apprentice type of education as medical education in the 1800s.

Other early chiropractors were instrumental in securing footing for chiropractic to be a health care profession. John F. A. Howard, DC, graduated from Palmer in 1906 and opened the National School of Chiropractic that same year in the same building where Palmer had adjusted Harvey Lillard.[7] Howard then moved his school to the Chicago area, where it remains today as the National University of Health Sciences (NUHS). Howard incorporated physiotherapeutic agents into the chiropractic curriculum to address the broader definition of health care, beyond the removal of vertebral subluxations. For this reason, some regard NUHS as the birthplace of this broad approach to chiropractic care.

Thomas H. Storey, DC, graduated from Palmer in 1901. Upon his return to Los Angeles, he was instrumental in training Charles Cale, DC, who opened the Los Angeles College of Chiropractic (currently Southern California University of Health Sciences).[7] Many others founded chiropractic colleges of their own in a multitude of places across the country. By 1910, it was estimated that 2,000 to 5,000 chiropractors were practicing in the United States.[3]

D. D. Palmer's son, Bartlett Joshua Palmer, graduated from the Palmer School and Cure in 1902. Being one of the early graduates, he was also encouraged to teach and practice chiropractic. Eventually, B. J. Palmer took over the Palmer School, which was in financial trouble. He worked diligently to promote the school and developed it into the largest chiropractic school at that time.

B. J. Palmer was flamboyant and known for assimilating popular culture into his management style. Over the years, he introduced changes into the Palmer curriculum and seemed to expect the entire profession to follow suit, even though there were many other schools by this time. In 1908, he claimed that he had developed a new chiropractic adjustment that was more specific than the procedures taught previously. He introduced the use of diagnostic X-rays in 1910, and he started a radio station at the Palmer School to spread the message of chiropractic.[9] B. J. Palmer and other chiropractic pioneers did much to promote chiropractic and encourage the growth of the profession. By the 1950s, an estimated 13,000 chiropractors were practicing in the United States.[3]

Early Challenges for Chiropractic

Legal challenges haunted the chiropractic profession from the beginning. Throughout the 1900s, orthodox medicine attempted to eliminate chiropractic by legal prosecution and jailing chiropractors for practicing medicine without a license. Under B. J. Palmer's guidance, the first nationwide legal defense system was created for chiropractors who were sent to jail for practicing chiropractic. This system would soon become an important feature in securing the profession while at the same time defining it as different from medicine.

A landmark legal case that greatly influenced the chiropractic profession was held in Lacrosse, Wisconsin, in 1907. Shegataro Morikubo, DC, a graduate from the Palmer School of Chiropractic, was accused of practicing medicine without a license. In this case, the lawyer who was provided by B. J. Palmer's defense team argued that since chiropractic was a distinct profession and had its own science, philosophy, and lexicon, the chiropractic profession should not be judged as if it were osteopathy or medicine. Early legal defense had much to offer the shaping of how chiropractic is perceived currently. The early legal defense was built upon the rationale that chiropractic was separate and distinct from orthodox medicine; therefore, chiropractors should answer to different licensure. A separate lexicon that was distinct from orthodox medicine was therefore created for legal defense purposes,[10] including terms such as "subluxation."[11] For years following, legal defense of chiropractors would use the "separate and distinct" argument in order to win their cases.[5]

Chiropractic education has evolved since D. D. Palmer took his first class of students in 1897. Initially, the educational program was only several months long, which was similar to medical education at that time. However, as health professions' education and licensing evolved, chiropractic education did as well. In 1910, the landmark Flexner report pressured medical schools to raise their standards and increase the focus of their curricula on science. The Flexner report caused a shift in orthodox medicine as it stimulated the closure of proprietary schools and emphasized an increase in scientific medicine. This event carried over to the chiropractic colleges by creating the expectation that health care should be based in science.[12]

Over the years, the requirements to matriculate were elevated and the quality and length of chiropractic programs increased. State laws licensing chiropractic first passed in Kansas in 1913 and in the last state, Louisiana, in 1974. Chiropractors fought for licensure in each of the 50 states over the years. Because each state had its own set of circumstances, licensure in each state became slightly different. Some states limited chiropractic practice to a narrower focus, which could be described as a focus on "adjustment of subluxations," discouraging diagnosis, staying separate from medicine, and not integrating into mainstream health care. Other states supported a broader scope of practice, including a wide variety of conservative treatments in addition to diagnosis, patient comanagement, and integration within the health care system. Today, chiropractors are licensed in all 50 American states and have the right to practice in over 80 countries internationally. Based on the unique licensing history in each state, the scope of practice currently varies across the United States.

In addition to the pressure from early licensing laws, chiropractic graduates were required to pass basic science examinations in order to practice. Basic science laws were an additional attempt by organized medicine in the early 1900s to regulate practice and keep nonmedical practitioners, such as chiropractors, out of business. The purpose of the basic science laws was to determine if chiropractors had sufficient basic science knowledge to practice. Chiropractors, medical doctors, and osteopaths were required to take and pass these exams in order to receive a license in their state.[7] Over time, the chiropractic profession gained the responsibility to administer its own examinations. Finally, the National Board of Chiropractic Examiners (NBCE) was created in 1963. The NBCE develops and administers various examinations, the results of which are among the criteria used by state licensing agencies to determine if a chiropractor has satisfied that particular state's minimum qualifications for licensure. At present, there are many sections to the NBCE exams in addition to the basic science topics, including diagnosis, patient management, physiotherapeutics, and a practical examination to test skills, knowledge, and proficiency in clinical care.

Early chiropractic educators recognized that improving the quality of education was essential. In the early 1930s, Dr. Claude O. Watkins of the National Chiropractic Association (NCA), which is now the American Chiropractic Association (ACA), introduced a Committee on Education.[7] At this same time, the Council of State Chiropractic Examining Boards was improving chiropractic education, and in 1938, these two groups established the Committee on Educational Standards. In 1939, the Committee on Educational Standards provided educational criteria to serve as guides for the nearly 40 chiropractic educational programs of various sizes that existed at the time. Following this, in 1941, the Committee on Educational Standards recognized the first 12 provisionally approved colleges. In 1947, the NCA Council on Education was formed by institutional representatives and members of the Committee on Educational Standards, which was the precursor to the Council on Chiropractic Education (CCE).

From 1941 to 1961, the NCA Council on Education focused on strengthening chiropractic programs. Weaker institutions merged to create stronger academic programs, and substandard schools were closed. By 1961, there were only 10 chiropractic programs and an estimated 13,800 chiropractors in the United States.[3] In 1971, the council incorporated as an autonomous national organization, the CCE.[3]

In 1952, the CCE's parent organization made initial contact with the U.S. Department of Education, and in 1959, an application for recognition was filed. Recommendations were made for strengthening academic standards and unofficial filing of materials was made in 1969, which resulted in further suggestions for improvement. In 1972, the CCE filed a formal application, and later that year, the CCE was listed as a "nationally recognized accrediting agency" by the U.S. Commissioner of Education.[3] In 1974, the CCE was recognized by the U.S. Department of Education to accredit doctor of chiropractic (DC) degree programs, which was crucial to the advancement of the profession. The mission of the CCE is to "to ensure the quality and integrity of its accredited doctor of chiropractic degree programs."

For the majority of the 20th century, the AMA continued its efforts to prevent other professions from being included in its monopoly of health care. For decades, it attempted to contain and eliminate the chiropractic profession. The AMA put legal and political pressure on other professions to prevent them from engaging in mainstream care. The AMA sought to prevent chiropractors from being recognized as health care providers for Medicare, from gaining membership in the American Public Health Association,[13] and from being allowed to practice in hospitals.[3] One of these efforts was the AMA disallowing members to refer patients to, or accept patients from, chiropractors. It was not until years later, in 1987, that the final decision of the *Wilk v. AMA* trial removed the barrier that implied that a medical doctor was not ethically allowed to refer a patient for chiropractic care.[14]

Chiropractic Today

Description of Chiropractic

Doctors of chiropractic focus on the relationship between human structure and function and wellness. Central to the philosophy of chiropractic is the belief that the body is a self-regulating organism capable of healing itself if barriers are removed. Doctors of chiropractic focus on correcting dysfunctional areas of the spine and other parts of the body, especially as these are relevant to the body's structure and function. It is thought that the correction of such dysfunctions stimulates reflexes mediated in the spine and nervous system that affect health.[15] While it is known that a diseased organ may cause symptoms in distant body parts,

DCs propose that neurological disturbances in the spinal column and other areas may cause dysfunction to appear in remote organs and tissues. The nervous system has an influence on all functions of the body. Thus, by addressing dysfunction in the nervous system, it is thought that all functions of the body may benefit. Terms associated with the entity that is addressed include "joint dysfunction," "chiropractic subluxation complex," and "vertebral subluxation complex."[15]

Most doctors of chiropractic recognize the importance of the interplay between biomechanics of the body, especially those of the spine and the nervous system, which may influence important body functions. Because chiropractors are interested in the relationship between the spine, the nervous system, and overall health, and they are experts in managing these problems, the public sometimes only views chiropractors as back and neck pain doctors. However, chiropractors may have more to offer patients seeking care. *Chapter 2 gives an inside look at the typical chiropractic clinical encounter, and Chapter 3 outlines the characteristics of a typical chiropractor.* Patients seeking chiropractic care may learn how to better maintain their health, in addition to achieving relief from common problems, such as neck and back pain, headache, sports injuries, and nonmusculoskeletal disorders.

Doctors of chiropractic address patients' health and wellness by using conservative and natural methods; for the most part, they do not use prescription drugs or surgery. This sets chiropractors apart from some other professions, such as medicine and osteopathy. Most common among chiropractic methods are chiropractic manipulations, also known as adjustments. Chiropractic manipulation is when the chiropractor applies specific and controlled movements to the various joints of the body to help normalize structure and function. *Chapter 4 gives details about chiropractic manipulation.* In addition to manual therapy, such as manipulation and mobilization, most DCs also provide education (e.g., in lifestyle, habits, environment), home exercises to support manual care, therapeutic modalities (e.g., electrical stimulation, traction, and cold and hot packs), and advice on nutrition.[1] *Chapter 5 discusses the most commonly used additional services provided by chiropractors.*

Chiropractic in the Health Care System

The U.S. government and state laws recognize doctors of chiropractic as portal-of-entry health care providers. Therefore, chiropractors may be the first provider to see a patient presenting with a particular complaint. DCs practice as portal-of-entry doctors because they are trained in diagnosis and management of a wide variety of health issues[1] and provide preventive services.[13] In the United States, there are three healing arts licensed to provide such care, which, in order of both numbers of practitioners and public use, are the orthodox medicine, chiropractic, and osteopathic professions. Chiropractic is the second-largest doctoral-level portal-of-entry health profession, accounting for over 190 million office visits in the United States each year.[16]

The number of chiropractors practicing in the United States has grown steadily over the decades. In 1980, it was estimated there were 19,700 chiropractors, and by 1991, there were nearly 50,000.[3] According to the Federation of Chiropractic Licensing Boards, there were 62,300 active licenses for DCs in practice in the United States in 2015. It is estimated that there are approximately 7,000 students currently studying in accredited U.S. chiropractic training programs.

The percentage of people receiving chiropractic care each year continues to grow. A nationwide telephone survey estimated that approximately 11 percent of the American population received chiropractic care per year in the early 2000s.[16] A recent survey estimated 14 percent of the population sought chiropractic care in the past year, and based on a recent Gallup poll, nearly 50 percent of those surveyed had seen a chiropractor at some point in their life.[17,18]

Visits to CAM practitioners are very popular, and chiropractic visits account for about 30 percent of all visits made to complementary and alternative practitioners.[16] Chiropractic is part of the U.S. health care infrastructure and is included in various federal programs, such as Medicare and Medicaid. Chiropractic services are included in workers' compensation acts and health insurance policies as well as major international, national, and local unions, and industrial employers provide for chiropractic services in their health plans for their members and employees. Chiropractic care is also part of the health care benefits afforded to military members and veterans of the U.S. armed services.[19,20]

Chiropractic Education

According to the World Federation of Chiropractic, as of 2017, there were 16 accredited chiropractic degree-granting institutions in the United States and 28 programs in the rest of the world. Chiropractic education in the United States is accredited both through discipline-specific accreditation and regional accreditation. The Council on Chiropractic Education is discipline specific and continues to be recognized by the U.S. Department of Education. As of 2016, the CCE accredited all 15 DC degree programs in 18 locations within the United States. Most chiropractic programs are also accredited by regional accrediting bodies that confirm the integrity of the academic program. Accreditation by CCE and by regional academic accreditation bodies are separate processes.[21] DC programs in the United States are standardized, with a requirement of at least three years of undergraduate education prior to admission to a typical four-year chiropractic program.

Chiropractic programs are very similar to orthodox medical school curricula.[21] Early didactic training is followed by clinical encounters and internships. Students must pass examinations within the program and national exams, such as from the National Board of Chiropractic Examiners. The NBCE examinations are standardized, assessing skills and knowledge of chiropractic. All state licensing boards use the NBCE scores to determine licensure. In addition to NBCE certification, DCs may also engage in residency and postgraduate specialty programs, such as in orthopedics, sports medicine, radiology, nutrition, pediatrics, and other topics. *Chapter 13 reviews more information about special populations, including older adults, children, and pregnant women. Chapter 14 covers topics related to sports chiropractic.*

Federal student loan assistance is available to chiropractic students, and the president of the United States has authorized doctors of chiropractic to serve as commissioned health care officers in the U.S. armed forces.

Licensure

Doctors of chiropractic are licensed in each of the states in the United States and in numerous other countries. Each jurisdiction's law delineates the scope of practice for its chiropractors.[22] While there are many similarities in chiropractic practice across states, regions, and countries, it should be noted that variations in practice laws cause a range of practices. Regardless of the location, each DC is expected to practice within the scope of practice where licensed and to the extent to which he or she was trained, which includes diagnosis, referral, and management. How each state or province regulates its chiropractors is also typically written into the practice act or law for the region.

Practice Environments for Chiropractors

DCs can be found in solitary private practice, but many chiropractors work in collaborative practices and interdisciplinary clinics.[23,24] Chiropractic services have been included in large health care settings, such as private hospitals,[25] the Veterans Administration,[19,26,27] and the Department of Defense.[28,29] The Department of Veterans Affairs health care systems offer chiropractic care as a benefit for veterans at more than 50 locations as of 2015, and the U.S. Department of Defense provides active-duty military personnel chiropractic care at 65 locations.[19] In these systems, chiropractors are integrated as part of the medical staff and have hospital privileges in some of the most prestigious medical centers in the country, such as Walter Reed National Military Medical Center in Washington, D.C., and the Naval Medical Center in San Diego, California.[29] Chiropractors also provide care in military treatment facilities in countries outside of the United States.

Safety of Chiropractic Care

Chiropractic care is a recommended nonpharmacological means to reduce pain and improve function for patients in chronic pain and can assist in better managing these patients. While chiropractic care is generally regarded as safe and effective, there can be side effects.[30] These include soreness or discomfort, but this is typically a short-term effect. Rarely, severe adverse or unexpected consequences of care may occur, including injury or death, although these are considered very rare.[31–34] Even though they are rare, doctors of chiropractic include practices to reduce these occurrences, including performing a thorough history and physical examination and identifying any warning signs and referring or comanaging the patient with another health care provider if appropriate. Research into mitigating risk associated with chiropractic care is ongoing. *Chapter 6 discusses the safety of chiropractic treatment in depth.*

Evidence-Based Practice, Guidelines, and Best Practices

The application of research to clinical practice is part of a concept called "evidence-based practice."[35] This practice combines three areas in an attempt to provide the best patient care possible: (1) patient's needs and values, (2) expertise and clinical reasoning of the practitioner, and (3) best available research evidence. Evidence-based practice evolved over many years and continues to develop today. Research requires substantial resources and is one of the important ingredients in evidence-based practice. Without research, there would be no evidence to apply to patient problems. The chiropractic profession has worked diligently to produce research to form a base of evidence pertinent to chiropractic practice, but this has not always been the case.

For the first 80 years of its existence, the chiropractic profession could afford to give little attention to generating original scientific research. Instead, resources in the early years were necessarily dedicated to the legal battles between chiropractic and organized medicine, elevating educational standards, and establishing licensing laws.[3] There were also few trained researchers in the profession and little institutional infrastructure for conducting research.[36] These obstacles notwithstanding, the first chiropractic research to be included in the National Library of Medicine's *Index Medicus* was published in 1960.

In the early 1970s, the National Institutes of Health gave funding to a conference in order to evaluate if there was scientific validity to the concepts of manipulation that were being used in chiropractic care. The result was the National Institute of Neurological Disorders and Stroke (NINDS) conference, The Research Status of Spinal Manipulative Therapy, held at the campus of the National Institutes of Health in 1975. Research and theoretical papers were presented by 116 researchers from various backgrounds, including chiropractic, osteopathy, medicine, and basic sciences. Although most studies at the time were observational, not experimental, this conference provided momentum for chiropractic research. With greater awareness and the approval implied by the NINDS conference, more funding became available for chiropractic research and development. The first chiropractic scientific journal to be indexed in Medline was the *Journal of Manipulative and Physiological Therapeutics*, which was created in 1978 and first indexed in 1982.

During the time that the chiropractic research enterprise was beginning to gain momentum, the concepts and practices of evidence-based care were becoming not only more common but expected. Research evidence was being produced at a rate that outpaced the practitioner's ability to stay up to date and integrate important findings into practice. At the same time, health care costs were increasing, and there was a focus on how to contain costs and provide more consistent high-quality care. Since all of health care was moving toward evidence-based care, a group of leaders within the chiropractic profession recognized that guidelines were being used to determine use of chiropractic care but that no chiropractic input was given to develop these guidelines. Therefore, efforts were made to develop the first set of scientifically supported guidelines to help guide chiropractic practice. Known as the "Mercy guideline" (named for its location) the *Guidelines for Chiropractic Quality Assurance and Practice Parameters* was published in 1993. This document represented a combined effort from many different viewpoints within the profession. The

Mercy guideline ultimately helped to inform the Agency for Health Care Policy and Research recommendations pertaining to spinal manipulation and other future guidelines for the inclusion of manipulation for conditions such as back pain.

Since that time, various groups and institutions have continued to develop guidelines for chiropractic care to guide education and clinical practice (Table 1.1). *The following chapters discuss these topics at greater depth: back pain (Chapter 7); neck pain, headaches, and temporomandibular joint pain (Chapter 8); upper extremity and lower extremity conditions (Chapter 9); other musculoskeletal conditions (Chapter 10); nonmusculoskeletal conditions (Chapter 11); and health promotion and wellness (Chapter 12).*

Today, chiropractors are involved in conducting research at universities around the world. Major chiropractic scientific and academic meetings

Table 1.1   Chiropractic Guidelines and Best Practices Published in Peer-Reviewed Journals

Topic	Peer-Reviewed Journal Publication
Neck Pain and Whiplash	The treatment of neck pain-associated disorders and whiplash-associated disorders: a clinical practice guideline. Bussières AE, Stewart G, Al-Zoubi F, et al. *J Manipulative Physiol Ther.* 2016;39:523–544.
Low Back Pain	Clinical practice guideline: chiropractic care for low back pain. Globe G, Farabaugh RJ, Hawk C, et al. *J Manipulative Physiol Ther.* 2016 Jan;39(1):1–22.
Children	Best practices for chiropractic care of children: a consensus update. Hawk C, Schneider MJ, Vallone S, Hewitt EG. *J Manipulative Physiol Ther.* 2016 Mar–Apr;39(3):158–168.
Neck Pain	Evidence-based guidelines for the chiropractic treatment of adults with neck pain. Bryans R, Decina P, Descarreaux M, et al. *J Manipulative Physiol Ther.* 2014 Jan;37(1):42–63.
Health	Consensus process to develop a best-practice document on the role of chiropractic care in health promotion, disease prevention, and wellness. Hawk C, Schneider M, Evans MW Jr, Redwood D. *J Manipulative Physiol Ther.* 2012 Sep;35(7):556–567.

(Continued)

Table 1.1   (Continued)

Topic	Peer-Reviewed Journal Publication
Shoulder	Manipulative therapy for shoulder pain and disorders: expansion of a systematic review. Brantingham JW, Cassa TK, Bonnefin D, et al. *J Manipulative Physiol Ther.* 2011 Jun;34(5):314–346.
Headache	Evidence-based guidelines for the chiropractic treatment of adults with headache. Bryans R, Descarreaux M, Duranleau M, et al. *J Manipulative Physiol Ther.* 2011 Jun;34(5):274–289.
Older Adults	Best practices recommendations for chiropractic care for older adults: results of a consensus process. Hawk C, Schneider M, Dougherty P, Gleberzon BJ, Killinger LZ. *J Manipulative Physiol Ther.* 2010 Jul–Aug;33(6):464–473.
Chronic Spine Conditions	Management of chronic spine-related conditions: consensus recommendations of a multidisciplinary panel. Farabaugh RJ, Dehen MD, Hawk C. *J Manipulative Physiol Ther.* 2010 Sep;33(7):484–492.
Wellness	Consensus terminology for stages of care: acute, chronic, recurrent, and wellness. Dehen MD, Whalen WM, Farabaugh RJ, Hawk C. *J Manipulative Physiol Ther.* 2010 Jul–Aug;33(6):458–463.
Fibromyalgia	Chiropractic management of fibromyalgia syndrome: a systematic review of the literature. Schneider M, Vernon H, Ko G, Lawson G, Perera J. *J Manipulative Physiol Ther.* 2009 Jan;32(1):25–40.
Tendinopathy	Chiropractic management of tendinopathy: a literature synthesis. Pfefer MT, Cooper SR, Uhl NL. *J Manipulative Physiol Ther.* 2009 Jan;32(1):41–52.
Diagnostic Imaging Upper Extremity	Diagnostic imaging guideline for musculoskeletal complaints in adults—an evidence-based approach—part 2: upper extremity disorders. Bussières AE, Peterson C, Taylor JA. *J Manipulative Physiol Ther.* 2008 Jan;31(1):2–32.

Table 1.1 (Continued)

Topic	Peer-Reviewed Journal Publication
Diagnostic Imaging Spinal Disorders	Diagnostic imaging practice guidelines for musculoskeletal complaints in adults—an evidence-based approach—part 3: spinal disorders. Bussières AE, Taylor JA, Peterson C. *J Manipulative Physiol Ther.* 2008 Jan;31(1):33–88.
Diagnostic Imaging Lower Extremity	Diagnostic imaging practice guidelines for musculoskeletal complaints in adults—an evidence-based approach—part 1: lower extremity disorders. Bussières AE, Taylor JA, Peterson C. *J Manipulative Physiol Ther.* 2007 Nov–Dec;30(9):684–717.

occur several times a year, and educators and researchers share the results of their investigations and collaborate on research projects. Chiropractic scientists deliver lectures and scientific presentations at scholarly meetings of the highest caliber and regularly publish research in academic journals scrutinized by the leading authorities in spine care and education. Research is now being produced at a rate never before thought possible and is being published by interprofessional teams.

Chiropractic in the Future

In 2013, the Institutes of Alternative Futures completed a report that looked at the potential position of the chiropractic profession in the year 2025.[37] This qualitative report suggested that there were four possible futures for the profession that might be realized depending on what the chiropractic profession chose to do:

1. Scenario 1: marginal gains, marginalized field (i.e., the profession is isolated from mainstream health care and has limited growth)
2. Scenario 2: hard times and civil war (i.e., the profession fights within itself, resulting in restricted growth)
3. Scenario 3: integration and spine health leadership (i.e., the profession becomes increasingly integrated within mainstream health care)
4. Scenario 4: vitalism and value (i.e., the profession remains outside of mainstream health care as a marginalized profession).

The activities of the profession and the interests of its newest members will continue to define the profession in the future. Only time will tell if the profession will follow one of these four hypothesized paths.

If the past is any indication of the future, the use of chiropractic will increase and the profession will continue to grow internationally. Chiropractic is now established in more than 90 countries[1] and is poised to be an attractive low-tech health care option in countries with few resources to commit to health care. Just a few years ago, the predominance of chiropractic training institutions and practitioners was in the United States. Now, there are more chiropractic training programs outside of the United States,[1] and more continue to develop. The international growth of chiropractic has caught the attention of governing bodies and health organizations, and the World Health Organization recently issued a report on safety and basic training for chiropractic programs.[38]

As chiropractic training evolves, it has started to collocate with other health care training programs. Such is the case in several countries, including the United States, Canada, Switzerland, and Denmark. It is anticipated that this trend toward interprofessional education will further evolve in the future. Students in chiropractic, medicine, physical therapy, nursing, and other professions have opportunities to train side by side and develop a better understanding of each other's chosen professions. It is hoped that such interprofessional training will lead to interprofessional practices and, ultimately, enhance patient care and population health.[39]

Originating from the simple beginnings of one man's observations of the power of hands-on care during the challenging health care practices of the 1800s, chiropractic has evolved into a leading health care profession. Chiropractic continues to be a dynamic profession that fights to ensure that this powerful form of health care is available to people all over the world.

References

1. Christensen MG, Hyland JK, Goertz CM, Kollasch MW. *Practice Analysis of Chiropractic 2015*. Greeley, CO: National Board of Chiropractic Examiners; 2015.

2. Hamowy R. The early development of medical licensing laws in the United States, 1875–1900. *J Libert Stud*. 1979;3(1):73–119.

3. Wardwell WI. *Chiropractic: History and Evolution of a New Profession*. St. Louis, MO: Mosby-Year Book; 1992.

4. Cassedy JH. *Medicine in America: A Short History*. Baltimore, MD: Johns Hopkins University Press; 1991.

5. Keating JC, Jr. Chiropractic: an illustrated history. *J Manipulative Physiol Ther.* 1996;19(2):147.

6. Gaucher-Peslherbe PL, Wiese G, Donahue J. Daniel David Palmer's medical library: the founder was "into the literature." *Chiropr Hist.* 1995;15(2):63–69.

7. Keating JC, Callender AK, Cleveland CS. *A history of chiropractic education in North America: report to the Council on Chiropractic Education.* Phoenix, AZ: Association for the History of Chiropractic; 1998.

8. Johnson C. Modernized chiropractic reconsidered: beyond foot-on-hose and bones-out-of-place. *J Manipulative Physiol Ther.* 2006;29(4):253–254.

9. Keating JC. *BJ of Davenport: The Early Years of Chiropractic.* Phoenix, AZ: Association for the History of Chiropractic; 1997.

10. Johnson C. Reflecting on 115 years: the chiropractic profession's philosophical path. *J Chiropr Humanit.* 2010;17(1):1–5.

11. Johnson C. Use of the term subluxation in publications during the formative years of the chiropractic profession. *J Chiropr Humanit.* 2011;18(1):1–9.

12. Johnson C, Green B. 100 years after the Flexner report: reflections on its influence on chiropractic education. *J Chiropr Educ.* 2010;24(2):145–152.

13. Johnson C, Baird R, Dougherty PE, et al. Chiropractic and public health: current state and future vision. *J Manipulative Physiol Ther.* 2008;31(6):397–410.

14. Chapman-Smith D. The Wilk case. *J Manipulative Physiol Ther.* 1989;12(2):142–146.

15. Leach RA. *The Chiropractic Theories: A Textbook of Scientific Research.* 4th ed. Philadelphia, PA: Lippincott Williams & Wilkins; 2004.

16. Meeker WC, Haldeman S. Chiropractic: a profession at the crossroads of mainstream and alternative medicine. *Ann Intern Med.* 2002;136(3):216–227.

17. Weeks WB, Goertz CM, Meeker WC, Marchiori DM. Characteristics of US adults who have positive and negative perceptions of doctors of chiropractic and chiropractic care. *J Manipulative Physiol Ther.* 2016;39(3):150–157.

18. Weeks WB, Goertz CM, Meeker WC, Marchiori DM. Public perceptions of doctors of chiropractic: results of a national survey and examination of variation according to respondents' likelihood to use chiropractic, experience with chiropractic, and chiropractic supply in local health care markets. *J Manipulative Physiol Ther.* 2015;38(8):533–544.

19. Green BN, Johnson CD, Daniels CJ, Napuli JG, Gliedt JA, Paris DJ. Integration of chiropractic services in military and veteran health care facilities: a systematic review of the literature. *J Evid Based Complementary Altern Med.* 2016;21(2):115–130.

20. Lisi AJ, Brandt CA. Trends in the use and characteristics of chiropractic services in the Department of Veterans Affairs. *J Manipulative Physiol Ther.* 2016;39(5):381–386.

21. Coulter I, Adams A, Coggan P, Wilkes M, Gonyea M. A comparative study of chiropractic and medical education. *Altern Ther Health Med.* 1998;4(5):64–75.

22. Chang M. The chiropractic scope of practice in the United States: a cross-sectional survey. *J Manipulative Physiol Ther.* 2014;37(6):363–376.

23. Meeker WC. Public demand and the integration of complementary and alternative medicine in the US health care system. *J Manipulative Physiol Ther.* 2000;23(2):123–126.

24. Smith M, Greene BR, Meeker W. The CAM movement and the integration of quality health care: the case of chiropractic. *J Ambul Care Manage.* 2002;25(2):1–16.

25. Branson RA. Hospital-based chiropractic integration within a large private hospital system in Minnesota: a 10-year example. *J Manipulative Physiol Ther.* 2009;32(9):740–748.

26. Dunn AS. A survey of chiropractic academic affiliations within the Department of Veterans Affairs health care system. *J Chiropr Educ.* 2007;21(2): 138–143.

27. Dunn AS, Green BN, Gilford S. An analysis of the integration of chiropractic services within the United States military and veterans' health care systems. *J Manipulative Physiol Ther.* 2009;32(9):749–757.

28. Green BN, Johnson CD, Lisi AJ, Tucker J. Chiropractic practice in military and veterans health care: the state of the literature. *J Can Chiropr Assoc.* 2009;53(3):194–204.

29. Goldberg CK, Green B, Moore J, et al. Integrated musculoskeletal rehabilitation care at a comprehensive combat and complex casualty care program. *J Manipulative Physiol Ther.* 2009;32(9):781–791.

30. Johnson C, Rubinstein SM, Cote P, et al. Chiropractic care and public health: answering difficult questions about safety, care through the lifespan, and community action. *J Manipulative Physiol Ther.* 2012;35(7):493–513.

31. Boyle E, Cote P, Grier AR, Cassidy JD. Examining vertebrobasilar artery stroke in two Canadian provinces. *Spine (Phila Pa 1976).* 2008;33(4 Suppl):S170–175.

32. Cassidy JD, Boyle E, Cote P, et al. Risk of vertebrobasilar stroke and chiropractic care: results of a population-based case-control and case-crossover study. *Spine (Phila Pa 1976).* 2008;33(4 Suppl):S176–183.

33. Rubinstein SM, Leboeuf-Yde C, Knol DL, de Koekkoek TE, Pfeifle CE, van Tulder MW. The benefits outweigh the risks for patients undergoing chiropractic care for neck pain: a prospective, multicenter, cohort study. *J Manipulative Physiol Ther.* 2007;30(6):408–418.

34. Rubinstein SM, Knol DL, Leboeuf-Yde C, van Tulder MW. Benign adverse events following chiropractic care for neck pain are associated with worse short-term outcomes but not worse outcomes at three months. *Spine (Phila Pa 1976).* 2008;33(25):E950–956.

35. Johnson C. Highlights of the basic components of evidence-based practice. *J Manipulative Physiol Ther.* 2008;31(2):91–92.

36. Keating JC, Jr., Green BN, Johnson CD. "Research" and "science" in the first half of the chiropractic century. *J Manipulative Physiol Ther.* 1995;18(6):357–378.

37. Bezold C. *Chiropractic 2025: Divergent Futures.* Alexandria, VA: Institute for Alternative Futures; 2013.

38. World Health Organization. *Guidelines on basic training and safety in chiropractic.* Geneva, Switzerland: World Health Organization; 2005.

39. Green BN, Johnson CD. Interprofessional collaboration in research, education, and clinical practice: working together for a better future. *J Chiropr Educ.* 2015;29(1):1–10.

CHAPTER TWO

The Chiropractic Clinical Encounter

Robert A. Leach, DC, MS, CHES

Introduction

It has been said that every generation has an opportunity to reinvent itself. This has never been truer than in the case of modern-day chiropractors. During the past 25 years, the level of pre-chiropractic education has risen steadily. According to the most recent *National Board of Chiropractic Examiners' Practice Analysis of Chiropractic 2015* survey results, 95 percent of practicing chiropractors have had postsecondary training in addition to their chiropractic education. Of all respondents, 66 percent hold bachelor's, 6 percent master's, and 7 percent hold non-chiropractic doctoral degrees. Since 1991, the percentage of female chiropractors has doubled to 27 percent, as has the percentage of black chiropractors, although still underrepresented at only 1 percent. Meanwhile, Hispanic (2 percent) and Asian-Pacific Islander (3 percent) ethnicities have seen perhaps more representative growth. While characteristics and demographics of chiropractors will be explored in detail later (*see Chapter 3*), it is important to understand that modern chiropractors are better equipped by education and diversity to interact with, diagnose, and treat today's technology-savvy patient than were their predecessors just a quarter of a century ago. And that's a good thing, since during that time millennials were the first generation to grow up with cell phones replacing land lines, Google replacing library card catalog searches, and Wikipedia replacing *Encyclopedia Britannica*, with all these resources available in nearly all American households.

Beyond education and training, the chiropractic clinical encounter with a new patient varies according to the practice type, philosophy, and focus of the chiropractic physician. For example, chiropractors in solo practice may interact with patients differently than chiropractors in group practices, hospitals, or military installations, although some interactions will remain constant across those settings. Similarly, some chiropractors limit their focus to analysis and correction of subluxation, a process they consider central to the historical philosophy of the profession. However, the majority of practitioners embrace a more "holistic" approach to their care. In addition to giving spinal adjustments, these doctors prescribe nutritional supplements and herbs, treat with physiotherapeutic procedures, prescribe and teach stretches and exercise, and offer an interdisciplinary approach that may include massage therapy, acupuncture, or other practices. A limited number of practitioners favor limited prescription rights for chiropractors, although continuing with a focus of conservative spine care. The chiropractor's focus plays a role in the clinical encounter as well, since, for example, a great deal more dialogue is needed to work with the geriatric patient presenting with multiple comorbidities compared to the athlete being treated by a sports chiropractor for a simple strain. Similarly, dialogue is limited just to the mother or caregiver of the infant with colic, and just to the owner of the pet in the case of the animal chiropractor. In contrast, the chiropractor working on injured employees, athletes, or military personnel, or in an interdisciplinary practice working alongside orthopedists, physical therapists, or even family nurse practitioners, is required to learn to communicate verbally and through use of good medical notes. In the latter case, in addition to interacting with patients, chiropractors are required to communicate with stakeholders, such as employers, coaches, and other providers. In summary, while this chapter will focus on the clinical encounter that chiropractors have with patients in a typical chiropractic practice, it is important to understand that there is wide variation in what that "typical" encounter might look like, depending on the practice specialty, as we shall see in later sections of this work.

Studies of chiropractic patients suggest that they are not substantially different from the rest of the population, and chiropractors generally draw patients from all walks of life, education, and income strata. Typically, a patient presents to the chiropractor's office with a specific pain or problem, called the chief complaint. Sometimes there will be other problems, called secondary complaints. After an initial consultation and exam, the chiropractor will make a first assessment of what's wrong, called a preliminary diagnosis. The National Board of Chiropractic Examiners (NBCE) survey revealed that chiropractic patients are most often diagnosed with neurologic conditions, such as headache, arm or leg pain or numbness, neck or back joint pain, and muscle strain and inflammation. Chiropractors also regularly treat arthritis, whiplash, spinal disc herniation, and sprains of joints anywhere in the body. Problems like dizziness and rheumatoid or inflammatory arthritis, scoliosis, carpal tunnel syndrome, temporomandibular (TMJ) problems, tendon problems, widespread chronic pain and tenderness (fibromyalgia), osteoporosis, obesity, diabetes, pregnancy-related problems, menstrual pain, sinus issues, and nutritional and food problems are treated less frequently by chiropractors. In addition, chiropractors may rarely treat other problems. The most recent report by the U.S. Agency for Healthcare Research and Quality suggests an evidence basis for chiropractic treatment of acute and chronic neck and back pain and tension and migraine headaches. Research of chiropractic care for these problems will be discussed in detail later in this work. However, suffice it to say that there is growing evidence that chiropractic patients are satisfied with the care they receive and even that patients care about the quality of care they receive irrespective of costs.

The typical chiropractor is in private, solo practice (75 percent) with at least one or more full-time employees, and one in four employs a massage therapist in the practice. Staff members typically include a receptionist, who may also be a billing clerk, and at least one chiropractic assistant. Usually the chiropractic assistant has some training, and in a few chiropractic practices a licensed practical nurse or registered nurse is employed. In most states, some continuing education is required to maintain a license as a chiropractic assistant. However, some states require no licensure of chiropractic assistants and hence have no continuing education requirement for staff. Seven in 10 chiropractors have up to 99 patient visits each week, spending 30–39 (45%) or 40–49 (23%) hours either in direct patient contact or in related activity. While 9 in 10 chiropractors work in a private office setting, 8 percent of chiropractors now work in an integrated setting, including hospital (4%) and military (7%) facilities. The number of chiropractors working in a military setting grew 50 percent from 2009 to 2014, according to the NBCE survey results. There is a concerted push for doctors of chiropractic to work in interdisciplinary care coming from both within and outside the profession; examples of this include new federal health care provisions calling for community health centers and other forms of patient-centered medical home organizations that offer interdisciplinary care, as well as calls for such practices within the leadership of the American Chiropractic Association and among some of the profession's leading scientists. Hence, while the current chapter will focus on the routine new and continuing patient encounter as experienced by the typical doctor of chiropractic in solo private practice, in a broader sense, the rich milieu of modern-day chiropractic clinical encounters will vary from solo to group practices, from multidisciplinary clinics to research centers and hospitals, and from traditional chiropractic practice to specialty practice on humans or even animals.

The First Visit

Traditionally, upon entering a chiropractor's office for the first visit, the new patient would be handed a clipboard and asked to complete a case history and questionnaire requesting insurance and billing information. In contrast, today's new patient may be told to download and complete new patient forms online or even be directed to phone apps that collect information electronically prior to visiting the office. Rather than calling insurance companies for verification of benefits, as was typically the case in the past, today's chiropractic staff is often able to do this online. The role of the receptionist varies from office to office, but he or she is generally charged with gathering basic information about the patient, including demographic information (e.g., address and phone number); insurance, Medicare, or Medicaid coverage; and the reason why the patient is presenting to the office. For some doctors this is enough, but for others the receptionist may also screen emergency from non-emergency situations, working emergencies into an otherwise full schedule or referring to the emergency room as directed by the chiropractor. As such, the receptionist is an integral part of a thriving chiropractic practice, since he or she gathers essential information, keeps the practice schedule, acts to triage emergencies according to protocols established by the doctor, checks out patients, and collects fees.

In a new doctor's practice, when the patient volume is low, the receptionist may communicate with the doctor regarding nearly every phone call into the practice. There may be time, for example, for the receptionist to place the caller on hold while consulting with the doctor regarding questions about insurance coverage or when determining whether the caller's problem is routine, requires urgent work in, or needs immediate referral for emergency care. However, as the practice grows, most chiropractic physicians develop procedures and protocols for handling various issues so that they can maintain their focus on patient care while the

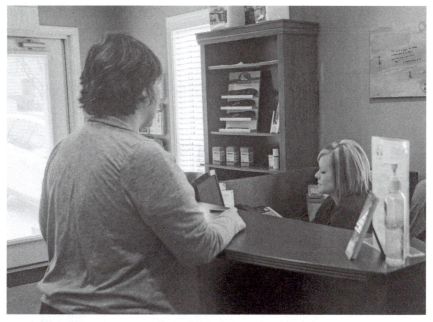

Figure 2.1 The receptionist is a focal point of a thriving chiropractic practice, in addition to scheduling appointments and collecting fees, acting to triage patients for emergency, urgent, or routine care. (Lisa Leach Photography)

receptionist handles the practice schedule. Seasoned doctors of chiropractic hold regular staff meetings where they review procedures. Because receptionist and assistant training in chiropractic may be limited, regular staff meetings and training is conducted in some chiropractic offices to teach staff a wide array of procedures, such as the following:

- identifying red flags for disease and emergencies
- verifying insurance coverage (workers' compensation insurance, regular insurance, Medicare, Medicaid, auto insurance)
- collecting paperwork regarding patient privacy
- obtaining written consent to treat
- collecting and assisting patients in completion of case history
- assisting patients with handicaps, disabilities, and foreign languages
- taking of vitals, such as blood pressure and pulse rate
- identifying other forms and questionnaires the doctor and/or insurance company may require given the patient's presenting complaints (e.g., back or headache questionnaires)

- rescheduling missed appointments
- answering the phone
- collecting fees at the end of the visit
- consulting with the doctor when necessary to triage patients to regular, urgent, or emergency care (perhaps the most important procedure)

The importance of receptionist training and having procedures in place to handle incoming calls is underscored during emergencies presenting both on the phone and in the office. The receptionist or chiropractic assistant who is trained in handling emergencies (e.g., has CPR training and understands red flags for disease) is in a far better position to serve the patients and practice compared to the employee without such training, who may panic and make a critical error, placing the patient in jeopardy. For example, the receptionist may want to triage calls to the doctor when the patient presents with red flags, such as unexplained cough or low-grade fever; reproductive system, bowel, or bladder problems associated with onset or worsening of spinal pain; numbness, tingling, or weakness of limbs; or lumps, masses, or unusual discharge. If the patient with such new symptoms cannot be immediately seen by the doctor, the reception-ist may interrupt the chiropractor so she or he may direct the patient to an emergency room (ER) or to an urgent care center, if indicated. Ulti-mately, while each situation is unique, it is up to the chiropractor's judg-ment whether referral is indicated or chiropractic consult and treatment is appropriate. And it is the receptionist who must make the call as to whether to interrupt the doctor to make such a decision. With protocols in place, the receptionist will either schedule the patient for the next available regular appointment, work in the patient as an emergency, or refer the patient to the ER with follow-up to the office when an appoint-ment is available, should the problem continue.

Once an appointment has been made or the patient has been worked into the schedule, the chiropractic assistant (CA) or therapist (in some cases, a single employee acts as receptionist, CA, therapist, and insurance clerk, while in larger offices these jobs are handled by different individu-als) typically collects new patient forms and insurance information and starts the chiropractic examination by collecting the patient's vital statis-tics. Many offices also have staff start the case history, so the therapist or CA would usher the new patient into a room and ask him or her how the problem started, what makes it better, what makes it worse, whether the patient has seen another doctor, and so on. Such a history is also referred to as the new patient consult and collection of symptoms or subjective findings, or the "S" of SOAP notes. ("SOAP" refers to *subjective* measures, such as rating of pain or pain scores; *objective* measures, such as how a joint motion has been restricted by pain; *assessment* being the diagnosis or at least possible diagnoses; and *plan*, or what adjustments and other in-office or in-home treatments should be completed to gain maximum improvement.) Regardless of whether he or she assists with an initial interview, the chiropractic physician personally consults with each patient, reviewing the work of staff and clarifying and asking further questions of the patient as indicated. Certainly, the patient consult is one of the most important elements of any office visit and is essential for the new patient visit. It is widely held throughout medicine that perhaps 90 percent of the information needed for making the correct diagnosis and directing patient care is obtained during the initial consultation. Perhaps 4 in 10 medical physicians and 1 in 10 chiropractic physicians in the United States use electronic health records and the Medicare "Meaningful Use" protocols. In these offices, this information is stored digitally on specific software in a format approved by the government and the Department of Health and Human Services and may be electronically accessed by patients as well as other providers.

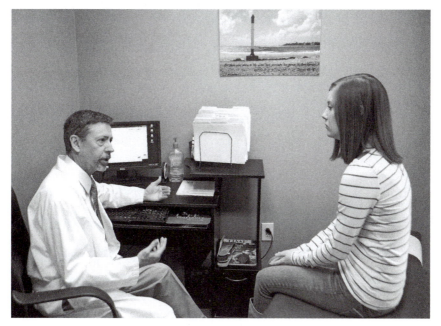

Figure 2.2 The new patient consult is one of the most important elements of the first office visit, essential to arrive at a correct diagnosis and prescribe optimal care. (Lisa Leach Photography)

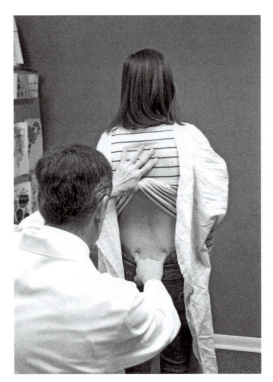

Figure 2.3 Observing gait, posture, and checking for tight muscles during the chiropractic exam provides clues to the presence and location of spinal and joint lesions. (Lisa Leach Photography)

After the initial consultation, the chiropractor typically begins a new patient examination, consisting of a problem-focused approach, although a wellness-oriented chiropractor may approach the exam with more global instruments and questionnaires. For example, in a problem-focused exam, the patient presents with a history of migraine headaches, and the doctor proceeds to examine the neck and shoulder region for signs of spinal dysfunction or "subluxation," lesions that may trigger or predispose patients to this form of headache. In contrast, a more wellness-oriented or "holistic" chiropractor may examine literally everything from the patient's diet to the patient's feet, prescribing nutritional supplements as well as orthotics if foot problems are present, arguing that if the foundation is not right, everything above it will not be right either.

The doctor will usually begin by examining the patient's gait and ability to stand erect, visually observing problem areas and looking for tissue texture changes and firm muscles that may indicate spasm or other problems. Checking range of motion and looking for areas of stiffness, tenderness, and pain during motion is a key focus of the exam, since these may be the best predictors of spinal or extremity joint inflammation and problems. In addition, the doctor will search for clues of more serious problems during the exam. She or he will note signs or so-called "red flag" symptoms, such as vomiting, imbalance, dizziness, slurred speech, difficulty holding the arm up, and inability to smile, that may indicate presence of a more ominous cause of the migraine headache (e.g., tumor, cancer, or stroke). Chiropractic physicians are trained to immediately triage such emergencies to the ERD, and it is the standard of care in literally all U.S. states for such referral to be made. However, the vast majority of chiropractic new patients have symptoms and signs of problems well within the scope of chiropractic treatment, and the exam includes chiropractic and orthopedic tests that manually provoke pain responses that help identify not only the presence of spinal or joint dysfunction but also its location, so treatment may be specific to the site of the problem. Many chiropractors still use radiographs

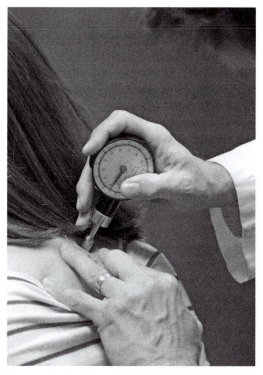

Figure 2.4 Chiropractic exam can include use of a force gauge to measure tender points, that may indicate areas of muscle spasm and inflammation. (Lisa Leach Photography)

(X-rays) to determine the course of adjustments for new patients presenting to their offices. However, a more evidence-based approach that has gained traction since the turn of the new century suggests that such films are not indicated in most cases unless the patient has been exposed to trauma, or examination reveals red flags for disease and X-rays will be used to further rule out complications or comorbidities, or in cases where the patient has failed to respond to conservative care and imaging has not previously been performed.

Once the exam confirms that both (a) no significant red flags for disease are present, and (b) mechanical maneuvers reproduce the patient's pain in joints or tissues in the problem area, then treatment may begin. Many chiropractors will offer a treatment—after briefly reviewing the patient's problem, exam findings, preliminary diagnosis, and obtaining the patient's verbal consent, including review of pros and cons of suggested treatment as well as other medical treatments and

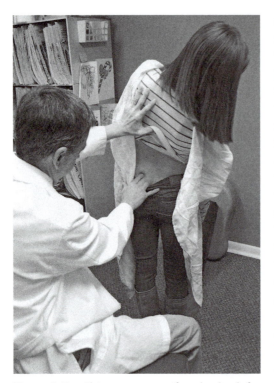

Figure 2.5 Chiropractors uniformly check for restrictions in range of motion, and for motion triggering a worsening of the presenting pain, as indicators of joint or muscle inflammation associated with the patient's problem. If range of motion and movement does not aggravate the problem, other causes of pain such as disease may need to be ruled out. (Lisa Leach Photography)

options—toward the end of the patient's very first visit. In other cases, chiropractors will order X-rays, if indicated, and/or have the new patient sign releases to obtain records from prior chiropractors or physicians and defer treatment until a second visit. Many chiropractors apply various treatments to prepare patients for the main chiropractic treatment, spinal manipulation or "adjustment." These supportive treatments to reduce inflammation, muscle spasm, and pain include heat or cold therapy, using a cold pack or heating pad; electrical muscle stimulation, in which electrodes placed on the skin send mild pulsations; ultrasound, which uses sound waves; and laser. All of these procedures are safe and painless.

As we shall see in subsequent sections of this work, there is evidence that spinal adjustments are as at least as effective for back problems as other typical physiological therapeutic procedures, exercise alone, or medications alone, based on a fairly large body of research. That said, most chiropractors use a variety of procedures to relax patients for the chiropractic adjustment and emphasize the role of exercise and stretches in helping prevent recurrence of spinal lesions (also termed "subluxations"). Regardless of whether an adjustment is provided toward the end of the first visit, the new patient will typically be provided with home care instructions that may include, for example, stretches and use of ice applied to the problem area at regular intervals and a recommendation to stay active and avoid prolonged sitting, standing, or even prolonged bed rest, which has been shown to contribute to disability. Before leaving the office, the new patient usually schedules a follow-up visit.

The Second Visit

Even prior to the patient returning for follow-up, the chiropractic physician will often prepare by calling the patient the evening after the first adjustment to check on the patient's progress, reviewing findings from examination, labs, and X-rays, if made. At this time, many chiropractors also prepare a written "report of findings,"

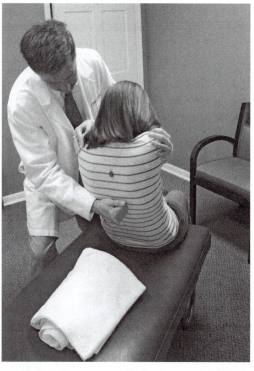

Figure 2.6 A so-called "anterior dorsal" adjustment can provide relief for middle back pain. (Lisa Leach Photography)

to be handed to the patient on presentation for the follow-up visit, which typically includes a chiropractic analysis (i.e., chiropractic joint problems, such as intervertebral subluxation or joint dysfunction) and an explanation of what is wrong with the patient (preliminary medical diagnosis or differential diagnosis). The chiropractor will update the diagnosis based on the patient's response to initial in-office and/or in-home treatment. If the patient responded well to the initial recommendations, or in the case of more chronic or more serious conditions at least obtained "temporary" relief, then the diagnosis is firmed up. On the other hand, since a strong predictor of future chiropractic results is the patient's response to the first two weeks of care, if after one to several treatments the patient is not seeing a good response to treatment, the chiropractor may order additional tests such as advanced imaging (e.g., magnetic resonance imaging or computed tomography), refer to another medical provider or specialist, or seek to "comanage" the patient with the help of the patient's own primary care provider physician or a medical specialist. After the chiropractor notes the initial response to treatment, the preliminary diagnosis is either changed or reaffirmed and is now referred to as the "working diagnosis" (i.e., the initial diagnosis made stronger by a positive treatment response, or a new diagnosis, or even a list of possible conditions to be ruled out instead of or in addition to the preliminary diagnosis). In this way, the chiropractor may recommend continuing chiropractic care for treatment of spinal lesions even while referring the patient for medical comanagement of other non-chiropractic problems.

When the patient arrives for the second visit, unless she or he already received care at the end of the first visit, some chiropractors will provide the patient with a written new patient report of findings, show the patient his or her X-rays, and review findings. It has been said that patients really have only a few simple questions they want answered by their health care provider, be it a chiropractic physician or other provider: (a) What's wrong with me? (b) Can you fix it? (c) How long will it take? and (d) How much will it cost? Perhaps a fifth question all patients have is (e) Will it hurt to fix? Addressing these basic questions through a brief written and oral report of findings, including review of X-ray and lab findings if included, will ensure optimal compliance and satisfaction with care, if not with the clinical outcome. The chiropractor who addresses these issues and has staff that will address insurance and financial questions and considerations will have greater odds that the patient will comply with the treatment recommendations, perform the exercises, follow the home care instructions, and make the indicated lifestyle modifications that will help achieve optimal

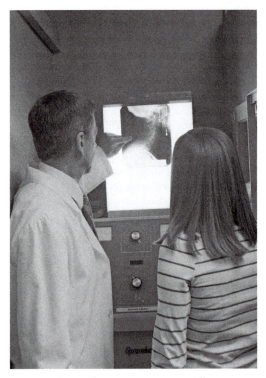

Figure 2.7 Chiropractors typically review exam and X-ray findings with their patients prior to starting a care plan. (Lisa Leach Photography)

clinical outcomes. If the patient is getting his or her adjustment on the second visit after the report of findings, then the doctor obtains written and verbal consent to treat after reviewing the diagnosis and imaging findings (if indicated) and proceeds with the adjustment and/or other treatment.

Another important issue addressed by the new patient report of findings pertains to gaining the patient's confidence to proceed with care. It is critically important that the patient is engaged and that any questions have been answered. Verbal consent to treat is a process whereby patients are made to understand the preliminary diagnosis and both the best and worst things that might happen to them should they obtain the suggested treatment or should they seek alternative treatments. While a written consent to treat can cover the most common problems and reactions patients might experience after chiropractic care, a verbal consent can fill in the gaps and provide an explanation of realistic problems that particular patients might experience given their own particular diagnosis and comorbid conditions. Patients can also be reassured by this process. When patients are engaged and looking forward to the care, they are more relaxed and typically get a better treatment and have better first visit outcomes, although these observations have not yet been validated through clinical research. In contrast, chiropractors who try to

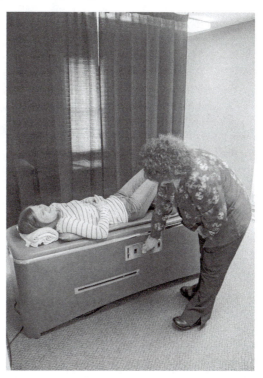

Figure 2.8 Intersegmental traction is often used by chiropractors to improve circulation and aid in relaxing patients prior to providing the chiropractic adjustment. Traditionally ice, moist heat, ultrasound, muscle stimulation, and other physiological therapeutic procedures have also been used by chiropractic physicians to prepare patients for and enhance the effects of chiropractic techniques. (Lisa Leach Photography)

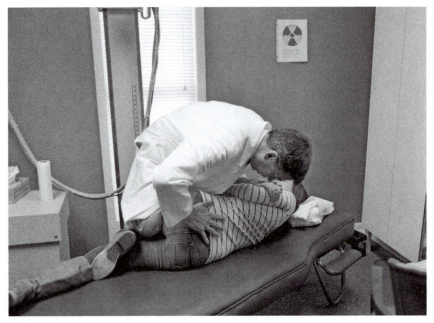

Figure 2.9 The side-posture diversified adjustment is perhaps the most commonly used chiropractic procedure for treatment of low back and sacroiliac joint pain. There is a large body of research evidence regarding the effectiveness of the technique, which will be reviewed later in this work. (Lisa Leach Photography)

strong-arm patients into receiving care that they are afraid of, don't really want, or don't think they can afford may find their patients less compliant and more likely to quit prior to receiving the recommended care. The recommendation may involve chiropractic care, immediate referral for medical care, immediate referral for medical comanagement with chiropractic care, or a brief trial of chiropractic care. When chiropractors refer to other physicians, usually staff will call to coordinate the referral, and a copy of the chiropractor's notes with preliminary diagnosis and rationale for referral will be faxed or e-mailed to the doctor receiving the referral. When a trial of care is indicated, patients might be told that further imaging or other medical tests might be indicated if satisfactory progress was not made.

Chiropractors typically use therapies to help patients relax, ranging from simple application of cryotherapy (e.g., a reusable ice pack wrapped in insulation and applied to the spinal area or joint being manipulated), to electrotherapies, ultrasound, or various forms of traction. Adjustments in a chiropractic office range from simple manual manipulations involving high velocity and short levers (e.g., the typical side posture low back or

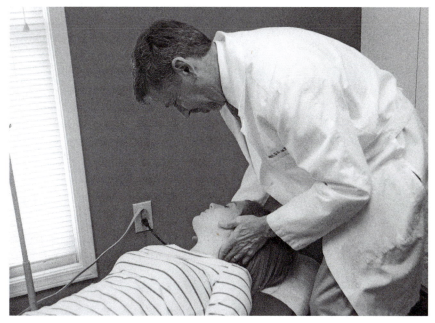

Figure 2.10 For headaches and neck and upper back pain, chiropractic physicians typically use the rotary or cervical break procedures. There is compelling evidence for both the effectiveness and safety of the adjustment, which will be reviewed in later sections of this work. (Lisa Leach Photography)

rotational neck procedures), to instrumented techniques involving manual (e.g., Activator) or even computer-assisted (e.g., PulStar) devices. Indeed, there are several dozen major chiropractic techniques used by chiropractors, and discussion here is beyond the scope of this chapter, but some will be discussed in later sections of this work.

The Routine Visit

Research suggests that there is a dose-response relationship between chiropractic treatments and clinical outcomes. Simply put, if for whatever reason a patient can only go to the chiropractor 9 or 12 times (e.g., because of a lack of available time or money), then it is important for treatments to occur in a condensed time period, three times per week instead of weekly, for example. Although the research that validated this approach to patient care was just published recently, chiropractors have traditionally scheduled their patients for daily or three-times-per-week adjustments, at least initially. Most chiropractic physicians gradually withdraw care after four weeks and a good response to treatment has been observed by both the patient and chiropractor. Chiropractors judge whether a good response to treatment has been achieved through clinical measures and standardized patient statements about pain collected during each visit. Tracking these measurements makes it obvious to both the doctor and patient (and to insurance companies or third-party payors if reviewed later) when the patient has improved, indicating that less frequent care is indicated, for example. Or, in a worst-case scenario, when these same clinical measures indicate that the patient is unimproved, or that the problem is worsening, tracking the course of these variables clearly reveals that a different treatment approach, medical comanagement, or referral is indicated. The standardized format chiropractors use to track clinical measures in this way is referred to as SOAP note reporting (SOAP refers to *subjective* measures, such as rating of pain or pain scores; *objective* measures, such as how a joint motion has been restricted by pain; *assessment* being the diagnosis or at least possible diagnoses; and *plan*, or what adjustments and other in-office or in-home treatments should be completed to gain maximum improvement).

In modern clinical health care, doctors rely on scientific studies to tell them what clinical measures are best to monitor to help them provide optimal care for their patients. In the past, we referred to a chiropractor who relied on modern scientific evidence to inform her or his opinions and practices as a "scientific chiropractor," but in modern terms we call this an "evidence-based" or "evidence-informed" chiropractic physician. As an example of a subjective measurement, in the past, chiropractors asked patients how they felt and recorded qualitative words, such as "better" or "the same." In contrast, today, based on modern scientific evidence, more quantitative data is recorded by chiropractors, such as a verbal pain score from 0 to 10 (where 0 is no pain and 10 is unbearable pain), which scientists have found can be used reliably between doctors and visits, and which has more validity for tracking progress.

Similarly, an example of an objective clinical measure traditionally used by almost all chiropractors to determine whether their patients needed an adjustment was the so-called "leg check." But modern chiropractic research showed that although the leg check was reliable, there were questions about its validity to measure clinical progress. Therefore, many chiropractors today use other objective measures to track progress, such as pain provocation tests, range of motion, or algometry by use of a force gauge to measure tenderness that might suggest muscle spasm and inflammation.

Regardless of the philosophy that the chiropractor brings to his or her practice, patients expect that minimum standards and safeguards will be in place to protect their welfare. Although some chiropractors and other types of "wellness" providers may wish to deny responsibility for making the correct diagnosis or differential diagnosis, courts and licensing boards generally mandate that the primary responsibility of the chiropractor is to "do no harm" through either acts of omission or commission. Simply put, having patients sign a waiver to the effect that the chiropractor does not have to diagnose the patient's problems and make appropriate referral does not relieve the doctor from her or his statutory duty to do just that. Moreover, saying you are a "wellness chiropractor" in your signage, website, intake, and consent-to-treat forms does not relieve you of responsibility for failure to immediately refer a patient presenting with a stroke in progress to the emergency room. Hence, modern chiropractors who embrace their portal-of-entry status as health care providers by taking appropriate SOAP notes and using evidence-informed clinical measures to track progress are more likely to live up to their statutory responsibilities while providing optimal chiropractic care. Further, they know when to make referrals for medical comanagement or specialist care because they track clinical measures on every visit.

There is an exception to this rule, however, that can still leave the chiropractor liable even though he or she had been initially providing care, perhaps even using evidence-based guidelines. The chiropractor can be found liable if a patient quits care without order of the chiropractor and staff fail to make appropriate follow-up contact. In the modern era, it is not enough that chiropractors provide optimal care. Most disease processes, for example, are not readily apparent on the first visit to a chiropractor or primary care provider. No one realistically expects that the patient who presents one time with just one sign of a serious spinal disease will get a correct diagnosis on the first visit. Instead, patients often have to be monitored over the course of several visits until more obvious symptoms present or their presenting condition fails to improve with typical conservative chiropractic care. When such patients fail to keep appointments or quit care, staff must make every effort to contact the patient, determine whether he or she is still hurting, and if so attempt to reschedule the missed appointment. If this is not possible or the patient does not respond to phone calls, the doctor must formally discharge the patient since she or he is unwilling to follow through with the agreed-upon care plan, such as a trial of two weeks of treatment followed by advanced imaging if improvement is not observed.

It is not uncommon for patients to quit chiropractic treatments because they were not getting "immediate" relief. Then, when their condition worsens or new symptoms develop, the patient's primary care physician or a specialist makes the correct diagnosis, and the chiropractor is sued for failure to diagnose and refer. In these cases, the chiropractic physician is protected when she or he has thorough notes showing that the patient agreed but failed to follow a plan of care and establishing that the staff made phone calls and followed up with a mailed written notice discharging the patient for quitting care without order of the doctor. In these cases, optimal treatment actually includes discharging a noncompliant patient from care.

Progress and Final Exam Visits

In the United States, the federal Medicare program is an example of a third-party payor that expects regular updating of patient care progress. The Physician Quality Reporting System requires regular reportage of whether, for example, the chiropractor is updating treatment plans and goals and recording pain and activities of daily living disability and other important clinical measures at 30-day intervals. A number of chiropractic "best practices" guidelines have been developed since 1993 to guide chiropractors, and they universally advocate tracking clinical measures, regularly setting clinical goals for establishing when progress has been achieved, and administering progress exams at regular intervals to determine when optimal care has been achieved. The guidelines help ensure that chiropractic patients receive the best possible care from chiropractors and that procedures are standardized so that various chiropractic physicians will all provide the same level of quality care.

Chiropractic physicians who adhere to these best practices receive higher levels of Medicare reimbursement. These practices are likely to be implemented and required by all third-party payors in the future. To achieve these benchmarks, chiropractic physicians typically perform progress exams at least every 30 days on patients who have significant pain, disability, or yellow flags. Typically, chiropractic physicians refer patients with red flags for further diagnostic work-ups or imaging, such as X-rays or magnetic resonance imaging, if the patient is unimproved within a two-week trial of care. Final exams are typically used to evaluate for disability; determine whether discharge, referral, or continuing care is indicated; and/or make a recommendation for maintenance or preventive care. During these exams, the chiropractor has staff collect vital signs, pain rating, and disability scores, and then after a brief exam to check previously positive findings, compares the patient's symptoms and findings before and after chiropractic care. Armed with this information, the chiropractic physician is confident in making subsequent care recommendations.

It should be noted that a small minority of chiropractors in the United States do not regularly perform exams nor check on the progress of their patients, other than through the use of leg checks, X-rays, and other measures of subluxation or spinal dysfunction. They inform their patients that they do not "diagnose" disease but instead perform an "analysis to determine the existence of subluxation." They advocate chiropractic as a cure for the "cause of all dis-ease." However, in all U.S. states, chiropractors are required by law to at least perform a differential diagnosis to determine whether patients require medical intervention, including emergency procedures, for their health care complaints. Legal experts generally believe that merely informing a patient that exam and diagnostic procedures are not used, or informing patients that if they want a medical diagnosis they must go to a medical doctor, does not relieve a chiropractor from the responsibility to avoid harming her or his patients. Generally, legal experts say all doctors, including chiropractic physicians, may harm their patients through either acts of commission (e.g., adjusting a spine that is pathologic due to disease) or acts of omission (e.g., failing to recognize referred pain from disease and refer to an appropriate specialist). In summary, jurisdictions in the United States charge chiropractors with providing for the "safety" of their patients, including knowing when adjustments are indicated and when referral is indicated instead of chiropractic and providing such referrals promptly.

Some chiropractors do not bill or accept insurance on assignment, often in areas where the quality of insurance benefits for chiropractic is poor. In the United States, chiropractors are required by federal law to bill for services when they treat patients with Medicare coverage. They may not opt out of this requirement, although they may be a "nonparticipating" chiropractor and ask patients to pay for their care as it is rendered—rather than waiting for Medicare reimbursement—by accepting a lower reimbursement rate. In contrast, probably a majority of U.S. chiropractors accept some or most insurance payments on assignment, so that patients only pay a portion of their care when seen, while the insurance pays the remainder of the amount owed directly to the chiropractic physician. These chiropractors submit health care claims by mail or electronically that include the diagnosis and other relevant information. Not all insurance plans pay for chiropractic once a patient is no longer in pain. So, when progress or final exams reveal that maximum chiropractic improvement has been achieved and spinal problems are improved to the highest level achievable, the chiropractor will generally dismiss the patient from passive "acute" care and recommend follow-up or "maintenance care." This is care designed to avoid deterioration of the patient's condition, so the patient can maintain optimal spinal function and health. Most chiropractors offer discounted plans that make maintenance care more affordable. In summary, exams and diagnosis are best practices that provide the foundation for decisions that help determine the optimal level of care or provide direction for referral for other diagnostic procedures or to other health care providers.

Similarities and Differences between Chiropractic and Physical Medicine, Osteopathy, Massage, and Physical Therapy Procedures and Practices

In addition to chiropractic, there are other health care professions that may also use adjustments, or spinal manipulation, the primary treatment provided by chiropractors in the United States. Medical doctors who specialize in conservative, nonsurgical treatment of spine, joint, and muscle problems are termed "physical medicine" specialists. Physicians who advocate a more holistic approach to health but also provide medicine and surgery when indicated are referred to as "osteopathic physicians." Physical therapists offer a range of conservative nonsurgical treatments for muscle and joint problems and other disorders that traditionally did not include manipulation. However, in the wake of increased research and the 1994 *Acute Low Back Pain Treatment Guidelines* developed by the U.S. Agency for Healthcare Policy and Research, which advocated for spinal manipulation, the profession has begun to endorse and undergo additional training for a doctor of physical therapy degree, to qualify providers with skill in diagnosis and manipulation. A profession that employs a variety of bodywork procedures, including stretching, light and deep touch, and friction applied to muscles, tendons, and ligaments, is massage therapy. Massage therapists, however, are not trained to provide spinal or joint manipulation services.

With the exception of massage therapy, these professions compete with chiropractors in the delivery of spinal manipulation for the treatment of spine and joint pain. However, chiropractors are unique in advocating it as a primary focus of their health care practice, not only to reduce spine and joint pain but to improve overall health. For example, while the other providers may perform spinal or joint manipulation services occasionally, on some patients, and during some visits, chiropractic physicians provide these services to nearly every patient entering the practice, and in most cases during every office visit. Further, while not all chiropractors use the high-velocity, low-amplitude thrust procedures that typically result in the characteristic "popping" of the joint, it is probably more likely that a patient attending a chiropractor will receive this type of treatment than will a patient attending one of the other provider types just mentioned. In contrast with this distinction, what these providers have in common is advocating for exercise, smoking cessation, reduction in alcohol and drug dependence, and other goals espoused by the U.S. Centers for Disease Control and Prevention in Healthy People 2010 and 2020. Indeed, of the original 10 leading health indicators listed among the Healthy People 2010 goals, chiropractors generally advocate for all but immunizations (some chiropractors criticize immunizations due to possible side effects and reactions and the recent increases to the newborn immunization schedule in the United States). Based on the most recent survey research, it is likely that chiropractors in general would support 25 of 26 of the 2020 leading health indicators, with the majority supporting all 26. Hence, patients who seek the care of any of these provider types, including chiropractors, will likely be informed about healthy lifestyle choices that will improve their spine, joint, and overall health.

The fact that chiropractors are responsible for perhaps 95 percent of all spinal manipulation performed in the United States ensures that of all provider types, chiropractic physicians may develop expertise and finesse in its application that surpasses that of other providers. Chiropractors claim that they also obtain results not seen by other providers of manipulation. While these observations remain to be explored, let alone proven, what is not in dispute is that surveys of patients and self-reports of disability for the past 40 years point to greater satisfaction and less back pain disability associated with chiropractic than for many other treatments. So, it is not known whether chiropractors' purported technique expertise directly lends itself to better results, but there is evidence that among providers of spinal manipulation services, studies continue to suggest that chiropractor-treated patients are more satisfied and experience less disability. It should also be noted that there is greater collaboration with massage therapy within chiropractic practices in the United States than any other provider type.

Research and Practice in the Future: Pain, Wellness, and Prevention of Spine and Musculoskeletal-Related Disorders in Collaborative Care Centers and through Sharing of Digital Records

The Affordable Care Act of 2010 advocates for patient-centered medical homes, often evolving from community health centers (CHCs) that include multiple provider types working in collaborative settings to provide opportunities for improved outcomes and patient-focused treatments.

By 2010, there were 1,124 CHCs operating in more than 8,000 locations, serving nearly 20 million patients in the United States. Three-quarters of the patients had low or poverty-level income ($22,050 for a family of four), and only 40 percent of the patients were covered by the federal Medicaid program. The federal legislation in the United States specifically includes chiropractors as a provider type eligible to participate in patient-centered medical homes. While such provocative associations remain elusive in common practice, it is indisputable that collaboration between medical and chiropractic providers continues growing. Today chiropractors practice in hospitals alongside other physicians in more than half the U.S. states, and they perform their duties alongside medical physicians at military installations and veterans' treatment centers, where patient-centered, problem-focused care allows chiropractic to be used for spine and joint pain and other musculoskeletal problems, if not for prevention and wellness care. These advances all occurred in just the past four decades, coinciding with the U.S. Supreme Court decision to let stand a landmark federal court ruling that prevents medical doctors from acting together to boycott chiropractic services and with the exponential rise in a chiropractic research enterprise during those same decades.

Further, new mandates regarding electronic health records from the U.S. Centers for Medicare and Medicaid Services suggest that all health care provider types will, for the first time, communicate in a common format, sharing information electronically in ways not heretofore envisioned. Sharing of accurate records between provider types ensures that the providers will not have to rely on the memory of the patient to describe what conversations have been had and what tests and treatments have already been performed. While it does not guarantee that best care practices will ensue, it certainly removes one of the barriers to the attainment of optimal care. For full integration of chiropractic services into the American health care system, uniformity in communication and lexicon stand as hallmark first steps, and the fact that today patients can request records from their medical or chiropractic physician and, by use of a password and portal obtain them from the "cloud," suggests that one day sharing of important data between various provider types will be the rule rather than the exception. Certainly, this trend toward increased accessibility and transparency of medical records bodes well for patients, who in the future may be expected to benefit from health care providers, including chiropractors, whose musculoskeletal and wellness care is integrated and collaborative.

Suggested Reading

Leach RA. *The Chiropractic Theories: A Textbook of Scientific Research.* 4th ed. Baltimore, MD: Lippincott, Williams & Wilkins; 2004.

Leach RA, Cossman RE, Yates JM. Familiarity with and advocacy of Healthy People 2010 goals by Mississippi Chiropractic Association members. *J Manipulative Physiol Ther.* 2011;34(6):394–406.

National Board of Chiropractic Examiners. *Practice Analysis of Chiropractic.* Greeley, CO: National Board of Chiropractic Examiners; 2015.

Weigel PA, Hockenberry J, Bentler SE, Wolinsky FD. The comparative effect of episodes of chiropractic and medical treatment on the health of older adults. *J Manipulative Physiol Ther.* 2014;37(3):143–154.

Weigel PA, Hockenberry JM, Wolinsky FD. Chiropractic use in the Medicare population: prevalence, patterns, and associations with 1-year changes in health and satisfaction with care. *J Manipulative Physiol Ther.* 2014;37(8):542–551.

CHAPTER THREE

The Typical Doctor of Chiropractic

Shawn Hatch, DC; Cami Stastny, DC; Francis J. H. Wilson, DC, MSc, PhD; and Lyndon Amorin-Woods, BAppSci(Chiropractic), MPH

Introduction

The purpose of this chapter is to present the characteristics of a typical doctor of chiropractic and a typical chiropractic practice in the United States. It begins with what is required in order to become a chiropractor, including educational and licensure requirements. It will also discuss the scope of practice for chiropractors (what they are legally able to do and not do within a region). Although there is a wide variety of practice styles and types, this chapter will discuss the kind of experience one might have when visiting a chiropractor, including what an average visit might entail and the types of treatments that are commonly used by chiropractors. It will then outline some of the criteria that might be used in order to select a chiropractor that best fits the needs of a potential patient and explain some of the conditions and injuries that are commonly treated by chiropractors. Although chiropractic education and practice originated and is most well established in the United States, the practice is growing quickly around the world. Therefore, brief descriptions of typical chiropractic practice in the United Kingdom (U.K.) and in Australia are also included to provide an international perspective.

Chiropractic Practice in the United Kingdom

The title "chiropractor" is protected under law in the United Kingdom, so that only those who are judged to be suitably qualified and of good health and character may use it. In this way, the public is safeguarded from poor standards in chiropractic practice. The statutory regulation of chiropractic in the United Kingdom is the responsibility of the General Chiropractic Council (GCC), a body that was established following the Chiropractors Act of 1994.[1] In the United Kingdom, it is illegal to call oneself a chiropractor, or to claim to practice chiropractic, without being registered with the GCC.

In addition to maintaining a register of chiropractors, the GCC also works to protect the public from poor practice by assessing and ensuring the standards of chiropractic education. There are currently three schools in the U.K. with chiropractic training programs that are recognized by the GCC. They are the Anglo-European College of Chiropractic, the McTimoney College of Chiropractic, and the Welsh Institute of Chiropractic. These schools offer master's degrees in chiropractic validated by British universities.

There are approximately 3,100 chiropractors in the U.K., with an almost equal number of males and females. Although they are fewer in number than their colleagues in the United States and Canada, the number of chiropractors practicing in the U.K. has roughly doubled in the last 15 years. There are more chiropractors practicing in the U.K. than in any other European nation.

To represent their interests and to provide professional and personal support, chiropractors in the U.K. have organized themselves into four voluntary associations, the British Chiropractic Association, the McTimoney Chiropractic Association, the Scottish Chiropractic Association, and the United Chiropractic Association. These associations act for the different branches of the profession. The oldest of them is the British Chiropractic Association, which was formed in 1925. Another body of note is the Royal College of Chiropractors, an organization that was granted its royal charter by Queen Elizabeth II in 2012 and that works to promote excellence, quality, and safety in chiropractic.

As in many other parts of the world, in the U.K., new patients coming to see chiropractors can expect that the chiropractor will obtain and record a case history and perform a physical examination, using the findings of these to reach a diagnosis and/or rationale for care.[2] Sometimes there will be a need for further investigation (e.g., ultrasound or X-ray studies) or referral to another practitioner. The Chiropractors Act did not define the scope of chiropractic practice and neither has the GCC, but the GCC does require chiropractors to employ a patient-centered, evidence-based approach to clinical practice. This involves thoughtful consideration and use of research evidence in making clinical decisions and working in partnership with patients. Patient choice is fundamental to the process of sound clinical decision making. Good practice involves not only taking account of a patient's values and circumstances, the practitioner's expertise, and the best available research evidence, but also recognizing that patients should be allowed to make decisions about their own care.

Following media debate about the scope of chiropractic practice and claims for its value in nonmusculoskeletal conditions, the GCC funded a study into the effectiveness of manual therapies, which was published in 2010.[3] In 2014, the evidence from that U.K. report was extended and updated by Clar et al.[4] Although, as both reports indicated, there is evidence to support the use of manipulation for conditions such as back pain, neck pain, some forms of headache, and a number of upper and lower extremity joint conditions, there is much that we still do not know about the benefits and harms of different manual treatments. The value of manual therapies in nonmusculoskeletal conditions, such as asthma, infantile colic, and ear infections, has not been demonstrated beyond reasonable doubt. Clar et al. concluded that there were considerable gaps in the evidence relating to the use of manual therapies, inconsistencies, and issues of generalizability to the range of settings in which manual therapy is practiced in the U.K. The lack of clear evidence presents a challenge for those working in chiropractic practice. The best practitioners do not make bold, unsubstantiated claims for chiropractic care, appreciating that chiropractic does not offer the panacea envisioned by its founders. Instead, they take a more modest stance, openly and honestly discussing areas of uncertainty with patients in order to facilitate understanding and inform decision making.

Chiropractic Practice in Australia

Australia's complex health care system includes a universal safety net coverage called Medicare (not to be confused with the United States' version of Medicare, which covers only Americans aged 65 and older), which can be optionally augmented by private insurance coverage. To receive primary care, which includes most health care providers, including chiropractors, a referral is not usually required. Although other types of primary care may be available in many different settings, currently, chiropractic care is only available in private practice settings. Australians are not required to purchase private health insurance, but those who do can use it to have more choices in selecting a provider.

As in other countries, Australia's health system has shifted toward more patient-centered and holistic care. Australian chiropractors in general strongly support a "natural approach" to health and healing, emphasizing a healthy lifestyle, and represent a position within the health care system described as "nonpharmacological, nonsurgical spine care."

In 2010, chiropractic joined other regulated health professions in national regulation, which was previously state based. Currently, most Australians who visit chiropractors do so for spine-related pain and other musculoskeletal complaints, including headaches. Most seek chiropractic care after being referred by family, friends, or other word-of-mouth sources; referrals from other health care providers are infrequent. Although most private health insurers include some level of coverage for chiropractic care, reimbursement is limited and patients are required to pay an often-substantial gap between fees and insurance reimbursement. Australia's federally funded health care system does provide limited coverage for treatment (five visits annually) and diagnostic imaging (X-rays). Workers' compensation and traffic injury insurance also cover chiropractic care, but these are regulated by the various states and not uniform nationally. See Box 3.1 for an example of typical chiropractic care in Australia.

Box 3.1

Example of Typical Chiropractic Care in Australia

Typically, new patients visiting the office of a practicing chiropractor may expect to spend about 10 minutes filling out initial forms, followed by about 30–45 minutes for the consultation, history, examination, and hands-on treatment. The history and physical examination are focused on the patient's presenting complaint, with written informed consent obtained only after the chiropractor explains the patient's condition and appropriate management options. Spinal manipulation is often included, and the chiropractor selects the technique most appropriate for the individual patient's needs. The chiropractor will also give active care instructions, including lifestyle advice for home and work and any special exercises. It is common for subsequent visits to be recommended over a period of several weeks. Along the way, the chiropractor will reassess the patient's progress and modify the management if needed. When the patient's initial complaint has been resolved, the chiropractor will often discuss measures to prevent recurrence and promote a healthy lifestyle.

Education

In the United States, the education required to become a chiropractor starts at the undergraduate level and is completed by graduating from an accredited doctor of chiropractic program (DCP). Before being admitted into a DCP, a student must first complete the equivalent of three academic years of undergraduate study (90 semester hours) at an accredited college or university with a GPA for these 90 hours of at least 3.0 on a 4.0 scale. The 90 hours must include a minimum of 24 semester hours in life and physical science courses to provide an adequate background for success in the DCP. At least half of these courses must have a substantive laboratory component. The undergraduate preparation also includes a well-rounded general education program in the humanities and social sciences and other coursework that helps students successfully complete the chiropractic curriculum.[5] A bachelor's degree is not required to be admitted into most DCPs; however, there are states that require applicants for licensure to have earned a bachelor's degree either before enrolling into the doctor of chiropractic program or prior to applying for a license in that state.

After the undergraduate requirements have been met, the student must then successfully complete an accredited DCP. In the United States, the Council on Chiropractic Education (CCE) is granted authority by the U.S. Department of Education to accredit doctor of chiropractic programs and institutions. Currently 17 chiropractic training programs in the United States are accredited by the CCE. There are also 17 programs outside of the United States that are accredited through affiliated chiropractic education councils, including three in Australia; two each in Canada, France, South Africa, and U.K.; and one each in Denmark, Japan, Malaysia, New Zealand, South Korea, and Spain. The chiropractic curriculum consists of either four or five academic years of instruction.[5] This includes courses in basic science (anatomy, physiology, biochemistry, microbiology, etc.) as well as clinical science (pathology, neurology, biomechanics, orthopedics, cardiology, gastroenterology, etc.). It also includes education in physiotherapy, nutrition, pediatrics, and geriatrics, among others. A significant portion of the curriculum is dedicated to the evaluation and treatment of joints and muscles. Although chiropractors are most known for treating the spine, they are educated in the clinical examination and diagnosis of the entire body.

Like other primary health care students, chiropractic students spend a significant portion of their curriculum studying clinical subjects related to evaluating and caring for patients. Typically, as part of their professional

Table 3.1   Example of First-Year Curriculum (12-Quarter Program)

Quarter 1	Quarter 2	Quarter 3
Spinal Anatomy	Gross Anatomy II	Neuroanatomy
Gross Anatomy I	Biochemistry II	Gross Anatomy III
Biochemistry I	Histology	Physiology I
Cell Biology	Philosophy and Principles of Chiropractic II	Human Development
Philosophy and Principles of Chiropractic	Biomechanics/Palpation II Lecture	Adjustive Technique I Lecture and Lab—Thoracic Spine
Biomechanics/Palpation I Lecture and Lab	Adjustive Psychomotor Skills	Philosophy and Principles of Chiropractic III
Clinical Topics I	Biomechanics/Palpation II Lecture and Lab	
Radiographic Anatomy I	Information Mastery	
	Radiographic Anatomy II	

training, they must complete a one-year clinical-based internship dealing with actual patient care. In total, the curriculum includes a minimum of 4,200 hours of classroom, laboratory, and clinical experience. Government inquiries, as well as independent investigations by medical practitioners, have affirmed that today's chiropractic training is of equivalent standard to medical training in all preclinical subjects, including anatomy, physiology, biochemistry, and microbiology among others.[6] This extensive education prepares doctors of chiropractic to diagnose health care problems, treat these problems when they are within their scope of practice, and refer patients to other health care providers when appropriate. Tables 3.1–3.4 are examples of a chiropractic curriculum from an accredited chiropractic college in the United States that has a 12-quarter program. After graduation from a DCP, an individual may use the title "doctor of chiropractic," "DC," or, in some states, "chiropractic physician."

   Once licensed to practice, a chiropractor must complete continuing education each year in order to maintain a license. The specific number of hours and acceptable content of the continuing education is dictated by the state, province, or country in which the DC practices. This helps to ensure that DCs stay up to date on the latest research and treatment methods and continue their education throughout their careers. It is also a way for chiropractors to learn new techniques and treatments or obtain specialty certifications or advanced degrees in order to better serve their patients.

Table 3.2 Example of Second-Year Curriculum (12-Quarter Program)

Quarter 4	Quarter 5	Quarter 6
Neurophysiology	Nutrition	Neuromusculoskeletal (NMS) Diagnosis and Treatment I Lecture and Lab
Physiology II	Genetics	Adjustive Technique IV Lecture and Lab—Cervical Spine
Microbiology, Immunology, and Public Health	Clinical Microbiology and Public Health	Biomechanics/Palpation IV Lecture and Lab
General Pathology I	General Pathology II	Adjustive Technique V Extremities
Soft Tissue Therapies/ Rehabilitation I	Adjustive Technique III Lecture and Lab—Lumbar Spine	Clinical Topics III
Adjustive Technique II Lecture and Lab—Pelvis	Philosophy and Principles of Chiropractic IV	Physical Diagnosis II Lecture and Lab
Clinical Topics II	Biomechanics/ Palpation III Lecture	Clinical Lab
Evidence-Informed Practice I	Physical Diagnosis I Lecture and Lab	Radiographic Technique I
Radiographic Anatomy III	Patient/Practice Management I	
	Evidence-Informed Practice II	
	Dermatology and Infectious Disease	

Licensure

Along with obtaining a doctor of chiropractic degree, a potential chiropractor must also pass all the required board examinations before being granted licensure. In the United States, a series of exams provided by the National Board of Chiropractic Examiners (NBCE) must be completed before applying to a U.S. jurisdiction for a license to practice. The NBCE is also the international testing agency for the chiropractic profession. It develops, administers, and scores standardized examinations that assess a candidate's knowledge and other abilities in various basic science and

Table 3.3   **Example of Third-Year Curriculum (12-Quarter Program)**

Quarter 7	Quarter 8	Quarter 9
NMS Diagnosis and Treatment II Lecture and Lab	NMS Diagnosis and Treatment III Lecture and Lab	Adjustive Technique VII Lecture and Lab
Taping and Splinting I	Soft Tissue Therapies/ Rehabilitation II	Clinic Phase III
Adjustive Technique V Advanced	Taping and Splinting II	Clinical Internship III
Adjustive Technique VI	Chiropractic Physiological Therapeutics II	Clinical Neurology
Chiropractic Physiological Therapeutics I	Clinical Internship II	Genitourinary Survey
Cardiorespiratory Diagnosis and Treatment	Clinic Phase II	Jurisprudence and Ethics
Clinic Phase I	Clinical Nutrition and Botanicals I	Clinical Nutrition and Botanicals II
Clinical Internship I	Gastroenterology Diagnosis and Treatment	Introduction to Pharmacology
Clinical Pathology	Radiographic Technique III	Patient/Practice Management III
Patient/Practice Management II	Bone Pathology II	Bone Pathology III
Emergency Care		
Radiographic Technique II		
Bone Pathology I		

clinical areas. NBCE examinations are administered at 25 test sites in the United States, Canada, England, France, Australia, New Zealand, and South Korea. These examinations consist of a series of four different parts. Part I includes subject examinations in each of six basic science areas: general anatomy, spinal anatomy, physiology, chemistry, pathology, and microbiology. Part II includes examinations in each of six clinical science areas: general diagnosis, neuromusculoskeletal diagnosis, diagnostic imaging, principles of chiropractic, chiropractic practice, and associated clinical sciences. Part III addresses nine clinical areas: case history, physical examination, neuromusculoskeletal examination, diagnostic imaging, clinical laboratory and special studies, diagnosis or clinical impression,

Table 3.4   Example of Fourth-Year Curriculum (12-Quarter Program)

Quarter 10	Quarter 11	Quarter 12
Clinical Psychology	Adjustive Technique X	Clinical Internship VI
Adjustive Technique VIII	Evidence-Informed Practice IV	
Bone Pathology IV	Philosophy and Principles of Chiropractic VI	
Evidence-Informed Practice III	Adjustive Technique IX	
Clinical Pediatrics	Correlative and Differential Diagnosis	
Patient/Practice Management V	Patient/Practice Management IV	
Philosophy and Principles of Chiropractic V	Soft Tissue Interpretation	
Clinical Geriatrics	Obstetrics	
Clinical Internship IV	Clinical Internship V	

chiropractic techniques, supportive interventions, and case management. Part IV tests individuals in three major areas: radiographic interpretation and diagnosis, chiropractic technique, and case management. The NBCE also offers a physiotherapy exam, which some states require in order for a chiropractor to be able to treat patients with physiotherapy modalities, such as ultrasound and electrical muscle stimulation.[7]

Other countries may require a candidate to successfully complete board exams taken in that country or they may accept board exams that have been successfully completed in other countries. The NBCE has also expanded its standardized testing services globally through the creation of the International Board of Chiropractic Examiners (IBCE). The IBCE has conducted pilot examinations of chiropractors and students in Brazil and Spain and currently assists chiropractors in Thailand, Japan, and Portugal with customized registration and testing. It also cofounded the International Chiropractic Regulatory Collaboration to promote international mobility.[7] Students typically complete all of the required examinations before graduation from a chiropractic college.

Once national board exams have been successfully completed, the final step is getting licensed in the individual state or states in which one wants to practice. The regulatory agency that exists in each state has a regulatory board that is typically composed of doctors of chiropractic, consumer members, and other healing arts professionals. The chiropractic regulatory board is charged with protecting the public. Although the majority of states are similar, many states have their own unique requirements for licensure. Since the scope of chiropractic practice varies from state to state, most states require an applicant to pass an exam that covers the laws and regulations pertaining to chiropractic practice in that state. Additional exams are required in some states where the scope of practice is broader in order to ensure that the chiropractor is adequately trained in everything that lies within the scope of practice of that state. Individual states may also require an applicant to have passed certain national board exams with a minimum score that is higher than a general passing score. Once licensed, a DC must pay an annual or sometimes biannual fee to each state in which he or she is licensed in order to maintain an active license.

Demographics

According to a 2014 survey administered by the NBCE, 73 percent of chiropractic practitioners are male and 27 percent are female. At the time of survey, the number of female chiropractors had almost doubled since a previous survey, which was done in 1991.[7] The same survey found that about 90 percent of respondents identified themselves as white, while multiethnic, Asian, Hispanic, African American, Native American, and other ethnicities comprised the remaining respondents.

About 95 percent of DCs hold a postsecondary academic degree in addition to their DC degree. About 65 percent have bachelor's degrees, about 6 percent have master's degrees, and about 7 percent have doctorate degrees in nonchiropractic fields. About 16 percent of the surveyed chiropractors reported that they had attained an advanced certification in a specialty within chiropractic.

Survey respondents reported that about 59 percent of their patients were female. The highest percentage of patients (about 29 percent) is in the age range of 31 to 50 years old, followed by 51-to-64-year-olds (23 percent) and under-18-year-olds (about 18 percent).

Like other small businesses, there tend to be more chiropractic clinics in more populated areas. In the same NBCE survey, 34 percent of the chiropractors reported that their office is located in a city, 31 percent reported practicing in a suburb, and 19 percent reported practicing in a small town. Only about 15 percent reported that their practice was located in a rural area.[7]

Scope of Practice

Chiropractic is licensed and regulated in every state, but the chiropractic scope of practice varies from state to state and from country to country. "Scope of practice" is the regulation of professionals in a specific jurisdiction and is used to create legal boundaries by restricting the allowed activities for a specified profession. Its purpose is to protect the public by setting legal limits for what a provider can and cannot do, and it can be used as a means to define a profession in a particular area.[3] Statutes and regulations determine the scope of clinical procedures chiropractors may legally perform in the state in which they practice. Diagnosing and treating joint and muscle conditions using manipulation as a primary intervention is within the legal scope of chiropractic practice in all 50 states. In many states, this includes the treatment of animals, as long as the proper certification and learning is completed. Some states may also require a chiropractor to work under the direction of a veterinarian in order to treat animals. Giving nutrition and lifestyle counseling is generally within a chiropractor's scope; however, some states have restrictions regarding the prescription of dietary supplements. Therefore, it is important for DCs to have a good relationship with other professionals, like naturopathic doctors or nutritionists, in areas where the nutritional scope is limited.

Beyond this, there is considerable variation between states. In states with the narrowest scope of practice, chiropractors are limited to the treatment of the spine or other musculoskeletal conditions related to a spinal condition. This means that any joint in the upper extremities (the shoulder, elbow, wrist, hand) or lower extremities (hip, knee, ankle, foot) cannot be treated unless it is related to a spinal condition that is also being treated. In states that have a broader scope, they may be able to perform minor surgery or have limited rights to the prescription of medications.[8]

All states allow DCs to perform orthopedic and neurologic exams of the spine and extremities related to the care of their patients, but there is variation among states as to whether a DC may perform preparticipation sports physicals, school physicals, or occupational physicals. Although a chiropractor who has graduated from an accredited chiropractic school has been trained to perform a thorough health history and physical exam, some states would prefer that patients be referred to a medical provider for these types of exams.

Chiropractors are allowed by law to perform gender-specific examinations in most states but must be sure to properly document the appropriateness of the exam since these are not routinely performed by most chiropractors. Many states also specify that the patient must sign a written informed consent prior to the examination.

In some states, chiropractors are allowed to draw blood for the purpose of laboratory testing, and in all states, they are able to order blood tests, analyze the test results, and discuss the results with the patient. Chiropractors in all states can take their own X-rays or order and interpret X-rays taken elsewhere. They are also permitted to order computed tomography (CT scans) and magnetic resonance imaging (MRI), but some states limit this to the spine only. A few states authorize chiropractors to sign birth and death certificates.

Since chiropractors work with the nervous, muscular, and skeletal systems, physiotherapy modalities often play an important role in the treatment they provide. The most common therapies include therapeutic ultrasound, various forms of electrical muscle stimulation, and low-level light therapy, also known as cold laser therapy. These treatments are valuable in reducing pain and inflammation and relaxing muscles and are within the chiropractic scope of practice in the vast majority of states, but there are a few that prohibit their use by chiropractors. Since there are varying types of laser therapies, if laser is permitted it is generally limited to a specific type of therapeutic laser that does not include the types that are used for hair removal or dermatological procedures.

Physical rehabilitation is another important and specialized form of treatment that chiropractors can perform in almost all states and is a major focus of many chiropractic clinics. Massage, and a variety of other methods of manual muscle therapy, is within the chiropractic scope in almost all states. Since there are procedures and treatments that may be within the scope of practice of chiropractors in some jurisdictions but are not taught at all chiropractic schools, it may be helpful for potential students to research the scope of practice in the state or states in which they want to practice before selecting which school to attend.[8]

Practice Setting

Once licensed to treat patients in a chosen region, there are a variety of settings in which a DC may choose to practice. The most common setting is in a private practice owned and operated by the chiropractor. In this case, the chiropractor is a self-employed small business owner who manages the business and its employees along with providing care for patients. About 40 percent of DCs in the United States are self-employed.[9]

A typical chiropractic office generally consists of a waiting room/reception area, treatment room(s), a doctor's office, and sometimes an office for support staff, such as billing personnel or an office manager. Many chiropractic clinics also have additional rooms for massage therapists or other health care providers who are employees of the clinic or who work as independent contractors renting the space. The size of the office and number of staff vary depending on how many providers work in the office and the volume of patients. Like other small businesses, a chiropractic clinic may be located in a stand-alone building or in a building with other businesses. Many clinics are located in buildings with other health care providers.

New chiropractors who want to get experience before opening their own practice, or others who do not want to have to run a business, may choose to work for another chiropractor. In this situation, they generally work in a private practice as an employee of the chiropractor who owns the practice. DCs who work in this type of situation are typically referred to as "associate" chiropractors and generally receive a salary, a percentage of the income that is collected from services they provide, or sometimes a combination of the two. DCs may also choose to work out of a private chiropractic practice or other type of health care facility as an independent contractor. In this situation, the DC generally pays either a monthly rate or a percentage of collections to the owner of the facility. This can be financially advantageous since as an independent contractor the DC does not have to worry about paying all the expenses involved in running a clinic but generally has use of the full facility and staff. A situation where the independent contractor pays a percentage of collections is often helpful for DCs who are just starting out. Since they only pay a percentage, if they don't earn a lot they don't have to pay a lot, rather than having to pay a specific amount of rent per month regardless of patient volume.

Many chiropractors work in group practices with multiple DCs working out of the same clinic. In this situation, they may be business partners or they may be separate businesses sharing the same space. They will often work at the same time if the space is large enough, or they may work opposite schedules if there are not enough treatment rooms. One advantage of this type of situation is that it allows DCs to share the overhead costs of the clinic, so they can afford a larger, more expensive space. Another advantage of DCs working together is that they can cover for each other when someone is sick or goes on vacation.

Many chiropractors choose to work in multidisciplinary clinics or health centers with other types of health care providers, including acupuncturists, naturopaths, and massage therapists as well as medical doctors, nurse practitioners, and physical therapists. In this type of clinic, the providers may also be business partners or may be separate businesses sharing the same space and working under the same clinic name. This type of situation provides the advantage of being able to refer patients to other providers within the same clinic and receiving referrals from them as well. It facilitates better communication between providers when comanaging patients. This often provides a better experience and better outcomes for patients.

Although not as common, a growing number of chiropractors work in integrated medical clinics and hospitals. They are generally employees of the facility and work as part of a health care team, comanaging patients with other providers. A small percentage of these DCs are currently employed under contract to provide chiropractic care to active or retired military personnel.

The amount of time a chiropractor spends engaged in the various activities required to maintain a practice can vary significantly. A 2014 survey of chiropractors in the United States showed that those chiropractors who responded spent about 60 percent of their time, on average, performing direct patient care. They reported spending about 30 percent of their time documenting the care they provided and the rest on business management and marketing.[7]

About 37 percent of chiropractors report that they treat between 50 and 100 individual patients per week, and about 35 percent say they treat fewer than 50 per week. The rest reported that they treat more than 100 per week with some reporting more than 150.[7] In general, the more patients the chiropractor sees, the less time he or she spends with each patient. If the chiropractor is treating the patient with adjustments only, the patient may only have 5 to 10 minutes with the doctor. If the patient is receiving other types of treatments as well, the appointment may take as long as an hour.

Practice Styles

There is a wide variety of practice styles among chiropractors. Some treat the spine only, while others also treat the extremities. The amount of time each patient spends in the office can vary considerably; it all depends on the style and methods of treatment the doctor uses. Some only treat their patients with adjustments, while others incorporate soft tissue work or massage, rehabilitation and exercise, or nutritional and lifestyle counseling as part of their treatment.

In order to arrive at a diagnosis and determine what type of treatment will be best suited to the patient, the chiropractor will first take a medical history. The extent of this history will vary depending on what the patient is presenting with, and may vary somewhat among DCs, but it will likely include questions about the details of the symptoms that have caused the person to seek care. It will also generally include questions about whether the person currently has any other health conditions, is taking any medications, or has had any serious illnesses, injuries, or accidents; questions about family health history; and questions about the person's diet and lifestyle, including occupation, exercise routine, and personal habits like consuming tobacco and alcohol. All this information helps to guide the type of examination the chiropractor will perform.

As part of the physical exam, height, weight, and vital signs (blood pressure, pulses, temperature, respiration rate) are often measured. If indicated, the DC may also listen to the patient's heart and lungs with a stethoscope; look into the eyes, ears, and throat; or manually examine the lymph nodes or abdomen. A large part of the physical examination will be a musculoskeletal exam. This will include assessment and often measurement of the ranges of motion of the joints involved. It will also generally include orthopedic tests to determine if there has been any injury to the various tissues of the body (muscles, ligaments, tendons, etc.). A neurological exam is often included as well. It consists of measuring reflexes, the strength of muscles, and evaluating different types of sensation, including pain, temperature, pressure, and position. The chiropractor will usually examine the muscles in the area of complaint or related areas to determine if there is any pain, tenderness, or tightness in these muscles. Part of the examination will include an assessment of the movement and position of the joints of the spine and/or extremities in order to determine if they are moving properly or are in proper alignment. Some DCs primarily use their hands to assess joint motion and alignment by feeling the position of the bones relative to others or by putting the joint through its range of motion and feeling for restriction of movement. Other chiropractors may take X-rays to visualize joint alignment. Some chiropractors use other methods, such as postural analysis, functional movement assessments (to see how the body moves as a whole), muscle testing, or leg length assessment to help them determine how to best treat the patient. Depending on the results of the history and physical exam, laboratory studies (bloodwork, urine tests, etc.) or imaging (X-ray, MRI, etc.) may be ordered or performed in the office.

The majority of chiropractors use manual adjusting as a primary method of treatment to improve the motion of the joints. After completing the examination to determine which joints need to be adjusted, the patient is placed in a specific position and the chiropractor places his or her hand on a specific spot and applies a quick impulse to create movement in the joint. This often results in the patient feeling or hearing a pop or crack.

Chiropractors use a wide variety of diagnosis and treatment techniques. The main differences between them have to do with the way the chiropractor determines where to perform adjustments and how the adjustments are delivered. Although most chiropractors use their hands to adjust, the position the patient is put in and the forces and directions used during the adjustments can vary considerably between different techniques.

The equipment that the chiropractor uses is also variable. This often includes the type of table that is used. There are many different types of chiropractic tables. Some have functions that aid in the specific technique that the chiropractor uses, and some have varying functions for the convenience of the provider using them or for the patient. A commonly used function in chiropractic tables is a drop piece. This type of table has one or more pieces that lift up slightly underneath the patient, about a half inch to an inch, and lock into place. When the chiropractor applies the adjustive thrust, the piece drops back to its original position. This allows the DC to use less force due to the momentum created by the drop piece. This type of adjustment is used exclusively by some DCs, but others may use it along with other types of adjustments.

Another type of table, commonly known as flexion-distraction, has an end piece (the part on which the patient's legs rest) that may go up and down or side to side in order to move the patient in different ways during the treatment. They may be motorized or moved manually by the chiropractor. This allows the DC to treat the joints and muscles in the area without using a thrust adjustment.

There are also tables that stand up to allow a patient to simply step into place and be lowered into a prone position for treatment. The table lifts the patient back up to a standing position once the treatment has concluded. These tables are very helpful for patients who are in a lot of pain or have physical disabilities.

Besides using different tables, chiropractors may also use an instrument to perform the adjustments. This allows the DC to apply minimal force to the area being adjusted and often does not require the patient to be put into various positions. Instrument adjusting of many areas can be done from a single patient position. The type of instrument used to perform the adjustments can also vary. Many use a hand-held spring-loaded instrument with which the provider administers a single impulse per adjustment. There are other electronic instruments that administer repetitive impulses while the trigger is held down by the provider. Although there are chiropractors that use only manual adjusting or only instrument adjusting, there are many who use a combination of the two methods in order to cater to a wider variety of patients.

There are also various muscle work and massage techniques that may be used by the chiropractor or a massage therapist that works in the office. In addition to various techniques performed with the hands, some providers use metal or plastic instruments to treat the muscles and other soft tissues. It is also common for chiropractors to use various taping methods as part of their treatment.

Many DCs have specialty practices. Some specialize in the treatment of specific groups of people, such as pregnant women, children, athletes, or older adults. (*See Chapter 13 for details on chiropractic care for pregnant women, children, and older adults, and Chapter 14 for sports chiropractic.*) Others specialize in treating specific types of injuries or conditions, such as injuries from automobile collisions, work injuries, athletic injuries, or neurological conditions. Some specialize in specific methods of treatment, such as physical rehabilitation and exercise or nutrition counseling. There are also chiropractors who function as primary care providers and treat a variety of conditions through physical medicine as well as diet and lifestyle counseling. Many DCs who have these specialty practices have advanced training and certifications in these areas.

How to Select a Chiropractor

There are many factors to consider when looking for a chiropractor, so prospective patients should gather as much information as possible about each chiropractor they are considering before selecting one. It is usually a good idea to start with asking family and friends if they have been to any chiropractors in the area and what their experiences were like. Most people want to find a DC who is close to their home or work and convenient to get to, since generally the treatment plan will include multiple visits to the clinic. It is also helpful to call the chiropractor and talk over the phone or schedule a consultation to meet with the doctor and find out what the practice is like and the methods and techniques used. To follow are some questions a person may want to ask when searching for a chiropractor.

*Which chiropractic techniques does the DC use and why? How much
training and experience does the DC have in the specific techniques used?*

Most DCs are experienced in several techniques and will choose the one
technique or the combination of techniques that is best suited to the
patient and his or her condition. After finding out which techniques are
used, one should talk to the DC about why he or she chooses to use them
and why they might be helpful. It is also helpful to ask where to get more
information about these techniques to research them independently.

*Does the DC use manual, hands-on methods or an instrument for the
chiropractic manipulation?*

It is a good idea to find out how the DC performs adjustments. Ask the DC
to explain the type of adjustments that he or she generally performs. While
many people enjoy and get relief from the more forceful manual adjustments, some people may not prefer this approach and may want to find
someone who provides low-force manual techniques or uses an instrument to perform adjustments.

Is the DC experienced in treating the individual's type of problems?

Prospective patients should ask if the chiropractor has had experience and
success with treating cases like theirs so they can be more confident that
he or she will be able to help them as well.

What is the DC's typical practice pattern or treatment program?

It is important to find a DC who individualizes the treatment plan to each
patient and does not just use the same basic plan for everyone. Prospective
patients should ask for an estimate of how long the treatment plan would
be for an average person with a presentation similar to theirs.

Does the DC provide the recommended treatment plan in writing?

Some patients prefer this approach so that they can have all the information at hand to research and think about the recommendations.

What services does the DC offer?

Along with adjustments, some chiropractors offer additional services, such
as massage, exercise instruction, rehabilitation, strength training, and
nutritional and lifestyle counseling. They should discuss with each patient
whether those services are appropriate for him or her.

*What is the DC's recommendation if the treatment program isn't
helping?*

It is important to know that if the DC is not able to help an individual, she
or he can refer patients to other trusted providers. A good chiropractor will

recommend that patients consult another health care provider if other methods of treatment may be indicated.

Is the DC in the patient's insurance provider network?

Although there are some health maintenance organizations (HMOs) that require a referral in order to see a chiropractor, the majority of health insurance companies allow patients to see a chiropractor without a referral from another provider. The doctor or staff should be able to verify whether or not a patient's insurance will cover treatment in their clinic and if not, what the fees are for those paying out of pocket. Most clinics offer a time-of-service discount for those paying cash since they do not have to go through the process of billing the insurance company for the services rendered to these patients. Some clinics may also offer a sliding fee scale based on the patient's financial situation. Fees should be competitive and within the "usual and customary" range within the local area, so it is a good idea to compare the fees of several local clinics by calling and talking to the office staff. Some clinics may even post their fee schedule on their website. If the chiropractor offers specialty services, he or she may charge higher fees for those specialty services.

How long is the average wait time in the waiting room?

As with many medical practices, some have long wait times and some are quite prompt. Selecting one with a good fit for the individual may impact patient satisfaction with the chiropractor.

Does the DC have a specialty?

Although all chiropractors are trained to treat a wide variety of injuries, there may be one who specializes in the specific type of care a patient is seeking.

What do DCs treat?

Back and neck pain

Back and neck pain are among the most common conditions that chiropractors treat. In fact, a 2015 Gallup poll showed that 61 percent of Americans think that chiropractors are effective at treating back and neck pain.[10] A high percentage of people will experience neck and/or back pain at some point in their lives, and most of the time it can be treated without surgery. Chiropractors are experts at diagnosing and treating conditions and injuries that cause neck and back pain.

Due to the potential seriousness of injuries to this area, a detailed history and examination is performed. This is important since a chiropractor might be the first health care provider patients see for their spine pain, and damage to vital internal structures can cause what appears to be a simple ache or pain. If it is determined that the injury is severe or potentially needs treatment outside of what chiropractors generally treat, the chiropractor will refer that patient to the proper provider or even the emergency room. Even a patient who has been seeing a chiropractor for many years must be treated with care on every visit, because sudden changes in symptoms or severity can potentially be serious.

Muscle and joint injuries

Patients often see chiropractors because of pain in or injuries to muscles or joints. Causes of muscle and joint pain include joint sprains, muscle strains, and knots that develop in muscles (known as trigger points or muscle tension) due to repetitive activities or posture.

Sprains and strains are some of the more common injuries that chiropractors treat. Although they tend to see a lot of injuries in the back and neck, they also treat injuries to other areas, like ankles and shoulders. Sprains are caused when ligaments, the bands of tissue that hold bones together, become overstretched or torn. Strains involve damage to a muscle and/or a tendon, the tissue that attaches a muscle to a bone. These injuries can occur from lifting too much weight or lifting in a bad position, playing sports, car accidents, falls, or sometimes even bending or twisting improperly during regular activities. The chiropractor will use various methods to treat the injury and will also do an assessment to help determine how the injury occurred. This will guide the exercises that will be prescribed to the patient and help determine if any changes need to be made to the way the patient performs regular activities. Although many of these injuries seem minor and often get better on their own over time, if not treated they can often leave a person at increased risk for future injury. A chiropractor can help determine the severity of the injury and apply the proper treatment to reduce risk of reinjury.

Muscle pain, sometimes referred to as "myofascitis," is also commonly treated by chiropractors. A person's muscles can become tight and tender due to having constant stress on them, which can also lead to knots in the muscles, known as trigger points. The stress on muscles may be physical, due to daily activities or prolonged periods in poor postures, or it could be mental or emotional. People who have a lot of stress often have a hard time relaxing and tend to get very tight in certain areas. Chiropractors can treat the pain and discomfort that they are experiencing and help people improve their posture and the way they do things in order to decrease the stress on their muscles and joints.

DCs also commonly treat the symptoms of osteoarthritis. Since one of the main things that is beneficial in this type of arthritis is keeping the joints moving, chiropractic can be effective. Much of the treatment provided by DCs focuses on restoring and maintaining proper motion of the joints. Although the damage to the joints that causes them to become inflamed is generally not reversible, chiropractic care can help relieve the symptoms. A chiropractor may also counsel the patient on nutritional options that may help relieve the symptoms.

Headaches

Chiropractors also frequently treat headaches. There are many types of headaches with various causes. Two of the more common types that a chiropractor can effectively treat are called tension-type and cervicogenic headaches. Cervicogenic headaches are usually caused by problems in the joints of the neck, and tension-type headaches tend to be related to tension in the muscles of the neck and upper back. Tension-type headaches may be related to mental or emotional stress from the person's personal life, work, or even health, which leads to tight muscles, or they may be due to physical stresses from spending a lot of time sitting and doing other tasks for long periods with poor posture. Chiropractic is generally effective for these types of headaches and sometimes for others as well, such as migraines.[4]

Headaches can have many causes, including allergies, sinus problems, and hormones, but they can also have more serious causes. Chiropractors are trained to determine the cause of the headaches. Along with asking questions about what the headache feels like, the doctor assesses the muscles and joints in order to determine the kind of headache the patient is experiencing. If the headache is not a type for which chiropractic is effective, the DC will be able to refer the patient to a different provider who can provide the necessary treatment.

Dizziness

Patients who have dizziness can often get help with chiropractic care, and if the dizziness has a more serious cause, DCs will refer patients to the proper health care provider. Chiropractic can help when the dizziness is caused by problems originating in the joints and muscles of the neck (cervicogenic dizziness).[4] When the dizziness is caused by inner ear or other types of problems, it is less likely that chiropractic treatment will help.

Herniated discs

Herniated discs are another common condition treated by chiropractors. Typical symptoms of a herniated disc are back or neck pain. Often associated with the back pain are pain, numbness, and/or tingling going down the leg and into the foot. Often associated with the neck pain are pain, numbness, and/or tingling down the arm and into the hand. Discs are cartilage pads between the vertebrae, which are the bones in the back and neck that form the spine. There are different ways in which a disc can be injured. The center of the disc is a soft, gel-like substance. When the outer part of the disc gets damaged, due to accidents, repetitive motions, or other causes, the center part of the disc (the gel part) gets pushed through the outer layers and can put pressure on nerves. This can create the symptoms listed above as well as sharp or stabbing pain or a burning sensation. If the injury is severe enough, or has been ignored long enough before treatment, a patient can develop muscle weakness that can affect daily activities. In the leg, it can make even walking difficult and painful, and in the arm, it can weaken the person's grip and make it hard to lift or hold things.

The DC will take a thorough history and perform an exam to determine if a disc herniation is the cause of pain. Many disc herniations can be treated by a chiropractor without the need for surgery, although surgery is sometimes needed. Treatments from a chiropractor include adjustments and methods to relieve pressure on the discs. Treatment tables have been specifically designed to treat this issue, and they are often very effective. The treatment generally works best along with proper rehabilitation exercises and changes to the person's activities to prevent the stresses that caused the injury in the first place. It is often our daily activities done improperly that cause a continual stress on the discs that eventually leads to injury. It is important to understand that how we move plays a large role in how our muscles and other tissues develop, strengthen, or break down.

If a patient is not showing signs of improvement, or even worsening, a chiropractor may order an MRI to get a better view of what is going on inside the body and to visualize how healthy the discs are; if necessary, the DC will refer the patient to a specialist for a surgical consultation.

Athletic injuries

Many chiropractors specialize in treating athletic injuries. Two of the most common certifications that chiropractors receive in this specialty are the certified chiropractic sports physician and the diplomate of the American Chiropractic Board of Sports Physicians. These certifications include preparation for evaluating and treating athletes both on the sideline at athletic events and in office. The training also includes when to return athletes to play after they have recovered and additional training in the evaluation and management of concussion. Besides just treating athletic injuries, sports chiropractors are also trained in sports nutrition and strength and conditioning to help athletes improve their performance and reduce their risk for injury. (*See Chapter 14 for more information about sports chiropractic.*)

Since there are many different types of sports and athletic activities, there are many different types of sports injuries. Almost every joint and muscle, as well as the structures surrounding them, has the possibility of being injured during sport. Many of these injuries are sprains and strains as have been described above, but others can be more complicated. Since chiropractors are trained to treat not only the back and neck but also the extremities of the upper body (shoulders, elbows, wrists/hands) and lower body (hips, knees, ankles/feet), they are well equipped to treat a wide variety of sports injuries.

To be specialized in this field also requires knowledge about movement patterns, how the body functions as a whole, and how these things relate to the activities in which each individual participates. In some circumstances a chiropractor may even function as a team physician or as a member of the medical team for sports teams or athletic organizations.

Nutrition evaluations

Many DCs like to treat the body from the inside as well as the outside. While all DCs have training in nutrition, some choose nutritional counseling as a specialty and incorporate it into all patient treatments. Some people see these chiropractors specifically for nutritional reasons and not necessarily for treatment of pain or injuries. A DC can help patients understand what good nutrition is for them and develop healthy eating habits and can recommend supplements to help where their diet is lacking. A chiropractor may also work closely with a naturopathic doctor or other natural health care provider if nutrition is not a focus of his or her practice.

Children and the elderly

Children and the elderly are both groups that often need care but cannot always be treated in the same way as other people. They each have unique conditions and need specialized treatments and care. While all chiropractors have training in treating these patients, many take additional courses to improve their ability to meet the needs of these populations. Chiropractors will often modify the usual manual techniques they use to be more appropriate and comfortable with these age groups. To adjust these patients, a DC will often use an instrument or other lighter-force method to deliver adjustments and improve the motion of the joints. An adjusting instrument may use low force, and it can be very specific with the contact point on the body. This is particularly useful in older patients who may be at risk for osteoporosis, which makes their bones weaker. (*See Chapter 13 for more information about chiropractic care for these populations.*)

References

1. U.K. Parliament. *Chiropractors Act*, 1994. Ch. 17, Eliz. 2. London: Her Majesty's Stationery Office; 1994.

2. General Chiropractic Council. *The Code: Standards of Conduct, Performance and Ethics for Chiropractors*. London: General Chiropractic Council; 2015.

3. Bronfort G, Haas M, Evans R, Leininger B, Triano J. Effectiveness of manual therapies: the UK evidence report. *Chiropr Osteopat*. 2010;18:3. doi:10.1186 /1746-1340-18-3.

4. Clar C, Tsertsvadze A, Court R, Lewando Hundt G, Clarke A, Sutcliffe P. Clinical effectiveness of manual therapy for the management of musculoskeletal and non-musculoskeletal conditions: systematic review and update of UK evidence report. *Chiropr Man Therap.* 2014;22:12. doi: 10.1186/2045-709X-22-12.

5. Council on Chiropractic Education. *Accreditation Standards, Principles, Processes & Requirements for Accreditation.* Scottsdale, AZ: Council on Chiropractic Education; 2013.

6. Coulter I, Adams A, Coggan P, Wilkes M, Gonyea M. A comparative study of chiropractic and medical education. *Altern Ther Health Med.* 1998; 4:1078–6791.

7. National Board of Chiropractic Examiners. *Practice Analysis of Chiropractic 2015.* Greeley, CO: National Board of Chiropractic Examiners; 2015.

8. Chang M. The chiropractic scope of practice in the United States: a cross-sectional survey. *J Manipulative Physiol Ther.* 2014;37(6):363–376.

9. Bureau of Labor Statistics, U.S. Department of Labor. *Occupational Outlook Handbook, 2016–17 Ed., Chiropractors.* http://www.bls.gov/ooh/healthcare/chiropractors.htm. Accessed May 11, 2016.

10. Weeks WB, Goertz CM, Meeker WC, Marchiori DM. Public perceptions of doctors of chiropractic: results of a national survey and examination of variation according to respondents' likelihood to use chiropractic, experience with chiropractic, and chiropractic supply in local health care markets. *J Manipulative Physiol Ther.* 2015;38(8):533–544.

CHAPTER FOUR

Chiropractic Adjustment or Manipulation: The Therapeutic Intervention

Brian J. Gleberzon, MHSc, DC

Introduction

The most distinguishing feature of the chiropractic profession—what the public most commonly thinks of when they hear the word "chiropractic"—is its therapeutic intervention.[1] And the most common therapeutic intervention used by chiropractors is the type of procedure that puts a manual force into a targeted area of a patient, most commonly the spine, which results in a popping or clicking sound. The areas of the spine targeted by the chiropractor are usually ones the chiropractor has determined to be stiff or dysfunctional in some manner. Often, but not always, it is the same area that the patient points to when asked "Where does it hurt?" and the same area the patient reports to be painful when palpated by the chiropractor or during an orthopedic or provocative (meaning that it "provokes" the symptoms) test.

The therapeutic intervention chiropractors use for patient care is called either a "chiropractic adjustment" or a "manipulation" (when the spine is targeted, the term would then be "spinal manipulative therapy" or simply "SMT"). Although related, the terms "adjustment" and "manipulation" are not synonymous since they do have nuanced differences in meaning, and these differences remain an area of controversy within the profession itself.[2] From an outside perspective, these differences may seem trivial, but for some members of the profession they go to the very heart of what it means to be a chiropractor and underpin how they perceive the body to work.

In order to fully understand the chiropractic adjustment—what it is, how it is delivered, how students are taught to use it—this chapter will explore the following topics:

- chiropractic adjustment versus chiropractic manipulation
- spinal manipulative therapy
- Palmer Postulates and their relationship to the adjustment
- definition of "subluxation"
- operationalizing the term "subluxation"
- chiropractic technique systems
- finding the clinical target: training in how to perform spinal manipulation
- why spinal adjustment works
- issues of safety
- evidence of clinical effectiveness

Considerations about the Definition of "Chiropractic"

When asked to describe what an architect is, a layperson might respond, "A person who plans how to build a house or building." If a layperson is asked to describe a lawyer, the response might be, "A person who writes and interprets the law," and if asked to describe a dentist, a layperson might answer, "Someone who treats problems of the teeth, gums, and jaw."

This simple exercise illustrates several principles. First, each of these persons is part of a *profession*. A profession fills a niche in society based on its *cultural authority*.[3] Cultural authority is granted by society and is based on the recognition of a group's competency and legitimacy with respect to a domain over which it professes authority. It is a reflection of a profession's specialized knowledge, expertise, and skills.[3,4] With cultural authority comes a degree of autonomy and privilege but also a great degree of responsibility.

It is important to understand that there is a fundamental difference between the business world and the professional world. In the business world, participants are motivated by profit. There is a certain Darwinian principle in effect whereby only those businesses that are efficiently run, that successfully fill a share of the marketplace, and that are profitable will survive. While there are laws in place that regulate appropriate conduct, by and large consumers are expected to be educated and knowledgeable about the goods or services they consume. The burden of knowledge is on the consumer, not the seller. This general principle of the business world is captured by the Latin expression *caveat emptor*—"let the buyer beware."[3]

But the professional world is very different, and professionals have very different responsibilities. Among these responsibilities is a duty of fidelity;[3] that is, to only convey information to the patient or client that is true. There is also a duty of care owed to a patient, meaning that the professional is expected to act as would a reasonable member of that group under the same or similar circumstances. Lastly, unlike people involved in commerce, professionals are expected to act in their client's or patient's best interest at all times, setting aside any financial motivations. Monetary gain is expected to be subservient to the needs of the patient. This is captured by the Latin expression *credet emptor*—"let the buyer have faith."

Not only does the business world differ from the professional world, but chiropractors have historically tended to differ from other professionals. Specifically, unlike the example of architects, lawyers, and dentists discussed above, if a chiropractor were to be asked to describe him- or herself, we might see a unique feature among some groups of chiropractors: rather than describe *what they do*, they tend to describe themselves by *how they think*.[1,2]

It is important to understand this tendency among some chiropractors to self-identify by their ideology. This ideological perspective informs one's understanding of how the body works, how the term "subluxation" is operationalized (see discussion below), and, ultimately, this affects the chiropractor's preferred method of treatment. Relevant to this chapter, this semantic process also lies at the core of differentiating between a chiropractic adjustment and spinal manipulative therapy.

Chiropractic Adjustment versus Chiropractic Manipulation

In general, a chiropractic adjustment is any force a chiropractor delivers to a patient's joints for therapeutic purposes. A chiropractic adjustment may be delivered manually, or by use of adjusting instruments, or by the use of specialized equipment (padded wedges, mechanized or drop or mechanized-drop tables), or by a number of low-force techniques.[2] The World Health Organization captures this general idea in defining an adjustment as "any chiropractic procedure that ultimately uses controlled force, leverage, direction, amplitude and velocity, which is applied to specific joints and adjacent tissues. Chiropractors use such procedures to influence joint and neurophysical function."[3]

The distinction between an adjustment and a manipulation can be complex. Among those chiropractors who have a more traditional view of the profession, those members who embrace the Palmer Postulates (see discussion below), an adjustment can only be used if the chiropractor has detected a *subluxation* and has the therapeutic *intention* of removing or correcting it.[2,4] Thus, this definition is both broad in the sense that it captures any kind of force a chiropractor may impart with clinical purpose, and at the same time it is reductionist since it is only used for subluxation correction. And to make the matter even more complicated, some very traditional-minded chiropractors only use the term "adjustment" if they are applying a force to the spine, since by their definition a subluxation can exist nowhere else.[3]

The Palmer Postulates and Their Relationship to the Adjustment

The Palmer Postulates were developed by the earliest pioneers of the chiropractic profession, Daniel David (D. D.) and his son Bartlett Joshua (B. J.) Palmer. Traditionally, it is said that D. D. Palmer delivered the first chiropractic adjustment.[1] Specifically, on September 18, 1895, D. D. adjusted Harvey Lillard, a deaf African American janitor who had lost his hearing 17 years earlier. In Lillard's own words:

> I was deaf 17 years ago and expected to remain so, for I had doctored a great deal without any benefit. . . . Last January, Dr. Palmer told me that my deafness came from an injury in my spine. This was new to me; but it is a fact that my back was injured at the time I went deaf. Dr. Palmer treated my spine; in two treatments I could hear quite well. That was eight months ago. My hearing remains good.[5]

What must be emphasized is that it was D. D.'s intention to restore Lillard's hearing using a thrusting-type maneuver applied to his midthoracic spine.[2] D. D. himself acknowledges he was not the first healer to use thrusting procedures on the spine as a method of cure; bonesetters had been doing that in Eastern Europe for centuries.[2] But D. D. did claim he was the first to restore vertebral segments that were "racked out of place" by using the spinous process or transverse process of the vertebrae as levers, with the *intent* of affecting the nervous system. To quote D. D.:

> I am not the first person to replace subluxated vertebrae, for this art has been practiced for thousands of years. I do claim, however, to be the first

to replace displaced vertebrae by using the spinous and transverse processes as levers, wherewith to rack subluxated vertebrae into normal position, and from this basic fact, to create a science which is destined to revolutionize the theory and practice of the healing arts.[6]

Partly because he was experiencing financial challenges and partly because he had been jailed briefly for practicing medicine without a license, D. D. sold the chiropractic college he had established to his son B. J. in the early part of the 1900s. B. J. continued to develop, expand, and defend the profession until the end of his life in 1961.

The Palmer Postulates essentially distill down to the idea that a dysfunction between two adjacent vertebral segments can impinge an emerging nerve root, and this impingement can, in turn, result in a variety of neurological symptoms, including pain, numbness, and tingling as well as broader health problems depending on the specific nerve root affected.[4] According to Palmer's theory, this intervertebral dysfunction can be termed a "subluxation."[4] Although the specific theoretical models used to account for this intervertebral dysfunction and subsequent neurological impairment varied over time, the similarities outweigh the differences, and it is conventional to refer to this theoretical construct as the Palmer Postulates.

A chiropractor who embraces this approach would say he or she "corrects a subluxation" with a specific spinal adjustment, properly delivered.[4] A "manipulation" is too generic a term for advocates of this ideological approach, since it can be delivered by anyone (not just a chiropractor) to any area of the body (not just the spine) to mobilize joints. Not only that but, depending on the extent to which the chiropractor adheres to the Palmer Postulates, a traditional-minded chiropractor takes a more metaphysical approach to this type of healing and would say the specific spinal adjustment removes the nerve interference, and the *innate intelligence* of the body (essentially the natural recuperative abilities of the body, often referred to as "vitalism") corrects the subluxation, bringing the patient to a state of "ease."

Spinal Manipulative Therapy

A chiropractic manipulation is a type of chiropractic adjustment, delivered manually or using an instrument to the spine or peripheral joints; there is no requirement for the presence of a subluxation.[2] Many manipulative procedures, especially those performed when the patient is side-lying, require a great deal of coordination and choreography by the doctor, which requires substantial hands-on training. Thus, a manipulation can be defined as a "complex, bimanual motor skill involving various levels of interlimb coordination and postural control combined with a timely weight transfer . . . execution is highly adaptive and context-dependent, taking into account any coexisting pathological, structural weakness or other factors that may limit the approach to delivering manual maneuver."[7]

From a mechanical perspective, manipulation is usually described as a high-velocity, low-amplitude thrust into the paraphysiological space. The paraphysiological space is an area of joint motion beyond what the patient can achieve on his or her own (the active range of motion) and beyond the passive range of motion (those joint motions that exist within a joint that a person cannot voluntarily produce) but before the limits of anatomic integrity (the region of motion beyond which injury occurs).[8] A skilled therapist is able to bring the targeted joint beyond the passive range of motion to the paraphysiological space, but no further than that. This action typically results in joint cavitation (which causes the popping or cracking sound), which is caused by nitrogen gas being forcibly expelled from the joint. The World Health Organization[2] defines joint "manipulation" as a manual procedure involving direct thrust to move a joint past the physiological range of motion without exceeding the anatomical limit.

What this means is, from a semantic point of view, all manipulations are adjustments but not all adjustments are manipulations.

Defining "Subluxation"

Consider dentistry: the main therapeutic intervention used by dentists when they identify a problem that needs fixing is an amalgam filling. The filling is used to fix the diagnostic entity known as a cavity. Dentistry is an example of a very standardized profession, since dentists across the world perceive and identify the clinical target (the cavity) in much the same way and treat it virtually the same way, regardless of where they obtained their training or the jurisdiction in which they practice. This is not the case with chiropractic, since the chiropractic profession is less standardized, and the type of care you might receive from one chiropractor may be very different from the care you might receive from another chiropractor, even if the two chiropractors were neighbors and graduated from the same accredited chiropractic program.

The variability of chiropractic practice is reflected in the various definitions of the term "subluxation," definitions that are replete with and/or qualifiers. For example, the World Health Organization defines a subluxation as "a lesion or dysfunction in a joint or motion segment in which alignment, movement integrity and/or physiological function is altered, although contact between joint surfaces remains intact. It is essentially a function entity which may influence biomechanical and neural integrity."[2] Similarly, the Association of Chiropractic Colleges' 1996 definition defined a subluxation as "a complex of functional and/or structural and/or pathological articular changes that compromise neural integrity and may influence organ system function and general health."[9] In both definitions we see how these organizations, no doubt with the input of several different stakeholders, struggled to develop a definition that applied to different practice approaches.

Setting aside its semantic challenges, for many chiropractors the subluxation is the equivalent to the dental cavity: it is the clinical entity that needs to be fixed. Depending on the chiropractic technique system being used, a chiropractor may use any number of different diagnostic tests to identify a subluxation, and understanding how the term is operationalized allows for a better understanding of why a chiropractor may choose to use a particular diagnostic test and particular plan of patient care.

Operationalizing the Term "Subluxation"

Several years ago, it was proposed that one way to understand the differences and similarities among various chiropractic technique systems (there are several dozen of them) was to employ a Linnaean taxonomic method used to classify plants and animals.[7] Instead of using kingdoms, phyla, orders, and classes that differentiate organisms by their type of cellular structure or ability to move, chiropractic technique systems could be grouped by how they operationalize the term "subluxation"; specifically, whether the technique system was based on a *structural*, *functional*, or *tonal-based* model.[10]

In the case of a *structural* approach, the chiropractor is concerned about the architecture of the patient's spine; it should have what are theoretically believed to be "optimal" curves. These curves may be assessed visually during a standing postural examination or by performing various line markings from plain film X-rays. In the case of X-ray line markings, spinal curves are mathematically defined. The goal of care would be to restore or establish optimal spinal curves. Examples of this approach are Chiropractic BioPhysics and Pettibon technique, as well as Gonstead technique to a certain extent.[2] This approach is used by a minority of chiropractors.

The second major operational definition of "subluxation" is a *tonal-based* approach.[10] From this perspective, the spinal cord is thought to have a normal vibratory frequency, not unlike the vibratory frequency of a guitar string. Theoretically, in this approach, when a subluxation is present, there is impingement on neurological structures that ultimately result in an abnormal "tone" of the nerve system, which would detrimentally affect the organs, muscles, and other tissues innervated by those nerves.[10] Chiropractors who adhere to a tonal-based model would assess a patient using instruments thought to assess neurological function, such as thermography or manual muscle testing as used by applied kinesiologists.[2] Unlike postural observation or palpation, diagnostic methods used to identify the tone of the nervous system are usually more indirect. Examples of tonal-based chiropractic techniques would be network spinal analysis, torque release technique, and upper cervical chiropractic techniques (of which there are many).[2] Like the previous approach, this one is also used by a minority of chiropractors.

The approach to chiropractic assessment and treatment most commonly used by chiropractors is *functional*, which has as its intent the reestablishment of optimum ranges of motion of each vertebral segment or of the entire spine.[2] Patients are assessed by various types of palpation (static, motion, and joint play analysis) as well as various orthopedic tests that determine if a spinal or peripheral joint is moving to the limits of its inherent normal ranges of motion. A chiropractor may also assess the relative stiffness of one vertebral segment compared to others. The goal of this approach is to restore motion, reduce stiffness, or alleviate pain—or any combination of the three. Diversified technique is often cited as an example of a functional and pain-based chiropractic technique system.[10] Diversified technique is the most commonly used technique internationally and also the one most closely identified in the public's mind with the chiropractic intervention.

It is important to understand that not all chiropractors exclusively adopt only one theoretical approach. Many chiropractors use a combination of approaches. For example, chiropractors may consider both functional and structural components of the spine, or they may concern themselves with the structure of the spine and its effect on the tone of the nervous system.

It is also important to realize that some chiropractors superimpose other equally important concepts onto their operationalization of the term "subluxation," beyond the super-groupings of structure, function, or tone. Many chiropractors perceive their job to be to identify the "primary subluxation" that they believe is the basis for the patient's problem.[2,10] These chiropractors opine that, even though a patient may report pain or symptoms in many different areas of the body, once the primary subluxation is identified and corrected, all other "secondary" subluxations (also termed "compensatory subluxations") will self-resolve.[2,10] Chiropractors who focus primarily on the upper cervical spine (the neck) and use some upper cervical chiropractic technique systems theorize that subluxations of the occiput (base of skull), atlas (first cervical vertebrae), or axis (second cervical vertebrae) are primary and adjusting one of these segments will result in the best clinical outcomes. Similarly, there are chiropractors who focus on the pelvis and use Logan Basic technique; these chiropractors adjust the pelvis and believe that all other dysfunctional segments will self-correct.

Last, it should be mentioned that some chiropractors focus on the management of pain and other symptoms, whereas other chiropractors, typically traditional chiropractors, do not. As Owens observed, "Since presence or absence of symptoms of diagnosable disease is seen as not necessarily germane to the location and correction of vertebral subluxation by many objective chiropractors, they may place very little emphasis on the diagnosis of health conditions other than those that are life-threatening."[11]

Chiropractic Technique Systems

Different approaches to the application of manual procedures are often called "chiropractic technique systems."[2] A chiropractic technique system is essentially a step-by-step cookbook-type approach, from diagnosis to treatment, with a codified set of rules. Typically, chiropractic technique systems were developed by practitioners after some type of personal experience or serendipitous observation, and the practitioner then often (but not always) named the technique system after himself (examples include Gonstead, Logan Basic, and Palmer HIO techniques[2]). It is important to understand that the basis for the differences among chiropractic technique systems is not as much the type of application of biomechanical force but rather the explanatory model of how the body (especially the spine) should optimally function.[2]

Patient-Centered Reasons for Selection of Technique

There may be times when the use of spinal manipulative therapy is contraindicated. Perhaps the patient has advanced osteoporosis, and the chiropractor has judged it would be unwise to impart the type of forces generated during the delivery of spinal adjusting into a fragile spine. Perhaps the patient has not responded favorably to spinal adjusting in the past, or perhaps the patient simply doesn't like it. Perhaps there is a substantial difference in size between a small doctor and much larger patient. In these cases, there are many other chiropractic technique systems that can be used for patient care.

What is usually termed "diversified technique" is the technique most commonly used by chiropractors and most commonly associated with spinal manipulation in general. It is the one primarily characterized by high-velocity, low-amplitude thrusting procedures. The most commonly used chiropractic technique system after diversified technique is Activator methods chiropractic technique. The Activator is a hand-held instrument that allows the user to adjust the amount of force the device delivers to the targeted area. There are other very similar adjusting instruments developed after the Activator, so that this form of adjustment is commonly referred to as "instrument assisted." Some patients refer to the instrument as the "clicky device" based on its sound. There is a fair amount of evidence that demonstrates the clinical effectiveness of instrument-assisted adjusting, along with a very good safety record.[2]

Flexion-distraction is a technique system that makes use of specially designed tables that allow the operator to create axial distraction in a targeted area of the patient, typically the low back. That is, using the movement of the table sections, the chiropractor can stretch specific areas of the spine and thus widen the joint space. Table-assisted techniques like flexion-distraction are based on a sound physiological model and has been shown to be effective for patients with mechanical low back pain or back pain due to intervertebral disc instabilities. Other types of specialized table allow for the cervical, thoracic, or lumbopelvic piece to disengage or drop, which allows for the application of forces in a very controlled manner. Some chiropractors use these drop-piece tables on their own or along with a form of physical examination known as prone leg checking as part of a technique system called Thompson Terminal Point.[2]

Some chiropractors use pelvic wedges or blocks for patients with low back pain who may not be candidates for spinal manipulative therapy. SacroOccipital Technique (SOT) is a technique system that has developed a series of protocols for the use of pelvic blocks, but these devices can be used without following SOT protocols as well.[2] Using these padded wedges, the chiropractor positions the patient in such a way that his or her own body weight facilitates the joints of the pelvis and low back to gently settle into a more biomechanically normal position.

Other less commonly used technique systems are BioEnergetic Synchronization Technique (BEST) and Network Spinal Analysis. These are very low-force techniques that have their roots in a more tonal-based model. There have been a few studies conducted that have demonstrated the clinical effectiveness of these techniques, but for the most part their usefulness is unproven. Even so, they remain an option of use.

In addition to the use of various electrical modalities, such as TENS, ultrasound, or laser, some chiropractors have used acupuncture or cranial therapies to manage a variety of health problems.[1]

Finding the Clinical Target—Where Should the Patient Be Adjusted?

Starting in 2011, Triano and his colleagues[12] undertook a tremendously ambitious project: a comprehensive review of the studies that assessed the validity and reliability of all the diagnostic tests used by chiropractors to find the clinical target. This study, colloquially referred to as the "site of care study," also assessed the methodological strength of the studies found.

In general, the site of care study determined that the diagnostic tests that take a *direct* measure of the presumptive site of care—palpation for pain, static and motion palpation, palpation for stiffness, postural assessment—were more valid and reliable and had a more robust evidence base than did diagnostic tests that relied on an *indirect* assessment approach. Examples of indirect assessment methods include manual muscle testing, skin conductance, and thermography. It's noteworthy that high-quality evidence was found indicating that the use of X-ray analysis for locating the site of care is not appropriate (neither valid nor reliable).

Leg-length analysis, a diagnostic test used by many chiropractors, requires special mention. Leg-length analysis is a procedure that assesses the relative length of one leg to the other when the patient is prone, supine, or seated and the legs are moved into various positions. Activator methods, Thompson Terminal Point, and upper cervical techniques each use a type of leg-length analysis.[2] It should come as no surprise that the type of information the doctor is thought to be extracting using leg-length analysis differs depending on the technique system being used. For example, some technique systems use leg-length analysis as a measure of pelvic obliquity and would therefore be considered functional-based tests. Conversely, chiropractors who focus on the upper cervical spine use supine leg-length analysis as an indicator of neurological function; in this case, the test would be classified as a tonal-based test. The study by Triano et al.[12] reported that leg-length analysis had favorable evidence with respect to its validity as a test to assess the position of the pelvis (whether it was in a balanced position), but the relationship of leg-length analysis to patient symptoms has not been demonstrated.

Chiropractic Education: Learning How to Perform Spinal Manipulation

Chiropractors pride themselves on being experts in the diagnosis and management of conditions of the neuromusculoskeletal system, and this pride is not unjustified. The focus of chiropractic education is on those skills needed to diagnosis conditions of the spine and peripheral joints. Chiropractic students devote large amounts of time to learning how to perform soft tissue therapies, mobilizations, and, in particular, spinal adjustments and other manipulative procedures in order to conservatively manage spinal pain. Most chiropractic programs in accredited colleges or universities devote hundreds of laboratory hours specifically to the acquisition of chiropractic "technique" skills. At the Canadian Memorial Chiropractic College, for example, more than 300 hours are spent on acquiring psychomotor skills during instructional labs in the undergraduate program, followed by more than 1,000 hours of experience as an intern providing patient care under the direct supervision of a licensed practitioner.

Classroom instruction is aimed at performing manual therapies with a great deal of precision and skill. It is designed to approximate how a chiropractor would successfully manage a patient's chief complaint in the field, while reducing the likelihood of adverse reactions in either the patient or the doctor. Obviously, the likelihood of injury to medical doctors who manage spinal pain by referring patients to other health care providers or by prescribing medications is very low. However, the likelihood of chiropractors injuring themselves during the administration of a complex psychomotor skill such as spinal adjusting is much higher. And because relatively large biomechanical forces are being delivered to the patient in a short period of time, it is incumbent on the doctor to know how to modulate the forces being generated or to modify the method in which these forces are being delivered as clinical circumstances dictate (or both) in order to minimize the possibility of injuring the patient. Examples of when these issues become particularly important include situations in which there is a large anthropomorphic difference (height and/or weight) between the doctor and patient or when the patient has a comorbid condition, such as osteoporosis, or is simply frail, as may be the case with some elderly patients.

For generations, teaching of manual manipulation skills during chiropractic education has relied heavily on the evaluation of a learner's progress through the subjective observations of a content expert, who is almost always a chiropractor. Students are typically grouped into working pairs, such that one student acts as the "doctor" and the other student acts as the "patient," since it would be impractical to find a large enough group of volunteers in the community to perform this function throughout undergraduate education. Lesson plans are scaffolded in such a way that more complex procedures are introduced after simpler procedures are mastered. In the case of spinal manipulative procedures, learners start with the basic choreography of the skill and practice thrust patterns on a table or other inert object prior to attempting it on fellow students. Once these basic skills are mastered, the instructor subdivides a procedure into its constituent subskills and then observes the students' attempts to mimic each subskill back to the instructor, working toward the goal of assembling all the subskills into the entire procedure. Students continually rehearse the procedures demonstrated by instructors until they are thought to be able to perform them independently. Assessments are typically conducted at various intervals throughout the academic year and involve students demonstrating procedures for their instructors, who measure the demonstrated skills against a grading rubric.[9]

There are some challenges to this method of teaching and assessment, not the least of which is long-term skill retention and the subjective nature of grading by tutors. These pedagogical challenges using traditional learner-coach pairings may be further complicated by the need to teach students to avoid the minor injuries that chiropractic students are susceptible to while they learn psychomotor skills during technique labs.

In order to overcome these teaching and assessment challenges, some chiropractic programs have embedded the use of emerging technologies into their course curricula. One example is the use of a force-sensing table technology, which is a standard chiropractic table equipped with a series of force-sensing plates yoked to visual display screens. When a student thrusts on the table, or a specially designed mannequin, the force-sensing plates are able to measure the force-time profile of the manipulative thrust generated and instantaneously provide a visual image of it for review. In this manner, students are provided with real-time visual feedback as they learn to modulate and improve their thrust patterns before they try it on each other or on living, breathing patients.

Why Spinal Adjusting Works

On the surface, it seems counterintuitive to posit that a way to improve low back pain, possibly the result of a trauma, fall, or improper ergonomics, is to apply procedures that deliver biomechanical force to the exact same area that was traumatized in the first place. Patients may wonder aloud, "Why is the doctor visiting a form of controlled force on my body in order to fix it?"

In their 2002 seminal article describing the chiropractic profession, Meeker and Haldemann[1] listed the prominent theories used to explain why a chiropractic adjustment achieves positive clinical outcomes. These authors broke down the prominent theories into two proposed mechanisms: "mechanical/anatomic" and "neurological/mechanical." The theorized effects of mechanical/anatomic models include the alleviation of entrapped facet joint inclusions, reposition of annual material in the intervertebral disc, and alleviation of stiffness induced by fibrotic tissue from previous injury or degenerative changes. Neurological/mechanical theorized effects include inhibition of excessive reflex activity in intrinsic spinal musculature or reduction of compression of irritative insults to neurological tissue.

Years later, Wong et al.[13] conducted a nonrandomized controlled study of patients with and without low back pain who were treated using spinal manipulative therapy (SMT), in order to identify those patients who are most likely to respond to SMT and determine if responders differ biomechanically from nonresponders. The authors reported that responders to SMT displayed statistically significant decreases in spinal stiffness and increases in multifidus (and intrinsic spinal muscle) thickness ratio. In essence, Wong et al.'s[13] study was congruent with the models described by Meeker and Haldeman[1] over a decade earlier.

Over the past decade, other studies have demonstrated how spinal manipulation has biochemical effects (the release of endorphins or cytokines) and biomechanical effects (e.g., alteration of muscle spindle functions). The explanation of these biological changes are quite complex and beyond the scope of this chapter.

Other factors may equally account for patient improvements in symptoms following spinal adjusting. Psychosocial factors that may affect clinical outcomes include patient fear or anxiety about the treatment, patient and doctor expectations of recovery, and the depth to which a positive doctor-patient rapport has been established.

Lastly, as mentioned previously, some chiropractors rely on more metaphysical theories to explain why a chiropractic intervention can heal a patient. Chiropractors who strongly embrace the Palmer Postulates may default to the idea that the natural recuperative abilities of the body account for the healing process, in a mechanism referred to as "innate intelligence." Specifically, it is thought that the innate intelligence of the body can be optimally expressed once any nervous interference, caused by vertebral subluxation, is removed. Thus, the degree to which both the doctor and patient adopt this belief may have an effect on outcomes, perhaps through a placebo effect, as it is known that belief can influence outcomes.

Safety Issues

In general, adverse reactions to spinal manipulative therapy can be divided into two groups. The first group of adverse reactions are those that are minor in nature and self-limiting, meaning they resolve on their own within 24 hours or so. Hallmark studies from Scandinavia published in the 1990s reported that roughly half of patients under chiropractic care experienced minor unpleasant reactions during the initial phase of care, usually after the first treatment.[14,15] This should come as no surprise, since it is during the initial examination that chiropractors perform diagnostic tests designed to reproduce the patient's presenting chief complaint, which is typically low back or neck pain or headache. In other words, it is during the initial stages of patient care that chiropractors employ tests meant to elicit pain or other symptoms in order to determine the source of the problem. Additionally, the clinical encounter may represent the first time a patient has received spinal manipulative therapy targeting a vertebral segment that has been dysfunctional and/or lacking in mobility for days, weeks, or even years. As such, the doctor may not yet know which regimen of treatment the patient will best respond to, and the tissue being targeted may be especially sensitive to the forces employed.

At the other end of the spectrum, serious side effects of SMT, such as disc herniation or stroke, are very rare and unpredictable, and it is because of this rarity and unpredictability that quantifying the risk with any precision is impossible. For example, a 2009 review of the literature reported the incidence of serious events to SMT varies between 5 strokes/100,000 manipulations to 1.46 serious events/10,000,000 manipulations and 2.68 deaths/10,000,000 manipulations.[16] Obviously, although the range is not exact, it is clear that the risk of serious adverse events is extremely low. *Chapter 6 discusses safety issues in more detail.*

Since the early 2000s, Scott Haldeman, a chiropractor and medical neurologist, has authored several articles on the incidence of vertebrobasilar stroke subsequent to cervical manipulation (cSMT), and the overall theme of these articles is consistent.[17] Specifically, his group found that the incidence of stroke following chiropractic SMT is very rare.[17] They noted documented cases of stroke following such benign activities as yoga, prayer, sex, and going to the hairdresser and found there were no consistent risk factors in those cases where there was a temporal link between the application of cSMT and the development of stroke.[17] For example, the temporal occurrence between the two events was independent of whether or not the patient was a smoker or had high blood pressure and was unrelated to the type of cervical manipulation the doctor performed.[17] It bears stating that while smoking and having high blood pressure are certainly risk factors of experiencing a stroke, there is simply no evidence that this risk is increased if a patient receives a cervical adjustment as well.

Epidemiological studies indicate that there is no difference in the incidence of stroke among patients presenting with neck pain or headache who visited either medical physicians or chiropractors.[18] This has led to the consistent conclusion that patients in the midst of a stroke are experiencing neck pain or headaches and thus seek care from either medical physicians or chiropractors, and the outcome is the same.

From a mechanical point of view, it has been shown that the amount of force generated during a typical cervical manipulation is a magnitude smaller (that is, 10 times less) than the force required to mechanically disrupt vertebral artery tissue.[19] It is important to note that the tissue examined in measuring these forces was obtained from elderly cadaveric samples, meaning the sample tissue was less robust than tissue found in living persons. These results have been confirmed in additional studies in high-impact, peer-reviewed journals that each demonstrate the same result.[19]

Evidence of Clinical Effectiveness

The most comprehensive reviews of the literature pertaining to the clinical effectiveness of spinal manipulation were conducted in 2010[20] and updated in 2014.[21] These publications are known as the "UK Evidence Reports." They reported that the strongest evidence supports the contention that spinal manipulation is clinically effective for acute, subacute, and chronic low back pain, migraine and cervicogenic headaches, cervicogenic dizziness, and several conditions involving the peripheral joints, and there is strong evidence of the clinical effectiveness of thoracic manipulation and mobilization in the successful management of acute and subacute neck pain. Although much less robust, there is some evidence that spinal manipulation may positively influence some nonmusculoskeletal conditions, such as certain types of dizziness, asthma, infantile colic, and problems of the gastrointestinal system.[21]

Since chiropractors tend to be generalists in the sense that they treat patients of all ages and with a myriad of conditions, they have become very adept at modifying care plans to match the specific needs and clinical circumstances of their patients. Although many field practitioners may rely on their own clinical experience and learn which modifications to SMT work best in this or that particular case, there exist clinical practice guidelines and best-practice documents that outline how the doctor may modify the delivery of SMT for special populations, including children or older adults, and many chiropractors substitute other types of low-force spinal adjustments often embedded in different chiropractic technique systems.[2]

Summary

This chapter has explored the topic of the chiropractic adjustment from many different perspectives, essentially using the "5W and 1H" approach. This chapter described "what" an adjustment is, both in terms of semantics and biomechanical properties. From a semantic perspective, the chapter explored the distinction between an "adjustment" and a "manipulation," and it operationalized the term "subluxation." By doing so, this chapter was able to better discuss the different types of spinal adjustments and chiropractic technique systems chiropractors use for patient care.

This chapter discussed the topic of "where" to adjust (finding the clinical target) and "why" to adjust, in terms of clinical effectiveness, and "how" to adjust in terms of student education. Instead of discussing "when" to adjust, this chapter focused more on the question of "when *not* to adjust," discussing the risk of adverse effects of spinal adjusting and the manner in which chiropractors modify the delivery of this type of therapeutic intervention in order to decrease an already-low risk.

This chapter did not go into detail about "who" is performing spinal manipulation. *Chapters 2 and 3 provided detailed information about chiropractors' characteristics and typical practice.* Suffice it to say that, while chiropractors can legitimately claim they have cultural authority in the field of manual medicine, especially with respect to spinal manipulation training and use in clinical practice, other health care providers are authorized to administer SMT in many jurisdictions, including medical doctors, physiotherapists, and naturopaths. That said, students in these other professions do not receive the same amount of training as do chiropractic students, and the use of spinal adjusting is not the central focus of these other professions as it is for chiropractic.

Despite the fact that chiropractors use a wide variety of different types of spinal adjustments for completely different ideological reasons, perhaps the most important take-home message the reader should gain from this chapter is how central the chiropractic adjustment is to the collective zeitgeist of the profession.

References

1. Meeker WC, Haldeman S. Chiropractic: a profession at the crossroads of mainstream and alternative medicine. *Arch Intern Med.* 2002;136:216–227.

2. Cooperstein R, Gleberzon BJ, eds. *Technique Systems in Chiropractic.* Edinburgh, UK: Churchill-Livingston (Elsevier); 2004.

3. World Health Organization. *WHO Guidelines on Basic Training and Safety in Chiropractic.* Geneva, CH: World Health Organization; 2015.

4. Nelson CF, Lawrence DJ, Triano JJ, et al. Chiropractic as spine care: a model for the profession. *Chiropr Osteopat.* 2005 Jul 6;13:9.

5. Keating JC, Callender A, Cleveland CS III. *Chiropractic History: A Primer.* Montezuma, IA: Sutherland Companies; 2004.

6. Palmer DD. *The Chiropractor's Adjustor: The Science, Art and Philosophy of Chiropractic.* Portland, OR: Portland Printing House; 1910.

7. Triano J, McGregor M, Howard L. Enhanced learning of manipulation techniques using force-sensing table technology (FSTT). Toronto, ON: Higher Education Quality Council of Ontario; 2014.

8. Sandoz R. Some physical mechanisms and effects of spinal adjustments. *Ann Swiss Chiropr Assoc.* 1976;6:91–142.

9. Association of Chiropractic Colleges. Position Paper #1. 1996. http://www .chiro.org/chimages/chiropage/acc.html. Accessed October 29, 2015.

10. Cooperstein R, Gleberzon BJ. Towards a taxonomy of subluxation-equivalents. *Top Clin Chiropr.* 2001;8(1):49–58.

11. Owens, E. Theoretical constructs of vertebral subluxation as applied to chiropractic practitioners and researchers. *Top Clin Chiropr.* 2000;7(1):74–79.

12. Triano JJ, Budgell B, Bagnulo A, et al. Review of methods used by chiropractors to determine the site of applying manipulation. *Chiropr & Man Ther.* 2013;21:36.

13. Wong AY, Parent EC, Sukhvinder D. Do participants with low back pain who respond to spinal manipulative therapy differ biomechanically from nonresponders, untreated controls or asymptomatic controls? *Spine.* 2015;40(17): 1329–1337.

14. Senstead O, Leboeuf-Yde C, Borchgrevink C. Frequency and characteristics of side effects of spinal manipulative therapy. *Spine.* 1997 Feb 15;22(4): 435–440.

15. Leboeuf-Yde C, Hennius B, Rudberg E. Side effects of chiropractic treatment: a prospective study. *J Manipulative Physiol Ther.* 1997;20(8):511–515.

16. Gouveia LO, Castanho P, Ferreira JJ. Safety of chiropractic interventions. a systematic review. *Spine.* 2009;34(11):E405–E413.

17. Haldeman S, Kohlbeck FJ, McGregor M, et al. Risk factors and precipitating neck movements causing vertebrobasilar artery dissection after cervical trauma and spinal manipulation. *Spine.* 1999;24(8):785–794.

18. Cassidy DJ, Boyle E, Cote P, et al. Risk of vertebrobasilar stroke and chiropractic care. results from a population-based case-control and case-crossover study. *Spine.* 2008;33(45):S176–183.

19. Symons B, Herzog W. Cervical artery dissection: a biomechanical perspective. *J Can Chiro Assoc.* 2013;57(4):276–278.

20. Bronfort G, Haas M, Evans R, Leininger B, Triano J. Effectiveness of manual therapies: the UK evidence report. *Chiropr & Osteop.* 2010 Feb 25;18:3.

21. Clar C, Tsertsvadze A, Court R, Hundt GL, Clarke A, Sutcliffe P. Clinical effectiveness of manual therapy for the management of musculoskeletal and non-musculoskeletal conditions: systematic review and update of UK evidence report. *Chiropr Man Therap.* 2014;22(1):12.

CHAPTER FIVE

Other Chiropractic Services

Robert M. Rowell, DC, MS; and Robert Vining, DC

Introduction

Doctors of chiropractic (DCs) perform a variety of therapeutic activities using many different treatment options in their practices. Some treatments used by DCs include physiological therapeutics, which is the application of devices or physical agents for the purpose of helping the body to heal. The devices used are often referred to as "modalities." These devices include treatment with electrical stimulation, ultrasound, and laser light. Physical agents include ice, heat, and mechanical energy, such as traction, massage, and vibration. In addition, DCs will often prescribe exercise, supports, braces, and taping methods and engage in many other activities. DCs have used a multitude of therapeutic procedures since the beginning of the chiropractic profession.[1] Descriptions of physiological therapeutic use by the chiropractic profession date as far back as 1912. This chapter will discuss a variety of therapeutic methods and other activities used by DCs.

Thermal Agents

The word "thermal" refers to temperature, and the phrase "thermal agent" refers to the application of either heat or cold. The application of heat is called "thermotherapy" while the application of cold is known as "cryotherapy." Heat has the effect of increasing blood flow, metabolic activity in cells, and joint mobility, and decreasing pain, muscle spasm, and joint stiffness.[2] Cold decreases blood flow, cellular metabolic activity, pain, and muscle spasm. There are many ways to apply heat or cold to the body. No matter what method is chosen, the same basic principle of physics applies. Thermal agents transfer heat from a warmer to a colder surface. In the case of ice application, ice does not impart cold, rather it removes heat from body tissues.

Thermotherapy

Moist hot packs are the most common method of applying heat used by DCs.[3] Heat is transferred from canvas packs with pouches containing silica gel that are soaked in very hot water. The packs release heat and steam, typically for 15 to 20 minutes, warming the skin and deeper structures. Moist hot packs come in a variety of shapes and sizes to better deliver heat to different regions of the body. The main pitfall of these hot packs is that the temperature is very high, so there is a risk of sustaining a burn if not used properly. However, they are commonly wrapped in towels and terry-cloth covers to allow safe delivery of heat.

Hot whirlpools typically employ stainless steel tubs filled with warm water. A pump circulates warm water around the immersed body part. The constant water circulation helps make whirlpools very effective at heating the intended body part. Whirlpools can also be used to help patients perform exercises in water, especially when moving the heated body part has been determined to be beneficial.

Paraffin baths contain melted paraffin wax mixed with mineral oil, which lowers the melting point of the wax. These baths are mostly used to impart heat to the hands, which are dipped in the melted wax/ mineral oil mixture 7 to 10 times. The wax is then covered with a plastic bag and wrapped in a towel for insulation. This is left in place for up to 30 minutes. The hot wax delivers heat directly to the small joints of the fingers, hand, and wrist, promoting increased joint mobility and decreased stiffness and pain.[2] While the hands are the most common area treated with paraffin, the feet can also be treated. Alternatively, a paintbrush can be used to paint layers of warm paraffin wax on other body parts.[4]

Therapeutic ultrasound is a method of heat therapy that uses high-frequency sound waves to create heat within muscles, tendons, and ligaments.[4] Sound waves are generated by the vibration of a crystal within the applicator head of an ultrasound machine. Crystalline vibrations occur between 1 and 3.3 million times per second, creating sound waves with frequencies that are much too high for the human ear to detect. These sound waves cause vibration of the molecules within the soft tissues of the body, producing heat. Heat from ultrasound treatments penetrates deeply into muscles, ligaments, and tendons but can also be used to treat tissues close to the surface. Ultrasound is applied by first covering the area to be treated with a thin layer of conductive gel (to transmit the sound waves). Then the ultrasound head is moved, or rubbed, in small circles around the treatment area. Another common method of applying ultrasound is to place the body part into water along with the ultrasound head. The sound waves are transferred to the body part through the water. The last recommended method of ultrasound application is to place a special disc of a gel material over the body part to be treated. The gel disc method and the underwater method are often used when the part to be treated has an irregular contour, such as the side of the ankle. Ultrasound is a safe and effective method of heating tissue in the body, but there is a precaution to its use. It can cause heating of bones that are close to the surface and result in a burn. To prevent this, DCs typically don't apply the ultrasound directly over bony prominences.

Diathermy is a thermal treatment that can also heat tissues deep inside the body. Diathermy involves the production of shortwave radio waves that create either an electrical or a magnetic field.[5] The electrical or magnetic field causes molecules to rotate or oscillate back and forth, leading to friction and heat. The most commonly used diathermy devices in chiropractic practice have a round plastic drum on the end of a moveable arm. Within the plastic drum is a coil of wire that emits the magnetic field. The drum can be placed over virtually any body part to cause heating. A new method of diathermy application involves a cuff or sleeve that is worn over the body part.[4] For example, a cuff can be worn over the elbow or ankle. Wires inside the cuff emit the electrical or magnetic field. Because the sleeve surrounds the body part, it generates heat from all directions.

Infrared heat is a final method of applying heat to the body using infrared lamps (or heat lamps). An infrared lamp is simply a lamp with a light bulb that emits infrared rays. These light rays heat the surface of whatever they contact, much the way the sun heats the sand on a beach. Infrared lamps heat only the very superficial layers of the skin and have generally fallen out of favor. Consequently, they are not as commonly used as other forms of thermal therapies.[3]

Table 5.1 Summary of Common Thermal Therapies

Therapeutic Technique	Definition	Application	Intended Effects
Moist Hot Packs	Typically, canvas-covered packs of silica gel soaked in hot water	○ Applied directly to the skin through towels that transmit heat and moisture	Heat-related Modalities:
Hot Whirlpool	Warm-water-filled tub with circulator pump	○ Body part is immersed in warm circulating water	○ Increase local blood flow
		○ Exercises sometimes performed while immersed in warm circulating water	○ Relax muscles
			○ Reduce joint stiffness
Paraffin Bath	Container of warm paraffin wax mixed with mineral oil	○ Hands/feet or other body parts are dipped in wax and then removed from container	○ Increase cellular metabolic activity
		○ Wax then wrapped in a towel or other thermal insulator material	
		○ Wax conveys heat to body part over a period of several minutes	
Therapeutic Ultrasound	High-frequency sound waves that generate heat within body tissues	○ Transmitted through a round applicator head (2–5 cm diameter) using gel or water as a conductive medium	
		○ Usually applied while moving applicator head in small circles	
Diathermy	Radio waves creating an electromagnetic field, generating heat when contacting body tissues	○ Electromagnetic field generated by a drum-shaped device that can be oriented toward target body areas	

Infrared Lamps	Infrared-wavelength-emitting light	○ Infrared-emitting lights oriented toward a body part or contained within flexible pads placed on the skin
Ice Pack	Frozen water contained within a thin material to allow efficient thermal energy transfer	○ Typically applied directly on the area for several-minute periods
Gel Pack	Frozen gel contained within a thin material to allow efficient thermal energy transfer	○ Usually applied to the skin through wet towel for several-minute periods
Ice Massage	Local ice application using ice as the massage agent	○ Ice applied by hand in slow circular or linear movements
Cold Whirlpool	Cold-water-filled tub with circulator pump	○ Body part is immersed in cold circulating water
Ice Bucket	Container of combined liquid water and ice	○ Body part is immersed in ice and water

Cold-related Modalities:
- Reduce swelling
- Reduce blood circulation to the area
- Reduce cell metabolism and prevent secondary injury

Cryotherapy

Cryotherapy is the application of cold for therapeutic purposes.[4] As stated earlier, applying cold is more accurately described as the act of removing heat from body tissues. Cooling body tissues decreases the amount of blood flow through a process known as "vasoconstriction." It also decreases cellular metabolic rate. Both of these effects are desired when treating acute injuries. The swelling that can occur after acute injuries can cause increased tissue pressure, which can lead to cell death. This is called "secondary injury." Cells that were not injured in the actual injury can die as a result of swelling. Decreasing the metabolism of these cells allows them to survive longer, theoretically preventing or reducing the amount of secondary injury. Vasoconstriction caused by cryotherapy also leads to less swelling. Initially, during an injury, capillaries become very permeable, resulting in leaking of fluid and protein. By constricting the capillaries, less fluid leaks out, and less swelling results. There are many methods of applying cryotherapy.[4]

Ice packs are plastic bags filled with ice. The most common method of applying ice packs is to fill a plastic bag with crushed ice and place it directly on the skin of an injured area. Because the ice begins to melt as soon as it comes into contact with skin, there is almost always a layer of water between the ice and the skin, decreasing the risk of frostbite. Consequently, the cooling is much more rapid and efficient when the ice pack is applied directly to skin. There is no need to place a towel or other cloth on the skin first.

Gel packs are plastic bags filled with a gel and kept in a freezer. These are very common and very convenient for applying cryotherapy. Unlike ice packs, gel packs should not be placed directly on the skin. Gel packs are usually colder than ice because there is no layer of water between the gel and the patient's skin. Consequently, they should be wrapped in a wet towel. Without the wet towel, gel packs placed directly on the skin pose a greater risk of frostbite than ice packs.

Ice massage is an effective method used for cooling small areas while simultaneously applying a light massage. Ice massage can be done with a paper or Styrofoam cup of frozen water or with a specially made "cryocup." The cryocup is a plastic cup that has two parts. It is filled with water and then frozen. When used, the cup splits in half, leaving a plastic ring to hold while massaging the tissue. The advantage of ice massage is that it combines the mechanical effects of massage (see "Therapeutic Massage" below) with the cooling effects of ice.

Ice buckets/ice baths are containers of ice and liquid water that a body part can be placed into. This method is most often used to cool the extremities (hands, feet, arms, legs, etc.). Occasionally, the ice bath may be used for the whole lower body or even the whole body. Because cold water and ice completely surround the body part being cooled, it is a very efficient process for removing heat. This method is used to treat acute injuries, such as sprained ankles or other joints, and also for preventing delayed-onset muscle soreness that occurs following heavy or intense exercise.

Cold whirlpool is the final method of cryotherapy. Like warm-water whirlpools, cold whirlpools are stainless steel tubs filled with water that is circulated with a pump. The water temperature for a cold whirlpool is not as cold as an ice pack or an ice bath. Because the water is constantly swirling around the body part, it is very effective at removing heat and cooling the body part. Cold whirlpools can also be combined with exercise of the injured part. While the part is cooling in the water, it can be moved to preserve motion.

Electrotherapy

Electrical currents are used by many different practitioners to treat a variety of conditions. As long as electrical currents have been used for therapy, DCs have used them.[1] Electrical currents can be applied in a chiropractic clinic, or patients may use small portable devices to apply currents outside of the clinic. Electrical currents are applied through electrodes placed on the skin and are used for a variety of symptoms, such as pain, muscle spasm, and muscle weakness, and to promote healing.

Interferential current is one of the most common electrical currents used by DCs, usually applied to impart pain relief, though less commonly to strengthen muscles. Interferential current is named for the way in which the electrical current is formed. Two separate electrical currents interfere with each other, creating a distinct third therapeutic current. The interference of currents can happen within the patient by applying the two separate currents directly to the skin, or it can happen in the current-generating device before being applied to the patient. The current is typically applied over the area of pain, creating a light tingling sensation or a low-frequency tingling with possible light involuntary muscle contractions. Usually, when applied for moderating acute pain, a light tingling sensation is produced. When applied for chronic pain, the electrical current frequency is lower and may cause minor muscle twitching. These electrical currents interact with nerves in the body and create pain relief through natural neurological mechanisms.

TENS stands for transcutaneous electrical nerve stimulation. The electrical current of TENS is applied in pulses for the treatment of acute and chronic pain.[6] The current is applied over the area of pain either in the chiropractic clinic or at home using portable devices called TENS units. The current can be pulsed at a slow or fast rate just like with interferential current. Similar to interferential current, patients receiving TENS therapy may notice a light tingling and/or small muscle twitches in the area being treated.

NMES stands for neuro-muscular electrical stimulation, which is an electrical current applied to specifically targeted muscles to cause strong contractions. NMES therapies are sometimes applied to help strengthen weak muscles or to cause fatigue, thus reducing muscle spasm.[7] NMES is primarily used to retrain or reeducate muscles that have become weak due to disuse. An example might be muscle weakness following limb immobilization from casting a broken bone. Two types of currents are commonly used for NMES: Russian current and biphasic current. Interferential current can also be used for muscle strengthening but is not commonly used for this purpose.[8] Both Russian and biphasic current are applied to a muscle or muscles with the intent of causing a muscle contraction strong enough to exercise the muscle. Consequently, NMES treatments can be uncomfortable.

High-voltage current or high-volt pulsed current is an electrical current that aids in the healing of tissue and helps to decrease swelling.[9] When the skin is injured, a small electrical voltage can be measured between the site of injury and the normal skin next to the injury. This electrical signal is thought to stimulate cellular repair and the migration of healthy cells to the injured area. The specific cells that migrate to injured areas are called neutrophils and macrophages, which are attracted to positively charged current. These cells act as early responders and initiate healing early in the healing process.

High-voltage current is used to increase the voltage difference between the wound and the healthy skin in an attempt to speed healing. Epidermal cells and fibrocytes are attracted to negatively charged current and are active in later stages of healing as they form scar tissue and new skin. In addition to attracting cells for healing, negative charges repel negatively charged ions in body tissues, which cause water to move with them, thus reducing swelling.

High-voltage current has a very high peak voltage (150 volts or higher), but the electrical pulses are delivered so quickly that the total amount of current is low, which makes the current comfortable despite the high voltage. Patients typically notice a tingling sensation with this current. One advantage to using high-voltage current is its ability to penetrate more deeply into tissue than other electrical currents. Common complaints that are treated with high-voltage current are pressure sores, skin lacerations and abrasions, and swelling from acute injuries, such as sprains.

Microcurrent electrical stimulation is also used to promote healing of injured skin. Microcurrent is applied at such low amplitude that patients don't feel anything. It works in much the same way as high-voltage current by increasing the voltage difference between injured tissue and the surrounding healthy tissue. Treatment time with microcurrent can last up to two hours and can be applied two to four times per day.

Mechanical Energy

Mechanical energy is a category of therapy in which forces are applied to tissues. This can be in the form of stretching tissue, massaging, and vibration. These therapies use mechanical energy rather than electrical, thermal, or some other form of energy.

Traction is used by many types of practitioners, including DCs. It is the pulling apart of body parts or joints and is commonly applied to the lumbar and cervical spine. Traction can be applied with mechanical traction tables or by hand. Traction increases the space between joints, especially in the spine, where disc space narrowing can lead to neurological symptoms. Traction can also increase joint motion and decrease muscle tension, muscle spasm, and pain.[10] Traction tables are commonly used to apply intermittent traction in which the traction force is alternately raised and lowered. Total treatment time usually lasts for 15 to 20 minutes. Typically, patients lie on their back with straps holding the pelvis and the upper back in order to traction the low back, or with straps holding the head for traction of the neck. Patients with disc herniations and protrusions are commonly treated with traction. A unique form of traction, called spinal decompression therapy, uses special motorized intermittent traction machines. These treatments can be very expensive and are advertised for a variety of back and neck complaints. The motorized traction tables have brand names such as VAX-D and DRX900. The research that is available on these devices does not make strong recommendations for their use and suggests that there may be lower-cost and equally effective forms of treatment available.[11,12]

Therapeutic massage is the act of rubbing (usually by hand) specific muscles, ligaments, and tendons of the body for the purpose of inducing pain relief, lowering muscle spasm, and promoting relaxation. There are a number of different massage methods used by DCs. Some of the common methods include effleurage, petrissage, tapotement, and cross friction. Effleurage involves the application of long massage strokes that run

Table 5.2 Summary of Common Electrotherapy Techniques

Therapeutic Technique	Definition	Application	Intended Effects
Interferential Current	Two or three separate electrical currents that are combined either within the patient's tissues or within the machine, creating a separate current within a targeted body region	○ Applied directly to the skin through electrode pads connected to a current-generating device	○ Block nerve signaling, thus reducing perceived pain ○ Muscle stimulation or strengthening
Microcurrent	Electrical stimulation using very weak or low amperage	○ Applied directly to the skin through electrode pads connected to a current-generating device	○ Facilitate wound healing
Neuromuscular Electrical Stimulation (NMES)	Electrical stimulation of nerves that cause muscles to contract	○ Applied directly to the skin through electrode pads connected to a current-generating device	○ Muscle strengthening ○ Reduce muscle spasticity
High-Voltage Pulsed Current	Monophasic pulsed electrical current delivered at high voltage (up to 500V), but for short durations (less than 200 microseconds)	○ Applied directly to the skin through electrode pads connected to a current-generating device	○ Facilitate wound healing ○ Reduce swelling
Transcutaneous Electrical Stimulation (TENS)	Direct stimulation of the skin using electrical current	○ Applied directly to the skin through electrode pads connected to a stationary or portable electrical current-generating device	○ Pain relief by blocking nerve signaling underneath the skin

parallel to the muscle fibers. The massage strokes can be applied using deep or light pressure. Petrissage is defined as kneading, grabbing, or pinching tissue, while tapotement involves rhythmically tapping or slapping the body part.

Vibration therapy is usually applied using a hand-held machine or device, but it can be applied manually by grabbing the muscle and shaking it back and forth. Vibration therapy is used to relax muscles, increase flexibility and joint motion, and cause overall sedation or relaxation.[13] Mechanical vibration devices usually include rounded plastic cups or flat padded surfaces that vibrate either up and down or side to side. Vibration is thought to increase blood circulation to muscles and decrease muscle tension. Vibration can be used simply to relax muscles or it can be combined with stretching to increase muscle length and range of motion.

Light Therapy

Cold laser or low-level light therapy is the use of laser-emitting diodes along with light-emitting diodes to alter cellular metabolism. Laser therapy is often called "cold laser" because the energy of such lasers is low and does not generate heat. The most correct terminology, however, is low-level laser therapy or LLLT. Light photons from low-level lasers penetrate several centimeters into body tissues and are absorbed by cells, causing either stimulation or inhibition of those cells. Research evidence suggests that it can be beneficial for the treatment of skin wounds, tendinopathies, myofascial pain, rheumatoid arthritis, neck pain, low back pain, jaw joint pain, and carpal tunnel syndrome.[14] Though the energy level is low in cold laser devices, eye damage can occur, so both the DC and the patient should wear eye protection. Low-level light therapy is not appropriate for treating conditions such as cancer or epilepsy; nor should it be applied over the abdomen and pelvis of pregnant women, areas of hemorrhage, or the thyroid gland.[14]

Myofascial Therapies

Fascia is the tissue toward which a majority of the myofascial therapies are oriented. Fascia is a continuous, whole-body connective tissue system that surrounds and penetrates organs, muscles, bones, and nerves. Once thought to perform only a single role in connecting organs and tissues, fascia is now understood to be a vital whole-body interconnecting system composed of connective tissue containing many important sensory

Table 5.3 Summary of Common Myofascial and Neurological Therapies

Therapy	Description	Why Used	Treatment Use Goals
Friction-Based Myofascial Therapies			
Friction Massage	Firmly and repeatedly rubbing over specific areas of the body (muscles, tendons, fascia) with the goal of generating friction underneath the rubbed area	Break fibrous adhesions formed between neighboring body tissues Temporarily increase blood flow Sensory nerve stimulation to help reduce pain and relax muscle tone	Improve joint motion Break adhesions between tissues
Instrument-Assisted Soft Tissue Mobilization (IASTM) (e.g., Graston Technique, FAKTR)	Friction applied with special (stainless steel or plastic) tools to augment what can be applied with hands alone		
Nonfriction-Based Myofascial Therapies			
Active Release Technique (ART), Myofascial Release, Pin-and-Stretch Technique, and Soft Tissue Manipulation or Mobilization	Pressure to muscle or muscle-related tissues, usually combined with stretching and movement of nearby joints	Break fibrous adhesions that restrict movement or cause movements to be painful Stretch contracted tissue(s) Stimulate or improve lymphatic circulation	
Trigger Point Therapy, Nimmo Technique, Receptor Tonus Technique, Ischemic Compression	Short-term pressure applied to abnormally tight regions of muscle	Break a self-perpetuating reflex causing a region of a muscle to stay abnormally tight Increase circulation to help remove inflammation or waste products causing irritation to the muscle region	Reduce or stop pain originating from muscles

102

Proprioceptive Neuromuscular Facilitation (PNF)	Neurologically based treatment techniques focused on developing, improving, or rehabilitating areas needing increased muscular strength, endurance, and coordination	Influence nerves controlling muscle activity, thus altering muscle function	Improve joint stability Improve muscle control and strength Prevent injury
Neural Mobilization (Nerve Flossing)	Carefully controlled movement of the head, neck, spine, or one or more limbs while the patient remains relaxed, causing repetitive nerve stretching (or flossing) through constricted areas	Improve impaired nerve mobility and function by reducing abnormal tension, disrupting adhesions, and by improving blood and lymphatic flow	Improve function by reducing compression and fibrous entrapment of nerves
Acupuncture	Inserting very fine-gauge needles, electrical current, or manual pressure into or over the skin at certain points of the body	Traditionally thought to balance internal movement of energy or information within the body Stimulates sensory cells and anti-inflammatory activity May lead to pain reduction	Balance internal bodily functions Reduce inflammation Reduce pain Stimulate immune function

cells.[15,16] Fascia can play an important role in many disease processes by influencing the function of tissue with which it connects.

Myofascial therapies are applied to soft tissues around the spine and many other areas of the body, such as the shoulders, hips, upper and lower extremities, and the jaw area. These therapies may be used as stand-alone treatments or in combination with other procedures depending on the individual's condition and the goals of care.

Several friction-based myofascial therapies have been derived from a form of deep friction massage performed by firmly and repeatedly rubbing over specific areas of the body (muscles, tendons, fascia). The goal of these therapies is to generate friction underneath the rubbed area, which contributes to three suspected, though not fully understood, effects. First, the deep pressure and movement of the practitioner's hand is thought to disrupt adhesions formed between neighboring tissues (e.g., between muscles and nearby structures, such as other muscles and tendons) following injury, from disuse, or from other conditions, such as acute tendinitis or chronic tendinopathy.

Friction-based treatments also increase short-term blood flow, a phenomenon that is thought to promote recovery. Lastly, friction and pressure stimulate sensory nerves located within the skin and underlying tissues. Stimulation of special sensory nerves generates nerve impulses that can contribute to reducing perceived pain and altering muscle tone.

Friction-based treatments are performed manually, often with the aid of a cream or emollient primarily used to reduce skin irritation caused by rubbing and deep pressure. Some emollients contain additional ingredients, such as menthol to produce a skin-cooling sensation. Menthol also

---

Sidebar 5.1

SCAR TISSUE AND FIBROUS ADHESIONS

Scar tissue and fibrous adhesions can reduce the available motion between tissues and may cause pain by placing tension on structures that should otherwise be more freely moveable. For example, following injury or when a tendon becomes inflamed from overuse, a natural response to control pain is to reduce movement or use of that muscle or joint area. Reducing motion is often necessary to prevent further injury and allow recovery. However, reduced movement promotes the formation of fibrous adhesions in joints (similar to scar tissue).[17]

functions as a counterirritant, defined as a substance that reduces perceived pain by causing a separate and nonpainful sensation.

Several techniques used by DCs and other health care providers apply friction-based techniques with special tools designed to augment what could be applied with hands alone. These instrument-assisted techniques are called instrument-assisted soft tissue mobilization or IASTM. These techniques use handheld tools, usually made of stainless steel, specially shaped to facilitate treatment of many different body regions. A few organizations offer advanced training and certification in the use of their treatment protocols, such as Graston technique and FAKTR.

Although several case reports documenting the effectiveness of these friction-based techniques for individual or small groups of patients are published in the scientific literature, little experimental research has been performed. Therefore, the effectiveness and safety of these techniques is not yet thoroughly understood. Because friction-based therapies are designed to stretch internal tissues and break adhesions, they are not appropriate in some situations. All friction-based therapies are designed to cause minor tissue damage, which in turn initiates a natural healing response characterized by minor inflammation, possible minor bruising, and local discomfort. Because of these effects, it is important for the provider to have a thorough understanding of the overall health status of the patient, the condition being treated, and the appropriate pressure and duration of treatment to avoid unnecessary or unwanted side effects, including injury.

Like friction-based treatment, nonfriction-based myofascial therapies often focus on improving movement of joints and relieving symptoms caused by adhesions formed between muscles, ligaments, tendons, and fascia. Unlike friction-based therapies, nonfriction techniques use manual pressure combined with stretching or specific movements. Some techniques are passive; that is, they are performed without any movement initiated or controlled by the patient. Active techniques involve patients moving or contracting muscles while the practitioner applies direct pressure to a specific body region.

Nonfriction-based myofascial techniques are not rigidly defined, thus several subtypes exist with overlapping procedures and names. Some commonly used technique names include Active Release Technique or ART, myofascial release, myofascial release therapy, myofascial release technique, soft tissue manipulation/mobilization, and pin-and-stretch technique. As with some friction-based therapies, several organizations provide training and offer certifications for qualified practitioners.

Clinical research measuring the effectiveness of myofascial release therapy has demonstrated that it can be effective for some conditions, such as lateral epicondylitis (tennis elbow) and plantar fasciitis (a painful condition affecting the bottom of the foot). Additional research is needed to clarify where myofascial therapies are most effective and how they compare with other available treatments.

Other nonfriction-based myofascial techniques focus primarily on relaxing abnormally tight areas within a muscle, called "trigger points." Trigger points are tender when pressure is applied, sometimes painful, and can refer pain to remote areas. For example, trigger points in the neck region can refer painful sensations to the head, causing a pain pattern similar to that experienced by individuals suffering from tension-type headaches.[18]

Myofascial techniques designed to treat trigger points use manually applied pressure for short durations (usually several seconds). Short-term pressure applied knowledgably with trained and skilled hands is thought to help break a self-perpetuating reflex causing that region of a muscle to stay abnormally tight. Increased circulation following pressure removal may also help remove inflammation or waste products causing irritation to that region of the muscle. Common techniques focused on manually treating trigger points include Nimmo Technique, Receptor Tonus Technique, trigger point therapy, and ischemic compression.

Proprioceptive Neuromuscular Facilitation

Proprioceptive neuromuscular facilitation (PNF) is a group of neurologically based treatment techniques focused on developing, improving, or rehabilitating areas needing increased muscular strength, endurance, mobility, control, and coordination. PNF techniques recognize that muscles, in large part, simply function based on input they receive from nerve signals. PNF training and treatment procedures are primarily designed to influence the signaling patterns of nerves controlling muscle activity, thus altering muscle function.

A concept example of a PNF treatment could be represented by a soccer player experiencing a tight muscle in the front of the thigh. Taking advantage of a neurological phenomenon, excessive muscular tightness can theoretically be relieved by contracting a muscle that performs the opposite motion. In this example, a PNF treatment might be designed to capitalize on a process called reciprocal inhibition, which reduces (or inhibits) a muscle's ability to contract when another muscle performing the opposite task is active. In the case of the soccer player, because the several muscles in the front of the thigh work to straighten the knee, an appropriately positioned exercise that generates muscular effort to bend the knee might help relieve some tightness.

Sidebar 5.2

RECIPROCAL INHIBITION

Reciprocal inhibition is one of many simultaneously occurring processes influencing muscle function, making many PNF treatments more complicated than the example presented here.[19]

Most PNF therapies use specific stretches to accomplish the goals of balancing muscle tension and improving range of motion. However, some techniques are designed to improve muscle coordination, with goals of improving the stability and function of spinal, hip, shoulder, and other body joints. Coordinated muscle activity plays a dual role of producing controlled movement and preventing joint injury.

The concept of improving or maintaining joint stability is used by DCs and others who treat athletes focused on improving function and preventing, or recovering from, some injuries. PNF treatments are also used for patients recovering from illness resulting in poor joint stability.

There is a limited amount of clinical research showing the effectiveness of PNF therapies, perhaps due in part to the challenges with systematically studying a large set of available procedures variably applied toward individuals with a wide variety of conditions. Nevertheless, a few clinical studies have demonstrated that some PNF therapies can be effectively applied for patients with spine-related pain and those suffering from other conditions, such as reduced balancing ability experienced by some patients following a stroke.

Neural Mobilization

Nerves and the spinal cord stretch and bend as body parts move. However, nerve compression and fibrous adhesions from scar tissue can cause pain and impair nerve function by restricting the normal movement and stretching of nerves and/or the spinal cord. Understanding how nerves function when compressed, overstretched, or subject to inflammatory chemicals can sometimes help identify a diagnosis. Such is the case with an ailment called "sciatica," a painful condition causing symptoms in the back of the thigh and leg. By performing several examination tests designed to stretch or compress nerve components, a diagnosis can be confirmed or dismissed based on the symptoms produced (or not produced).

The concept of nerve movement and how such mobility relates to nerve function is also used to treat patients suffering from a variety of conditions. Neural mobilization treatments are employed under the working hypothesis that improving impaired nerve mobility helps restore nerve function. Improvement is thought to occur by reducing compression, abnormal tension, and adhesions, and by improving blood and lymphatic flow both in and around nerves. As with other therapies described in this chapter, neural mobilization is used by DCs, physical therapists, and other health care providers. A less formal, but perhaps more descriptive, term sometimes used to describe neural mobilization is "nerve flossing."

Neural mobilization therapies involve slow movements of the head, neck, spine, or one or more limbs guided by a provider while the patient remains relaxed. Some procedures can be employed as exercises patients perform on their own. The exercises often feel like slow, gentle stretches usually performed within the pain-free range of motion available to the patient in that area. These characteristics mean that neural mobilization therapies are applied individually to patients with many different conditions, making it challenging to systematically study their effectiveness in clinical trials. Nevertheless, some clinical studies have demonstrated beneficial effects of a few neural mobilization therapies. More research is needed to fully understand both the safety and effectiveness of the many treatments available.

Supports and Braces

DCs use a variety of supports and braces to help patients recover from joint injuries, reduce pain, and prevent injury or the worsening of a condition. The need for specialized supports is highly dependent on an individual's condition and activities. Because most joint supports are designed to limit movement, they are often recommended only when an alternative treatment is unavailable.

Like conventional braces, therapeutic tape is also used to support joints and other tissues. Taping typically allows more movement of the affected body part, while sacrificing some support when compared with bracing.

Kinesiology tape is a special kind of athletic tape manufactured by several companies under various names (e.g., Kinesio Tape, Kinesio Tex Tape, KT Tape, Rock Tape, SpiderTech, and TheraBand). Kinesiology tape is a breathable tape with an elastic component, usually containing a combination of cotton and synthetic fabrics. The characteristics of elasticity, breathability, and a strong adhesive allows kinesiology tape to be worn for several days before removal. The main proposed effects of kinesiology tape are (1) an increased awareness of the body region to which the tape is applied, (2) improved blood and lymphatic fluid flow beneath the skin, (3) supported contraction of weakened or overstretched muscles, (4) improved stability, without restricting normal motion, as an injury preventative, and (5) reduction of pain by stimulating the skin and acting as a mild support. Recent research has confirmed connective tissue deformation caused by kinesiology tape application. This suggests the proposed mechanisms may be responsible for some of the therapeutic effects. However, the actual mechanisms are likely far more complex.

Acupuncture

Acupuncture has been used as a therapeutic method for several thousand years, originating in China. It is considered either traditional or alternative medicine in different parts of the world. The name is derived from the Latin word *acus* for "needle," followed by the word "puncture." Acupuncture usually involves inserting very fine-gauge needles into the skin over certain points, which are thought to lie along important lines or meridians of the body.

Inserting acupuncture needles in specific patterns is traditionally thought to help balance processes within the body by affecting internal interactions and the movement of energy and/or information, which contributes to pain relief and helps restore function to diseased areas.

In part because of its long history and apparent effectiveness, numerous theories and modes of practicing acupuncture exist. Some acupuncture techniques use a small electrical current instead of needles, while others use manual pressure (acupressure) to stimulate the skin over acupuncture points. Some acupuncture techniques burn a very small amount of a substance formed from the leaves of an Asian plant called moxa near the skin over acupuncture points. This process, called moxibustion, may be therapeutic by acting as a counterirritant, relieving pain by causing a separate and nonpainful sensation.

To date, scientific study has provided a very limited understanding of how acupuncture contributes to healing. Several clinical studies have shown that different acupuncture treatments produce similar effects. These confusing findings might suggest that a key to the therapeutic effects reported from acupuncture treatment may be the penetration and stimulation of sensory cells in the fascia, the connective tissue system that links and permeates the entire body. Other recent research has established that the beneficial effects of needle acupuncture may be caused by stimulating several anti-inflammatory chemical pathways and cell receptors, leading to pain reduction and other immune system changes.[20]

Therapeutic Exercise for Treatment, Rehabilitation, and Prevention

"Therapeutic exercise" is a broad term with many components. The purpose of performing an exercise determines how frequently it should be performed, to what intensity, and for what duration. Exercises prescribed to strengthen weak muscles will differ from those focused on loosening joints, maintaining mobility, or improving the stability of a region. Therapeutic exercises performed for treatment, prevention, and rehabilitation purposes are used by many professions. For example, physical and occupational therapists commonly include therapeutic exercises as part of their care plans. DCs often prescribe exercises designed to support spinal function and stability. However, many other exercises are used depending on the condition and goals of care. Though exercise is only one part of the broader field of rehabilitation, it plays a relatively prominent role. In addition to the comprehensive and rigorous clinical education completed by all DCs, some take advantage of advanced training programs focused on rehabilitation, including graduate degrees and residency programs.

There is much evidence demonstrating that exercise in general results in numerous health benefits. Other evidence indicates some exercises can be equally or more effective than more traditional medical treatments for some conditions. Because the chiropractic profession is focused on non-surgical, nonpharmacological treatment and prevention of disease, especially of the spine, it is natural to see practitioners commonly using exercise to aid treatment intended for both symptom reduction and for prevention.

Properly prescribed and performed therapeutic exercise can supplement treatment provided during the in-office encounter with a practitioner. Simply performing therapeutic exercises may also play a dual role in healing. Patients may receive benefit both from the exercise itself and from being actively engaged in their own rehabilitation. Performing therapeutic exercises enables patients to actively contribute to their own recovery and manage symptoms. Many DCs encourage patients to play active roles in part by incorporating therapeutic exercise under a framework of team-based care.

Orthotics

"Orthotics" refers to the use of artificial devices as support, such as the use of braces and splints. Like many other health care professional groups, DCs may prescribe orthotics (or orthoses) for a wide variety of joint, muscle, and neurological conditions. Typically, the chiropractic scope of practice limits the treatment of ligament tears, fractured bones, and dislocated joints, meaning rigid braces or casts are rarely prescribed. However, a variety of less restrictive orthoses may be used for conditions involving the spine or upper and lower extremities.

Foot orthotics are commonly prescribed by DCs to treat foot conditions or as a supplemental treatment for lower extremity or spinal conditions. DCs often prescribe custom-made, removable insoles molded from the patient's foot using a laser scan or materials such as a foam or plaster cast.

Common foot conditions treated with orthotics may include high arches, plantar fasciitis (pain in the heel or bottom of the foot), and hallux valgus (when the base of the big toe protrudes toward the opposite foot). There is a relatively small amount of research examining the effectiveness of orthotics for these conditions. However, the research that is available suggests that orthotics can be effective in some instances.

The available research evidence suggests that orthotics alone are not particularly effective at preventing low back pain. However, a small amount of evidence suggests that some patients with low back pain may respond well to treatment with only foot orthotics.[21] In chiropractic practice, orthotics are not customarily used alone to treat low back pain. Instead, they are more commonly used to supplement other treatment(s) oriented toward the condition(s) causing the low back pain.

Nutrition and Lifestyle

Chiropractic is based, in part, on the idea that health is largely a natural process given properly functioning nervous and skeletal systems and adequate environmental and nutritional requirements. Therefore, DCs often address nutritional and other lifestyle elements as they relate to health maintenance and recovery goals.

Students in accredited chiropractic educational programs receive training through various courses in fundamental and clinical nutrition. Additional nutritional training can be obtained through a number of postgraduate continuing education and specialty certification programs.

Over 95 percent of DCs reported using some form of nutritional or dietary recommendations with patients in a national survey conducted in 2014. Recommendations for self-care strategies, exercises to promote fitness, stress reduction/relaxation advice, advice on changing risky or unhealthy behaviors, smoking cessation advice, and disease prevention screening are also commonly performed by DCs. The same national survey described above reported that DCs assess lifestyle components and render advice or recommendations several times per day as part of usual patient care practices.[3]

Collaboration

In most practice settings, DCs function as portal-of-entry health care practitioners, meaning patients have direct access without the need for a referral from another health care provider. Portal-of-entry status combined with privileges to order diagnostic tests and extensive clinical training creates opportunity for DCs to evaluate and monitor many health conditions not usually managed (at least primarily) with chiropractic care. For example, high blood pressure, or hypertension, is not commonly treated with chiropractic care. However, because chiropractic care often involves a sequence of treatments over a period of several weeks, serial blood pressure monitoring can readily be included in visits to measure the success of current medication management. When successful management is not achieved, follow-up recommendations can be provided.

DCs can play an important public health role by serving as an information resource and by recommending specific health care options for patients with conditions requiring management or comanagement with other health care specialties. DCs also have the capacity to function within collaborative care teams and to effectively communicate a patient's symptoms, examination findings, suspected diagnoses, and reasons for referral with other health care providers using a common "language" (medical terminology).

DCs can also play an important role in reinforcing care recommendations from other providers who are cotreating patients for separate conditions or when functioning within care teams. For example, DCs can support tobacco cessation efforts through education (e.g., helping patients understand the adverse effects of tobacco products on health), by reinforcing the education and care recommendations of another managing provider, through offering dietary and lifestyle advice and by affording the patient encouragement and support.

References

1. Ransom JF. The origins of chiropractic physiological therapeutics: Howard, Forester and Schulze. *Chiropr Hist.* 1984;4:47–52.

2. Cetin N, Aytar A, Atalay A, Akman MN. Comparing hot pack, short-wave diathermy, ultrasound, and TENS on isokinetic strength, pain, and functional status of women with osteoarthritic knees: a single-blind, randomized, controlled trial. *Am J Phys Med Rehabil.* 2008;87:443–451.

3. National Board of Chiropractic Examiners. *Practice Analysis of Chiropractic 2015.* Greeley, CO: National Board of Chiropractic Examiners; 2015.

4. Belanger A. *Therapeutic Electrophysical Agents: Evidence behind Practice*. 3rd ed. Baltimore, MD, Philadelphia, PA: Wolters Kluwer, Lippincott Williams & Wilkins; 2015.

5. Denegar CR, Saliba E, Saliba S. *Therapeutic Modalities for Musculoskeletal Injuries (Athletic Training Education)*. 2nd ed. Champaign, IL: Human Kinetics; 2005.

6. Johnson M, Martinson M. Efficacy of electrical nerve stimulation for chronic musculoskeletal pain: a meta-analysis of randomized controlled trials. *Pain*. 2007;130:157–165.

7. Herrero AJ, Martin J, Martin T, Abadia O, Fernandez B, Garcia-Lopez D. Short-term effect of strength training with and without superimposed electrical stimulation on muscle strength and anaerobic performance. a randomized controlled trial. Part I. *J Strength Cond Res*. 2010;24:1609–1615.

8. Kajbafzadeh AM, Sharifi-Rad L, Baradaran N, Nejat F. Effect of pelvic floor interferential electrostimulation on urodynamic parameters and incontinency of children with myelomeningocele and detrusor overactivity. *Urology*. 2009;74:324–329.

9. Houghton PE, Campbell KE, Fraser CH, et al. Electrical stimulation therapy increases rate of healing of pressure ulcers in community-dwelling people with spinal cord injury. *Arch Phys Med Rehabil*. 2010;91:669–678.

10. Beattie PF, Nelson RM, Michener LA, Cammarata J, Donley J. Outcomes after a prone lumbar traction protocol for patients with activity-limiting low back pain: a prospective case series study. *Arch Phys Med Rehabil*. 2008; 89:269–274.

11. Macario A, Pergolizzi JV. Systematic literature review of spinal decompression via motorized traction for chronic discogenic low back pain. *Pain Pract*. 2006;6:171–178.

12. Daniel DM. Non-surgical spinal decompression therapy: does the scientific literature support efficacy claims made in the advertising media? *Chiropr Osteopat*. 2007;15:7.

13. Rabini A, De SA, Marzetti E, et al. Effects of focal muscle vibration on physical functioning in patients with knee osteoarthritis: a randomized controlled trial. *Eur J Phys Rehabil Med*. 2015;51:513–520.

14. Schindl A, Schindl M, Pernerstorfer-Schon H, Schindl L. Low-intensity laser therapy: a review. *J Investig Med*. 2000;48:312–326.

15. Schleip R. Fascial plasticity—a new neurobiological explanation. Part 1. *J Bodyw Mov Ther*. 2003;7:11–19.

16. Schleip R. Fascial plasticity—a new neurobiological explanation. Part 2. *J Bodyw Mov Ther*. 2003;7:104–116.

17. Cramer GD, Henderson CN, Little JW, Daley C, Grieve TJ. Zygapophyseal joint adhesions after induced hypomobility. *J Manipulative Physiol Ther*. 2010; 33:508–518.

18. Fernandez-de-Las-Penas C, Ge HY, Alonso-Blanco C, Gonzalez-Iglesias J, Arendt-Nielsen L. Referred pain areas of active myofascial trigger points in head,

neck, and shoulder muscles, in chronic tension type headache. *J Bodyw Mov Ther.* 2010;14:391–396.

19. Sharman MJ, Cresswell AG, Riek S. Proprioceptive neuromuscular facilitation stretching: mechanisms and clinical implications. *Sports Med.* 2006; 36:929–939.

20. McDonald JL, Cripps AW, Smith PK. Mediators, receptors, and signalling pathways in the anti-inflammatory and antihyperalgesic effects of acupuncture. *Evid Based Complement Alternat Med.* 2015;975632. 2015;2015:975632. doi: 10.1155/2015/975632. Epub 2015 Aug 3.

21. Chuter V, Spink M, Searle A, Ho A. The effectiveness of shoe insoles for the prevention and treatment of low back pain: a systematic review and meta-analysis of randomised controlled trials. *BMC Musculoskelet Disord.* 2014;15:140.

CHAPTER SIX

Safety of Chiropractic Practice

William J. Lauretti, DC

As it is for all health professionals, the safety and welfare of their patients is the top priority for doctors of chiropractic. There is currently good evidence indicating that chiropractic care is a safe and effective treatment option for many common musculoskeletal conditions, such as back pain, neck pain, and some types of headaches.

Doctors of chiropractic (DCs)—often referred to as "chiropractors" or "chiropractic physicians"—are highly trained health care professionals who focus on caring for disorders of the musculoskeletal and nervous systems. Traditionally, chiropractic treatment philosophy has focused on providing conservative care, highlighting hands-on treatments rather than medications and surgery. By limiting their treatments to noninvasive methods, DCs consistently enjoy some of the lowest malpractice insurance rates of any health care provider group.

Despite this track record, there continues to be some controversy surrounding the safety of chiropractic treatments. One reason for this is that there continues to be widespread misunderstanding about what exactly chiropractors do, even though the chiropractic profession has made great strides in gaining credibility and acceptance in recent years.

One of the most misunderstood aspects of chiropractic treatment is the safety and efficacy of the traditional *chiropractic adjustment*. The treatment that is often considered the signature therapy of doctors of chiropractic is a hands-on style of *spinal manipulation* using a high-velocity, low-amplitude

(HVLA) force. In these manipulations, the doctor typically applies a very quick (high-velocity) but very shallow (low-amplitude) movement to a patient's abnormally stiff joints to restore normal, pain-free motion.

It requires extensive training and practice to acquire the proficiency to apply these manipulations in a safe and effective manner. Most other health care professions have little or no training in the skills required and have little knowledge about the evidence supporting their use. As is often the case, ignorance can lead to misplaced fear and suspicion, and the high-velocity manipulation techniques used by many chiropractors are sometimes the focus of safety concerns from others.

While there is significant evidence supporting the safety and efficacy of these HVLA manipulations for a variety of conditions, they may not be appropriate for all patients. In consideration of this fact, most contemporary DCs also have training and experience in a variety of other techniques. In some cases, chiropractors may perform low-force *mobilizations* that slowly move joints in an oscillating manner. Other techniques may use a precision instrument (usually either spring loaded or electromechanically driven) to move joints with high speed and minimal force in a particular direction. Still other techniques may use forms of soft tissue massage, therapeutic stretches, or other exercise protocols. In addition, DCs may also use electric modalities, such as electrical muscle stimulation and therapeutic ultrasound, and physical modalities, such as heat and cold. The point is that most modern doctors of chiropractic have a range of therapeutic methods to apply to their patients and the training necessary to judge the safest and most effective treatment protocol for a wide variety of patients with a wide range of health conditions.

This chapter will address the issue of chiropractic safety and explore the evidence that indicates that most common chiropractic treatments are safe and effective options for a wide range of health problems. It will also compare the safety and effectiveness of other common treatments for similar conditions. In addition, it will explore several continuing controversies regarding the safety of chiropractic treatments in certain populations. Finally, it will discuss the public protections that are in place to ensure patient safety in practice.

Chiropractic Education: Diagnosis

The key to providing patients with safe and effective treatment is an accurate diagnosis. Contemporary chiropractic education includes extensive training in diagnosis, including physical examination skills, ordering and reading diagnostic imaging, and interpreting laboratory tests. However, one of the most important components of reaching a correct diagnosis is skillful history taking. A doctor who is an accomplished listener and observer, and who knows the key questions to ask, can more efficiently reach a proper diagnosis and have confidence that the patient is receiving the most appropriate care.

As far as ensuring patient safety is concerned, there is a strong emphasis on recognizing "red flags" in a patient's clinical presentation. Red flags are findings that suggest a patient may have a potentially serious underlying health condition that might require further diagnostic evaluation before

Table 6.1   "Red Flags" for Patients Seeing a Doctor of Chiropractic

Sign or Symptom	Condition to Be Ruled Out
History of a significant trauma, such as a fall or auto accident	Possible traumatic fracture
History of osteoporosis, corticosteroid use, or endocrine disease; age >50	Possible pathological fracture
Recent unexplained weight loss or malaise, history of cancer or other serious disease	Possible pathological fracture or metastatic disease
Pain pattern not related to movements or activities; constant, progressive pain with no relief with rest; or severe pain during the night	Possible metastatic disease or referred pain from organ pathology
Severe or progressive weakness or numbness in the legs or arms, particularly if it extends past the knee or elbow	Possible disc herniation with true radiculopathy (nerve damage)
Neck pain that causes shooting pains into the arms or legs, or an extremely rigid neck when bending forward	Possible cervical disc herniation or meningitis
History of recent bacterial infection (e.g., urinary tract infection); intravenous drug use or immune suppression from steroid use, transplant or HIV infection; recent fever over 100° F	Possible spinal infection or meningitis
Constant headache or neck pain accompanied by numbness, weakness, dizziness, nausea, or vomiting	Possible evolving stroke or brain/spinal tumor
Headache or neck pain accompanied by confusion, visual disturbances, difficulties in speech or swallowing, or alteration in consciousness	Possible evolving stroke or brain/spinal tumor
Severe or constant and progressive headache, or a sudden onset of "the worst headache ever"	Possible evolving stroke or brain/spinal tumor

beginning treatment, or timely referral to another specialist for advanced care. Some common red flags that a practicing chiropractor might see in patients are summarized in Table 6.1. The presence of one of these red flags does not always indicate that chiropractic care should be avoided for that patient. In many cases, it only indicates that further diagnostic study is necessary to rule out a potentially more serious condition. If that more urgent condition is excluded, chiropractic care may be appropriate.

Screening for Contraindications

Once it has been determined that no red flags are present in the patient's history or examination, the practicing chiropractor then screens for *contraindications* to conservative care. A contraindication is a finding in the history or examination that serves as a reason to withhold or modify a particular type of treatment because it may be inappropriate or harmful for that patient.

In many cases, these contraindications may be similar in nature to the red flags, except that they usually suggest a less urgent referral is necessary. A patient with contraindications to commonly used chiropractic treatments may still be an appropriate patient for a chiropractor to treat if the treatment is modified to meet that patient's specific needs. For example, a patient who has an acutely sprained joint would have a contraindication to having high-velocity manipulation to that sprained joint, but it might be appropriate to perform soft tissue massage around that joint, or high-velocity manipulation might still be appropriate if it is performed on another body area.

Chiropractic Treatment

Once red flags and contraindications have been satisfactorily ruled out, the treating chiropractor will design a treatment plan specific to the patient's condition. The majority of patients seen by practicing chiropractors have painful spinal conditions that are usually accompanied by spinal joints that are stiff and not moving properly, a condition many chiropractors refer to as a "vertebral subluxation." High-velocity, low-amplitude spinal manipulation is often the treatment of choice for these conditions, along with other treatments to address any accompanying muscular dysfunctions. Depending on the treating chiropractor's experience and preferences, as well as the patient's particular condition and preferences, other less vigorous treatments may be used instead, such as low-velocity joint mobilization.

Table 6.2   Some Contraindications to High-Velocity Manipulation

Condition	Potential Complication	Method of Detection	Modifications Required
Severe Sprain, Lax Ligaments, Joint Instability, Suspected Fracture	Sprain, tear	History, observation, palpation, radiographic findings	No high-velocity manipulation; only low-velocity mobilization or soft tissue treatment in area of injury; possible referral for further diagnosis and/or immobilization
Suspected Tumor	Pathological fracture, undiagnosed pathology	History, radiographic findings, advanced imaging, findings of laboratory tests	Immediate referral for further diagnosis
Suspected Osteoporosis, Fragile Bones	Pathological fracture, undiagnosed fracture	Postmenopausal female, history of steroid therapy, nutritional deficiencies, radiographic findings	No high-velocity manipulation; only low-velocity mobilization or soft tissue treatment to involved area
Bony Fusion (Congenital or Acquired)	Fracture	History, radiographic findings	No high-velocity manipulation; only low-velocity mobilization or soft tissue treatment to involved area
Unstable Bleeding Disorder (Congenital or Acquired)	Risk of severe bruising, possible spinal hematoma	History, findings of laboratory tests, radiographic findings	No high-velocity manipulation; only low-velocity mobilization or gentle soft tissue treatment

Many studies have demonstrated positive results for chiropractic treatments. The majority of evidence-based clinical guidelines have consistently recommended the basic conservative treatment approach used by chiropractors—manipulation, mobilization, soft tissue massage, and exercises—as a primary treatment approach for conditions such as back pain, neck pain, and some types of headache.[1,2] *Chapters 7 and 8 provide more detailed information about chiropractic treatment of back pain, neck pain, and headache.* The effectiveness of manual therapies for nonmusculoskeletal conditions is more controversial, and the evidence of effectiveness for most of these conditions is still inconclusive.[1] *Chapter 11 discusses the evidence for chiropractic care for nonmusculoskeletal conditions.*

There have also been a fairly substantial number of studies that have investigated the safety of chiropractic treatments. However, designing a study that can systematically examine the frequency of complications following chiropractic treatments presents numerous major challenges. It is generally agreed that the frequency of serious adverse events after chiropractic treatment is very low. Therefore, a well-designed controlled study would probably need to include a very large number of subjects to be statistically valid, making it both very costly and logistically difficult to perform. Currently, the literature on complications following chiropractic treatment consists mainly of case reports. Many of these case reports suffer from significant methodological weaknesses, such as a lack of detail regarding the treatment applied and specifics about the patient's condition when seeking care.

Among the serious adverse events following a chiropractic treatment that have been reported in the literature are pathologic fracture, herniated disc, cauda equine syndrome, stroke, spinal fluid leak, and diaphragmatic palsy. These complications have been reported in the literature through isolated and sometimes poorly documented case reports. It is not clear whether these are spontaneous complications (as in the case of stroke or spinal fluid leak) or adverse events due to misdiagnosis or inappropriate care. These individual case reports are rare, and they cannot be used to estimate the frequency of serious adverse events following chiropractic treatment.

One study that systematically examined the occurrence of adverse events resulting from chiropractic treatment was conducted across 12 chiropractic clinics in Perth, Western Australia.[3] The study included 183 adults with spinal pain. Ninety-two participants received usual chiropractic treatment, as individualized by the treating DC. Ninety-one participants received a sham intervention. Thirty-three percent of the sham group and 42 percent of the usual care group reported at least one adverse event. Common adverse events included increased pain, muscle stiffness, and headache. The relative risk was not significant for any adverse event occurrence between the group receiving usual chiropractic care and the sham treatment group. No serious adverse events were reported in either group. The study concluded that a significant portion of adverse events reported after chiropractic treatment may result from natural history variation and nonspecific effects.

Good evidence indicates that chiropractic care is beneficial for patients with musculoskeletal pain, such as neck or low back pain, and the risks of serious adverse events are near negligible.[1,2] In contrast with the small risk of harm from chiropractic treatments for spinal pain, the other types of treatments commonly used for these conditions may have significant risks.

Risks versus Benefits: An Analysis of Common Treatments for Neck and Back Conditions

In clinical practice, doctors of chiropractic and medical physicians often treat musculoskeletal pain syndromes differently, based on differences in their education, clinical experience, and practice philosophies. Doctors of chiropractic tend to emphasize "hands-on" therapies, which may include various forms of manual manipulation or mobilization, soft tissue massage and stretching techniques, and various exercises and lifestyle advice. Many medical physicians tend to emphasize pharmaceutical treatments.

These differences in practice style and philosophies sometimes lead to tension between the medical and chiropractic professions. In addition, the chiropractic profession has long been labeled an "alternative" medical profession. Some view that label as a judgment on the evidence supporting a particular therapy, with the presumption that a "mainstream" therapy must have significant evidence, whereas an "alternative" therapy must be lacking in evidence. While that may be true in some cases, it is not always the case, and it's important to judge the efficacy of all therapies based on the actual evidence available and not prejudge them based solely on how they are labeled.

In recent years, the health care field has been moving toward promoting care that is more "evidence based," emphasizing care that has clear evidence of safety and effectiveness based on scientific studies. In keeping with the spirit of evidence-based medicine, a review of the scientific evidence of effectiveness and risks of various commonly used treatments for spinal pain follows.

Evidence Review

Simple Analgesics

Simple analgesics (pain relievers), such as acetaminophen (paracetamol), are commonly seen as being the safest and most conservative pharmaceutical treatment for neck and back pain. Despite the fact that it is generally perceived as safe, acetaminophen is the largest cause of drug overdoses in the United States. This is because of the narrow range between therapeutic dose and toxic dose. Before 2012, the recommended adult dose of Extra Strength Tylenol (500mg) was two tablets every four to six hours, totaling eight pills per day (4,000mg). However, the generally recognized adult toxic dose is considered above 4,000mg/day, or above 1,000mg per single dose. So the recommended dose was right at the toxic limit. Acetaminophen overdose can cause potentially fatal liver damage, and alcohol consumption significantly heightens the risk of overdose. The generally recognized toxic dose in adults who drink alcohol moderately or heavily is over 2,000mg/day. In rare individuals, even a normally recommended dose of acetaminophen can cause toxicity.

Beginning in 2012, the maximum recommended dose was reduced to six pills per day (3,000mg). However, overdose is still a problem because acetaminophen is part of many popular over-the-counter (OTC) drugs and prescription combination drugs (for example, prescription combination pain medications like Percocet, Panadol, and Vicodin, and OTC cold and cough remedies). Acetaminophen toxicity is the leading cause of acute liver failure in the Western world. One study found that acetaminophen overdose was responsible for 751,552 emergency department visits from 1993 to 2007.[4]

Because of its widely perceived safety (despite the evidence that it causes a large number of significant complications), acetaminophen has been recommended as a first-line therapy in virtually all clinical guidelines for treatment of low back pain published in the last 20 years. These recommendations were based on the widely recognized effectiveness of acetaminophen as a general pain reliever. However, few studies have specifically looked at acetaminophen's effectiveness as a treatment for back pain. One comprehensive review found that "paracetamol [acetaminophen] is ineffective in the treatment of low back pain and provides minimal short term benefit for people with osteoarthritis."[5] While this summary specifically looked at acetaminophen's effectiveness for back pain, even fewer have looked at effectiveness for neck pain.

Nonsteroidal Anti-Inflammatory Drugs

Another common first-line treatment for most musculoskeletal pain syndromes is nonsteroidal anti-inflammatory drugs (NSAIDs). This category of drug includes popular OTC medications, such as aspirin, ibuprofen, and naproxen, and prescription drugs, such as celecoxib, piroxicam, and indomethacin. These are among the most widely used pain medications and are generally considered safe, but they have significant risks of potentially serious adverse effects.

NSAID use has been associated with bleeding and ulcers in the stomach and intestine, stroke, heart disease, kidney failure, life-threatening allergic reactions, and liver failure. Gastrointestinal ulcers can lead to fatal complications, such as hemorrhage and perforation. One large study[6] estimated that at least 103,000 patients are hospitalized per year in the United States for serious gastrointestinal complications due to NSAID use. This study estimated that 16,500 NSAID-related deaths occur among patients with rheumatoid arthritis or osteoarthritis every year in the United States. This figure is similar to the annual number of deaths from AIDS and considerably greater than the annual deaths from multiple myeloma, asthma, cervical cancer, or Hodgkin's disease. If deaths from gastrointestinal toxic effects of NSAIDs were tabulated separately in the National Vital Statistics reports, these effects would constitute the 15th most common cause of death in the United States.

In 2015, the U.S. Food and Drug Administration issued new warnings on NSAID use that warned of an increased risk of heart attack and stroke even with short-term use. The risk may begin within a few weeks of starting to take an NSAID, and it increases with higher doses of NSAIDs taken for longer periods of time. The risk is greatest for people who already have heart disease, though even people without heart disease may be at risk.

NSAIDS are clearly valuable drugs and appear to be effective for their pain-relieving and anti-inflammatory properties. They are generally considered safe. However, it is also important to emphasize that there is no evidence that they are any more effective for long-term treatment of acute or chronic musculoskeletal pain than conservative chiropractic care.

Skeletal Muscle Relaxants

Skeletal muscle relaxant drugs, including benzodiazepines such as Diazepam (Valium), are often used for treatment of acute or subacute musculoskeletal pain. Side effects most commonly reported were drowsiness, fatigue, muscle weakness, and uncoordination. Less common side effects include confusion, depression, vertigo, constipation, blurred vision, and amnesia. One comprehensive review of the evidence for noninvasive treatments for low back pain found only a fair level of evidence that benzodiazepines provided moderate relief for patients with back pain.[7] Benzodiazepines also carry significant risks of abuse and addiction.

Opioid Pain Relievers

Opioid analgesics are narcotics that have a similar effect on the body as opium by binding to the same receptors in the brain. They are based on the drug morphine, the painkilling chemical extracted from the opium poppy plant. Prescription opioids include drugs such as codeine, fentanyl, hydrocodone, morphine, methadone, and oxycodone. Various brand names for opioid drugs include OxyContin, Demerol, Percocet, and Vicodin. Heroin is the illicit, highly potent derivative of morphine.

Opioid drugs have long been recognized for their useful pain-relieving properties in patients with severe pain. However, they have a significant risk of addiction and abuse, and until recently they were generally limited to short-term use and rarely used for long-term treatment of musculoskeletal pain. Recent trends have seen opioids used more often to manage spinal pain. One study of insurance records revealed that nearly one-half of patients with low back pain were using prescription narcotics.[8]

According to the U.S. Centers for Disease Control (CDC), the sales of opioids tripled in the first decade of the 21st century. In 2014, there were 259 million prescriptions for opioids, equivalent to one for every American adult. Up to 20 percent of patient visits to physicians result in a prescription for one of these opioid drugs. Overdoses of opioid painkillers are responsible for some 15,000 deaths per year, more than the number of deaths from cocaine and heroin combined.

In the United States, the number of prescriptions for opioid painkillers for low back pain has increased, and opioids are now the most commonly prescribed class of drug for back pain. This despite evidence that opioids do not improve functional outcomes of acute back pain patients or lead to injured workers returning to work sooner. For chronic back pain, systematic reviews find scant evidence of efficacy for opioids, and there is evidence that long-term opioid use serves to increase pain sensitivity. With the significant risk of addiction and abuse, there is increasing criticism of the appropriateness of long-term opioid use for chronic musculoskeletal pain. Serious questions are arising about the risk-to-benefit ratio of using these powerful and potentially dangerous drugs in treating musculoskeletal pain. The increasingly widespread use of opioids for treatment of musculoskeletal pain is contrary to most evidence-based clinical guidelines for treating these conditions and contributes to worsening trends in management of back pain.

Invasive Interventions

Management of painful spinal conditions that includes invasive interventions, such as surgery and injections, has been widely criticized as being ineffective, overly costly, and potentially risky. Rates of spinal surgeries vary widely across different industrialized countries and even across various regions in the United States. There seems to be no explanation for this wide variation except that areas with more practicing spine surgeons consistently have a much higher rate of spine surgeries per capita than areas with fewer surgeons.

Nearly all evidence-based clinical guidelines recommend spinal surgery in only a small minority of cases, and guidelines often outline clear and specific circumstances in which surgery should be considered. Yet despite increasing evidence supporting the use of conservative care and less surgery, rates of spine surgery have increased significantly in the United States over the last few decades, and there is little evidence that many common spine surgeries lead to consistently improved outcomes for patients. For example, one review found no evidence that surgical treatment was better than a conservative approach for lumbar spinal stenosis (narrowing of the boney canal that the spinal cord and nerves pass through).[9] This is troubling considering that this study found the rate of adverse effects ranged from 10 percent to 24 percent in surgical cases, and no adverse effects were reported for any conservative treatment. It is also troubling considering the economic costs of these surgeries. For example, in 2007, there were 37,598 operations for a primary diagnosis of lumbar stenosis that were paid by Medicare, with an aggregate hospital bill that was nearly $1.65 billion.[10]

Recent years have also seen a significant increase in spinal injections for back pain. One common procedure is epidural corticosteroid injections (injections of anti-inflammatory medications into the lining of the spinal cord). These are sometimes performed for spinal stenosis or lumbar radiculopathy (irritation of the spinal nerves that pass down into the legs). The increase in these procedures is again troubling considering the cost and lack of evidence of long-term effectiveness. One review article found the benefits of epidural steroid injections for radiculopathy were small and not lasting, and in the long term they did not decrease the chances of patients having spinal surgery. Based on limited evidence, the authors also found no evidence of effectiveness for spinal stenosis.[11]

There is evidence that patients who go to doctors of chiropractic as their first provider are less likely to end up having invasive procedures like surgery. One study of workers' compensation patients found that 42.7 percent of injured workers with an on-the-job back injury who saw a surgeon as their first provider ended up having surgery in contrast to only 1.5 percent of those who began care with a chiropractor.[12] Studies like this demonstrate that doctors of chiropractic have an important role to play in directing patients with spinal pain toward safe, effective, and

Table 6.3   **Risks and Benefits of Commonly Used Treatments for Neck and Back Conditions**

Treatment	Effectiveness	Risks
Manipulation, Mobilization	Likely helpful (Worth considering)	Common: Minor, temporary discomfort or soreness
		Very rare: Stroke (causal relationship not established)
Manual Therapy (Manipulation, Mobilization, and/or Massage) Together with Exercises	Likely helpful (Worth considering)	Common: Temporary discomfort or soreness, dizziness
NSAIDS	Not enough evidence to make determination	Occasional: GI bleeding, heart attack, stroke
		Rare: Kidney failure, life-threatening allergic reactions, liver failure
Acetaminophen	Not enough evidence to make determination	Rare: Liver failure from overdose
Skeletal Muscle Relaxant Drugs, Including Benzodiazepines	Not enough evidence to make determination	Common: Drowsiness, fatigue, and muscle weakness
		Occasional: Confusion, depression, vertigo, constipation, blurred vision
		Rare: Abuse, addiction, dependence, potentially fatal overdoses
Narcotic (Opioid) Pain Medications	Not enough evidence to make determination	Common: Drowsiness, fatigue, and muscle weakness
		Occasional: Confusion, depression, vertigo, constipation
		Rare: Abuse, addiction, dependence, seizures, potentially fatal injuries to the liver, potentially fatal overdoses

cost-efficient conservative care and away from expensive and potentially hazardous invasive procedures that have unproven benefit.

Conclusions

The current scientific evidence indicates that all commonly used treatments for neck and back pain have limited evidence of effectiveness. All treatments come with fairly common but mild side effects, and some have rare but potentially serious side effects. In general, the physical treatments (including manipulation, mobilization, massage, and exercise) have fairly good evidence of effectiveness and are very rarely associated with any serious complications. Pharmaceutical treatments, although commonly used, have limited evidence of effectiveness for treatment of neck and back pain and infrequent but potentially serious complications. Invasive procedures like injections and surgeries also have little evidence demonstrating their effectiveness but have a significant risk of serious complications.

Rationally, we should look at a cost-to-benefit ratio that would demand that any procedures that are more expensive and risky should be supported by a stronger level of evidence to justify their greater potential shortcomings. Ironically, the reality is that these more aggressive treatments tend to have considerably less evidence supporting their use compared to many conservative options.

Although the evidence supporting most commonly used chiropractic treatments for back pain is still evolving, considering everything, the evidence in their favor compares very well to other treatments for similar conditions as far as scientifically demonstrated efficacy and safety.

Controversies

Safety of Chiropractic Cervical Manipulation

The relationship between cervical spine manipulation and serious complications is highly controversial. Numerous case reports have associated cervical spine manipulation with a rare type of stroke that results from a *dissection* (tear) of the *vertebral artery (VA)*, a blood vessel in the neck. The best current evidence indicates that these dissections are likely due to an underlying abnormality of the vascular system that usually can't be identified in advance and are probably not directly caused by the manipulation. The likelihood of a person having one of these rare vertebral artery strokes is about 2.5 to 3 per 100,000 people and is similar among both chiropractic patients and the general population. Unfortunately, the only early sign of an evolving dissection is neck pain and headache, symptoms that may lead people to seek treatment from a doctor of chiropractic or other health professional.

The vertebral artery is a small artery that runs through the sides of the lower and midcervical vertebrae, loops around the two upper cervical vertebrae, and runs up into the base of the skull into the brain. Due to its unusually tortuous course in the upper neck, and its close proximity to the highly movable cervical vertebrae, it was long thought that the artery may be vulnerable to stresses applied when the neck is turned to the end range, as sometimes occurs during a cervical manipulation. Stress to the artery may cause a splitting (dissection) of the normally smooth inner lining of the artery. That injury can create turbulent blood flow around the dissection, which can lead to a blood clot forming. In many cases, the injury may heal and the patient will have no significant lasting effects. In other cases, pieces of the blood clot may break off and travel upward into the smaller blood vessels serving the base of the brain. If the traveling clot completely blocks off a smaller blood vessel, it won't allow blood to reach the brain tissue past the blockage, leading to an ischemic stroke—death of brain tissue from lack of blood flow.

Although cervical manipulation has been associated with VA dissection, several biomechanical studies have found that the strains experienced by the vertebral arteries during cervical manipulation are significantly smaller than the strains the arteries experience during many everyday activities, or during routine diagnostic and range-of-motion testing.[13] These strains are much smaller than the strains required to cause the arteries to be damaged.

An increasingly accepted opinion is that an otherwise normal VA probably cannot be damaged by the minimal forces applied to the neck during a competently applied cervical manipulation. In cases where a dissection occurred following neck motion, it is likely the VA had a preexisting weakness that caused failure of the arterial structure. This hypothesis is supported by the fact that vertebral artery dissections have been reported as occurring after minor motions to the neck that take place during everyday activities, such as swimming, star gazing, or talking on the telephone. Also, VA dissections are rare even in cases of devastating trauma to the neck, such as traumas that cause cervical spine fractures. That suggests that a normal VA is quite robust and should not be susceptible to significant injury from the minor forces applied during cervical spine manipulation.

Several likely risk factors have been identified that seem to increase the probability of a person having VA dissection. They include having a congenital connective tissue disorder, such as vascular Ehlers-Danlos syndrome, Marfan's syndrome, or osteogenesis imperfecta. A previous history of longstanding migraine headaches seems to increase the risk as well. Well-recognized risk factors for more common types of stroke (high blood pressure, smoking, use of birth control pills) seem to only mildly increase the risk of VA dissections.

Although rare, strokes from arterial dissections are the most common type of stroke among younger people (under age 45). Early signs and symptoms that young people should be aware of that may indicate an arterial dissection is occurring and may foreshadow the onset of a full stroke include the sudden onset of a severe headache unlike any previous one or sudden severe upper neck pain unlike any previous pain. These are especially serious if accompanied by any visual disturbances, dizziness, vomiting or weakness, or numbness in the face or in the arms or legs. In these circumstances, medical care should be sought out immediately.

Cases of vertebral artery dissections following chiropractic cervical manipulation are sometimes widely publicized, and some people have been left with the impression that this is a significant risk from chiropractic treatment. However, several large-scale epidemiological studies have shown no excess risk of stroke in people who have recently received chiropractic neck treatment compared with patients who have recently received care from a primary care medical physician.

One large study[14] looked at the medical records of 11 million people in the Canadian province of Ontario over a nine-year period and concluded that any observed association between a stroke and a patient's visit to either a chiropractic physician or a family physician was not directly caused by any treatment performed. Instead, any association was likely due to patients with an evolving VA dissection seeking care for symptoms such as neck pain or headache that sometimes take place before the stroke occurs.

Another more recent epidemiological study[15] looked at the medical records of nearly 39 million members of a large health insurance plan and found no significant association between chiropractic visits and vertebral artery stroke, although there was a significant association found between a visit to a primary care physician and this type of stroke. This study also concluded that this association was likely due to patients with early symptoms seeking care before the actual stroke occurs.

Nearly every chiropractor is well aware of the controversy concerning cervical manipulation and VA dissection. However, the vast majority of chiropractors will go through an entire career performing tens of thousands of cervical adjustments and treating thousands of patients without seeing a single case of VA stroke. One large study of malpractice claims in Canada[16] concluded that the likelihood a chiropractor will be made aware of an arterial dissection following cervical adjustment is approximately 1 in 8.06 million office visits, 1 in 5.85 million cervical manipulations, 1 in 1,430 chiropractic practice years, and 1 in 48 chiropractic practice careers.

As for the effectiveness of chiropractic care for neck pain (including manipulation and exercise), one recent study found it to be more effective in both the long and short term than pain medication and other medical treatments.[17]

One landmark comprehensive analysis was supported by the Neck Pain Task Force of the International Bone and Joint Decade, an international multidisciplinary organization.[18] This study found that mobilization, manipulation, and clinical massage are effective interventions for the management of neck pain. In contrast, the same review concluded that there was "not enough evidence to make a determination" about the helpfulness of NSAIDs, opioids, and other drugs for treatment of neck pain.

In conclusion, there is good epidemiological evidence that the odds of having a stroke following a visit to a doctor of chiropractic are no greater than the odds of having a stroke following a visit to a primary care doctor. In addition, there is biomechanical evidence that cervical manipulation stretches the vertebral arteries less than routine examination procedures, making it unlikely that a cervical manipulation can physically cause an arterial dissection.

There is evidence that a manual approach to neck pain, including manipulation, is at least as effective as a conventional pharmaceutical approach using NSAIDs and/or opiates, with no greater risk of complications.

Chiropractic Safety in Special Populations

Doctors of chiropractic often claim the ability to treat a wide variety of patient populations, including people of all ages and health status. In contrast, many health care professionals who have limited experience of chiropractic training and methods will sometimes warn patients they see as vulnerable away from chiropractic treatment. Among the populations that provoke the most misgivings are pregnant women, children (particularly below age 12), and the elderly.

Chiropractic during pregnancy

Although few controlled studies on chiropractic treatment for pregnancy have been performed, a literature review found virtually no reports of significant complications following chiropractic treatment in pregnant women.[19] More than one-half of pregnant women experience back pain during pregnancy. Treating this pain is difficult because common medical treatments for back pain (such as NSAIDs, analgesics, muscle relaxants, and opioids) are generally avoided during pregnancy for fear they may cause damage to the developing fetus. Radiographic imaging is also avoided during pregnancy for the same reason.

Since chiropractic treatment for back pain focuses on nonpharmacological conservative care, it appears to be a good option for treating back pain in pregnancy. There is also anecdotal evidence that chiropractic treatment during pregnancy may make labor easier and claims that one specialty chiropractic technique is purported to offer a conservative means to turn a breech presentation; however, these claims have not been well researched and remain highly controversial.

Chiropractic care during pregnancy often includes similar high-velocity manipulation as in other populations, although the manipulations are often done with extra care and somewhat more gently on pregnant women. Chiropractors may also use nonforce manipulation or low-velocity mobilization, soft tissue massage, and gentle stretches on pregnant women. The use of electrical modalities, such as electrical muscle stimulation and therapeutic ultrasound, are usually considered to be contraindicated anywhere near a pregnant woman's uterus. *Chapter 13 provides additional information on chiropractic care of pregnant women.*

Chiropractic for children

Children are perhaps the most controversial population commonly treated by chiropractors. Critics sometimes view chiropractic care for children, infants, and even newborns with alarm and seem to envision aggressively reckless manipulations being performed on fragile developing bones. However, chiropractors with experience caring for children will insist that their treatments are cautious and gentle and forces used are appropriate for the patient's age and condition.

While it has been estimated that over 30 million chiropractic treatments are given to children annually, there is no evidence of widespread injury resulting from these treatments. One review article[20] examined all reported cases of serious adverse events caused by practitioners who apply manual therapies (i.e., chiropractors, physical therapists, medical physicians, doctors of osteopathy, and other manual therapists) when caring for infants and children. After a comprehensive literature review, they found a total of 12 published articles in the worldwide English-language literature, reporting 15 serious adverse events. Three deaths were reported to have occurred under the care of various providers (no deaths were reported after care from a doctor of chiropractic), and 12 serious injuries were reported (seven following care from chiropractors).

Underlying preexisting pathology was identified in a majority of the cases, suggesting that many of the complications were not the direct result of the treatment provided but were due to an inappropriate diagnosis of the patient.

Although one can presume a large amount of underreporting (most cases of injury probably will not result in a published article), the paucity of case reports in such a controversial and emotionally charged topic suggests that significant injuries following chiropractic treatment of children are extremely rare.

Although direct injuries appear to be very unusual, for many critics the most troubling aspect of chiropractic care for children is the types of conditions pediatric chiropractors sometimes treat and the unsupported claims of efficacy they sometimes make. Even some respected chiropractic organizations claim chiropractic care is effective for childhood conditions such as ear infections, colic, enuresis (bed wetting), attention deficit hyperactivity disorders, and other conditions that have no obvious connection to the musculoskeletal system. These claims are made based on some anecdotal support but very little scientific evidence. The few controlled studies that have been performed on chiropractic care for these conditions have had either mildly positive, ambiguous, or negative results.[21] While it may be appropriate to offer apparently safe alternatives for conditions such as these that lack a definitively effective "conventional" treatment, it is understandable why chiropractors' sometimes fanatical claims of effectiveness in the absence of persuasive evidence can lead critics to view pediatric chiropractic with apprehension and even derision. It is likely that chiropractic care for children will remain a controversial subject until significantly more evidence is obtained regarding its safety and effectiveness for a variety of childhood health conditions. *Chapter 13 provides additional information on chiropractic care for children.*

Chiropractic for the older patient

Some critics also raise concerns with chiropractic treatment of older patients, again expressing apprehension that the high-velocity manipulations often performed by chiropractors may injure patients with frail skeletal structure or other comorbid conditions. However, elderly patients make up a significant portion of many chiropractic practices. Chiropractic coverage is popular under Medicare, the U.S. national health care insurance that primarily covers people over age 65. In 2006, chiropractic physicians provided 18.6 million clinical services under Medicare.

One observational, practice-based research project[22] collected data on 805 patients aged 55 years and older in 96 chiropractic practices in 32 states and 2 Canadian provinces during a 12-week study period. Patients were seen predominantly for pain-related complaints, most commonly back pain. For two-thirds of patients, the doctor of chiropractic was the only provider seen for the current complaint.

Another retrospective cohort study[23] compared the injury rates for Medicare beneficiaries treated by chiropractic spinal manipulation versus those evaluated by a primary care physician. It found that among Medicare beneficiaries aged 66 to 99 with an office visit risk for a neuromusculoskeletal problem, risk of injury to the head, neck, or trunk within seven days was 76 percent lower among subjects with a chiropractic office visit as compared to those who saw a primary care physician. The study concluded that it is unlikely that chiropractic care is a significant cause of injury in older adults.

When treating elderly patients, experienced chiropractors are especially careful to screen for relevant red flags and contraindications (especially osteoporosis and undiagnosed pathology) and will adapt treatment methods to be appropriate to the patient's physical condition and any special needs. *Chapter 13 provides additional information on chiropractic care for older adults.*

Informed Consent: What Patients Should Know

Like all health care professionals, doctors of chiropractic have an ethical and legal responsibility to obtain their patients' informed consent before beginning care. This is in keeping with the basic ethical values shared by all health professionals:

- respect for patients' wishes and their individual autonomy
- beneficence, the duty of the practitioner to act in the best interest of the patient
- nonmalfeasance, the obligation to do no harm
- justice, the responsibility to uphold existing laws and care for all parties involved with integrity

True informed consent is a process of communication between the doctor and patient; it's more than simply requiring the patient to sign a standard form that enumerates a laundry list of possible risks. Ideally, informed consent should be an ongoing and personalized discussion between the doctor and patient that reflects any changing circumstances of the patient's condition or any evolution in the doctor's understanding of the patient's condition.

Informed consent requires four elements:

1. A discussion of the recommended course of action for the patient's condition, including the nature of recommended procedures, tests, and so on
2. A discussion of reasonable alternatives to recommended care
3. Information covering the benefits, risks, and options regarding the recommended care versus other alternatives
4. The patient's voluntary and competent acceptance of proposed treatment

Legal requirements for informed consent may vary among jurisdictions, either by legislation or by legal precedent. One relevant issue that may vary is the threshold that determines what degree of risk is meaningful. All health care procedures carry some degree of risk, and if health care providers were required to discuss every conceivable risk of every procedure in detail with every patient, it would be an unreasonably high burden on their time. It could also undermine the spirit of true informed consent because patients might be so overwhelmed that they cannot truly appreciate which risks are significant and worth discussing in detail.

This problem is the crux of the controversy regarding whether chiropractors should be required to discuss the possibility of vertebral artery dissection and stroke with all their patients. Some have argued that since the possibility of a stroke following a chiropractic visit is so miniscule, and the causal relationship between the chiropractic treatment and the stroke is so doubtful, that requiring a discussion on the topic is unreasonable and actually counterproductive to the doctor-patient relationship. Others have argued that patients have the right to know about any possible risk, regardless of how rare and how uncertain the causal relationship.

This continues to be an evolving legal issue. At least one state in the United States, Connecticut, has looked at this specific issue in detail. In 2010, after extensive public hearings and testimony from numerous experts, the Connecticut Board of Chiropractic Examiners issued an opinion that doctors of chiropractic are not required to routinely inform patients of the supposed association between cervical manipulation and stroke. They supported this finding by stating that a reasonable patient would not find this to be a "material risk" to the procedure. That is, a fully informed patient would not consider this information important in deciding whether or not to have the treatment. Other jurisdictions have more restrictive rulings requiring DCs to routinely inform patients of the possibility of stroke following cervical manipulation, while most jurisdictions have not issued explicit guidance or have no specific legal precedents.

The informed consent process can be made a more valuable experience if the treating doctor also educates the patient about potential red flags or symptoms that may develop that the patient should really worry about. For example, when treating a patient with headaches, red flags should be ruled out during the initial visit, but it may be helpful to mention possible warning signs that the patient should beware of, such as developing visual disturbances, difficulties in speech or swallowing, new onset of dizziness or severe headache, nausea, or alteration in consciousness. This seems like it would be a potentially more useful educational discussion than an in-depth conversation about the dubious relationship between cervical manipulation and stroke.

Protecting the Public

Professional Licensure and Discipline

Doctors of chiropractic are granted a license by the state that provides them certain privileges, for example, protection of title and exclusive scope of practice. In exchange for these privileges, chiropractors agree to abide by the minimum standards of competence established by the appropriate governmental regulatory authorities. In the United States, each individual state regulates chiropractic practice in accordance with its own specific laws. In most states, the body that is charged with enforcing the laws and standards is called the State Board of Chiropractic Examiners. In Canada, chiropractors are licensed in each province and regulated by the Provincial College of Chiropractors.

The responsibility of the state licensing boards is to enforce the laws and regulations regarding the practice of its profession and to protect the public from misconduct by members. State boards may enact regulations defining appropriate scope of practice, professional advertising, medical records policies, and other activities.

Members of state licensing boards are usually appointed by the state governor and function as a part of the executive branch of government. In most states, doctors of chiropractic make up a majority of the members of the chiropractic board. Most boards also include one or more non-DC members representing the general public.

State boards have the legal authority to approve or deny licensure to applicants and discipline licensees for professional misconduct. Most boards are "complaint driven" when it comes to investigating their members. They are required to investigate complaints from the public against one of their licensees. If the complaint cannot be resolved satisfactorily, formal hearings may be conducted to determine the facts of the case and whether sanctions against a licensee are appropriate. Sanctions against licensees may include a formal letter of reprimand, fines, probation, required retraining or reexamination, suspension of license, or revocation of license.

The Federation of Chiropractic Licensing Boards is an international organization that maintains a database of actions taken by chiropractic licensing boards. The database contains information on chiropractors who were disciplined by a state board and/or who are excluded from Medicare/Medicaid reimbursement by the U.S. Department of Health and Human Services because of fraud or misconduct. This database prevents chiropractors who lost their license due to misconduct in one state from simply moving to another state and getting another license there.

Chiropractic Malpractice Claims

The ultimate protection for the public against negligence from a practicing doctor of chiropractic is to sue the chiropractor for malpractice. "Professional malpractice" is defined as an act or continuing conduct of a professional that does not meet the standard of professional competence and results in provable damages to his or her client or patient.

Malpractice is a *tort*, which is a legal claim between two or more individuals. Torts are tried under the standards of civil law. Malpractice is not a criminal act, which is a violation of the laws of the state tried under criminal law. These two different types of law have different standards of judgment. In a criminal case, the standard for the defendant to be proven guilty is "beyond a reasonable doubt," whereas under civil law the standard is "a preponderance of evidence."

To have a successful malpractice claim, the patient (plaintiff) must prove all the following were present at the time of an injury:

1. *Doctor-patient relationship:* There must have been a contractual relationship between the two parties that was entered into willingly by both.
2. *Duty:* The treating chiropractor legally owes certain duties to her or his patients, including
   a. the duty to determine whether the patient presents a problem that is treatable through chiropractic means;
   b. the duty to refrain from further chiropractic treatment when a reasonable chiropractor should be aware that the patient's condition will not be responsive to further treatment;

    c.   if the ailment presented is outside the scope of chiropractic care, the duty to inform the patient that the ailment is not treatable through chiropractic means;

    d.   the duty to obtain the informed consent of the patient for the procedures performed; and

    e.   the duty to treat the patient in a manner consistent with the community *standard of care* for that profession. This standard is judged relative to scientific knowledge and to what is generally accepted within the profession. It is consistent with what is taught in academic and clinical training received in and through accredited chiropractic educational programs. In practice, standard of care is usually established through expert testimony in court.

3.   *Dereliction of duty:* The injury may have been caused by either an error of commission or an error of omission.

4.   *Direct causation:* "But for" the dereliction of duty, the injury would not have happened.

5.   *Damage:* The plaintiff must have suffered some demonstrable loss due to the injury, such as loss of income due to inability to work, costs of further medical treatments, or pain and suffering.

If any one of these elements is absent, the doctor (defendant) should prevail in litigation. Just because care of a patient leads to a bad outcome, it is not necessarily malpractice. If the treating doctor followed the accepted standard of care in treating the patient, no malpractice was committed even if the outcome of that care is tragic.

Conclusions

In considering the safety and effectiveness of a particular health care treatment, it is important to think broadly, comparing the range of available treatments, rather than looking at any one particular treatment in a vacuum. It is true that the evidence supporting the commonly used chiropractic approach for musculoskeletal pain is still evolving, but the evidence demonstrates that this approach is at least as effective as any other commonly used treatment. If one applies the same standard of evidence to other commonly used treatments for spinal pain, such as pharmaceuticals and surgical procedures, none of those other treatments have any more evidence of effectiveness than manual therapies; in fact, they often have far less evidence, despite risk profiles that are often significantly less favorable.

In chiropractic training and in postgraduate continuing education courses, doctors of chiropractic are taught to practice with a culture of patient safety. They are educated to recognize risk factors in patients and how to treat patients in the safest, most effective, and most responsible manner. Despite continuing controversies regarding the treatment of certain patient populations and the treatment of some conditions, the chiropractic profession continues to have a remarkably good record of safety in patient care. The public has various layers of protection against unsafe practices, including the civil courts for malpractice cases, and regulatory bodies that are charged with protecting the public from incompetent or unscrupulous practitioners.

Like all health care sciences, chiropractic methods will continue to be put under increased scrutiny for evidence of safety, effectiveness, and cost efficiency. Forward-thinking chiropractors welcome this scrutiny and see it as an opportunity to improve their practice in order to serve their patients better.

References

1. Clar C, Tsertsvadze A, Court R, Hundt GL, Clarke A, Sutcliffe P. Clinical effectiveness of manual therapy for the management of musculoskeletal and non-musculoskeletal conditions: systematic review and update of UK evidence report. *Chiropr Man Therap.* 2014;22(1):12.

2. Bronfort G, Haas M, Evans R, Leiniger B, Triano J. Effectiveness of manual therapies: the UK evidence report. *Chiropr Osteopat.* 2010;18(1):3.

3. Walker BF, Hebert JJ, Stomski NJ, et al. Outcomes of usual chiropractic. The OUCH randomized controlled trial of adverse events. *Spine (Phila Pa 1976).* 2013;38(20):1723–1729.

4. Li C, Martin BC. Trends in emergency department visits attributable to acetaminophen overdoses in the United States: 1993–2007. *Pharmacoepidemiol Drug Saf.* 2011;20(8):810–818.

5. Machado GC, Maher CG, Ferreira PH, et al. Efficacy and safety of paracetamol for spinal pain and osteoarthritis: systematic review and meta-analysis of randomised placebo controlled trials. *BMJ.* 2015;350:h1225.

6. Wolfe MM, Lichtenstein DR, Singh G. Gastrointestinal toxicity of nonsteroidal antiinflammatory drugs. *N Engl J Med.* 1999;340(24):1888–1899.

7. Chou R, Qaseem A, Snow V, et al. Diagnosis and treatment of low back pain: a joint clinical practice guideline from the American College of Physicians and the American Pain Society. *Ann Intern Med.* 2007;147(7):478–491.

8. Rhee Y, Taitel MS, Walker DR, Lau DT. Narcotic drug use among patients with lower back pain in employer health plans: a retrospective analysis of risk factors and health care services. *Clin Ther.* 2007;29 Suppl:2603–2612.

9. Zaina F, Tomkins-Lane C, Carragee E, Negrini S. Surgical versus non-surgical treatment for lumbar spinal stenosis. *Cochrane Database Syst Rev.* 2016;1:CD010264.

10. Deyo RA, Mirza SK, Martin BI, Kreuter W, Goodman DC, Jarvik JG. Trends, major medical complications, and charges associated with surgery for lumbar spinal stenosis in older adults. *JAMA.* 2010;303(13):1259–1265.

11. Chou R, Hashimoto R, Friedly J, et al. Epidural corticosteroid injections for radiculopathy and spinal stenosis: a systematic review and meta-analysis. *Ann Intern Med.* 2015;163(5):373–381.

12. Keeney BJ, Fulton-Kehoe D, Turner JA, Wickizer TM, Chan KC, Franklin GM. Early predictors of lumbar spine surgery after occupational back injury: results from a prospective study of workers in Washington State. *Spine (Phila Pa 1976).* 2013;38(11):953–964.

13. Herzog W, Leonard TR, Symons B, Tang C, Wuest S. Vertebral artery strains during high-speed, low-amplitude cervical spinal manipulation. *J Electromyogr Kinesiol.* 2012;22(5):740–746.

14. Cassidy JD, Boyle E, Cote P, et al. Risk of vertebrobasilar stroke and chiropractic care. *Spine (Phila Pa 1976).* 2008;33(4S):S176–S183.

15. Kosloff TM, Elton D, Tao J, Bannister WM. Chiropractic care and the risk of vertebrobasilar stroke: results of a case-control study in U.S. commercial and Medicare Advantage populations. *Chiropr Man Therap.* 2015;23:19.

16. Haldeman S, Carey P, Townsend M, Papadopoulos C. Arterial dissections following cervical manipulation: the chiropractic experience. *CMAJ.* 2001; 165(7):905–906.

17. Bronfort G, Evans R, Anderson AV, Svendsen KH, Bracha Y, Grimm RH. Spinal manipulation, medication, or home exercise with advice for acute and subacute neck pain: a randomized trial. *Ann Intern Med.* 2012;156(1 Pt 1):1–10.

18. Guzman J, Haldeman S, Carroll LJ, et al. Clinical practice implications of the Bone and Joint Decade 2000–2010 Task Force on Neck Pain and Its Associated Disorders: from concepts and findings to recommendations. *Spine.* 2008; 33(4 Suppl):S199–213.

19. Stuber KJ, Wynd S, Weis CA. Adverse events from spinal manipulation in the pregnant and postpartum periods: a critical review of the literature. *Chiropr Man Therap.* 2012;20:8.

20. Todd AJ, Carroll MT, Robinson A, Mitchell EK. Adverse events due to chiropractic and other manual therapies for infants and children: a review of the literature. *J Manipulative Physiol Ther.* 2015;38:699–712.

21. Ferrance RJ, Miller J. Chiropractic diagnosis and management of non-musculoskeletal conditions in children and adolescents. *Chiropr Osteopat.* 2010;18:14.

22. Hawk C, Long CR, Boulanger KT, Morschhauser E, Fuhr AW. Chiropractic care for patients aged 55 years and older: report from a practice-based research program. *J Am Geriatr Soc.* 2000;48(5):534–545.

23. Whedon JM, Mackenzie TA, Phillips RB, Lurie JD. Risk of traumatic injury associated with chiropractic spinal manipulation in Medicare Part B beneficiaries aged 66–99. *Spine (Phila Pa 1976).* 2015;40(4):264–270.

The Chiropractic Approach to Low Back Pain

Mark Pfefer, DC, RN, MS; and Jon Wilson, DC

Back pain and arthritis are among the most common and costly health conditions, costing more than $200 billion per year in direct and indirect costs.[1] Direct costs refer to money spent in treating the condition, and indirect costs refer to lost work time and other costs associated with the condition. In addition to high monetary costs, back pain may have psychological and social impacts for those individuals suffering from pain, especially when it is chronic or long-lasting.[2] Low back pain causes significant disability in a small percentage of the population, and new strategies are needed to prevent and manage this condition effectively.

Most back pain is likely caused by mechanical problems in joints and muscles, which is referred to as "functional pathology" (e.g., restricted joint movements, tightness, weakness, or painful areas in muscles), rather than structural pathology (e.g., diseases, tumors, fractures, disc herniation).

Often low back pain has a nonspecific cause and improves within several weeks with or without treatment. In the past, back pain episodes have been perceived as separate events, but this view is now being modified to consider back pain as a long-term or chronic condition.[3] Back pain can be present throughout life, affecting young as well as older adults, and some people have episodes of pain intermittently throughout their lifetime. Tobacco use, inadequate sleep, and obesity have been associated with back pain and general musculoskeletal pain.[4–6] A number of factors may predict back pain at different stages of life, but more research is needed to improve our understanding of the development and fluctuations in back pain.

The causes of back pain are varied. Research has evaluated multiple epidemiologic categories related to the development of low back pain. The categories include environmental factors, human factors, and psychosocial risk factors. Jobs that require high levels of physical exertion—including lifting, bending, twisting, prolonged sitting, and prolonged standing—are often related to the development of low back pain. Human risk factors include gender, body size, muscle strength, and physical fitness. Psychosocial factors implicated in low back pain include attitudes toward pain, depression, emotional distress, and drug addiction.

The development of low back pain is complex and individually variable, with a complex balance of adequate activity—not too much or too little. Some investigators report similar incidences of low back pain with sedentary workers versus those engaged in heavy labor, although a majority of the evidence points to a role of physical overuse as a frequent cause of low back pain. Recently there has been a focus on prolonged sitting and lack of exercise as a precursor to a variety of negative health effects, including the possibility of low back pain. Exposure to repeated vibration may also contribute to the development of back pain, as has been found in over-the-road truck drivers. Just as prolonged sitting is associated with low back pain, prolonged standing at work has also been implicated in a number of potentially serious health outcomes, including lower back and leg pain.[7]

Age is often thought to be a risk factor for low back pain, but this association is not entirely clear. As people age, they do tend to develop some degenerative changes in their spinal and extremity joints, yet many people with degenerative changes at any given time will not experience pain. There is little association between abnormal X-ray findings and low back pain, so the degeneration-pain relationship as it relates to aging is quite complex. Low back pain incidence peaks in middle-aged adults and declines somewhat with aging. Advanced age and being male are often associated with chronic back pain, but this may relate to the number of years exposed to certain types of work, overuse, or lack of physical conditioning.

Obesity is associated with increased prevalence of low back pain within the last 12 months, seeking care for low back pain, and chronic low back pain. Compared with people of a healthy weight, overweight people have a higher prevalence of low back pain but a lower prevalence of low back pain compared with obese people.[8] This is a complex relationship because other physical fitness factors may be partly responsible for this association, such as overall physical fitness, muscle strength, and muscle endurance factors. It is also important to keep in mind that decreased physical fitness and being overweight may be risk factors for development of low back pain or may be a secondary effect of chronic low back pain. That is, decreased physical fitness and extra weight may contribute to having low back pain, or low back pain may contribute to decreased physical fitness and extra weight.

Psychosocial factors are associated with disability related to low back pain. Patients experiencing back pain may develop fear and anxiety related to activity and exercise. This leads to deconditioning and ongoing pain. People with chronic pain can develop depression, and this may also lead to lack of physical activity and exercise. Depression has also been linked as a risk factor for the development of low back pain.

Although back pain often improves over time and with little or no treatment, it also tends to have high rates of recurrence. Research has demonstrated that many people with back pain have repeated intermittent bouts of pain and disability. However, this research has limitations, because people's recall of episodes of back pain in the past may not be reliable. Few studies have followed large numbers of back pain patients over many years.

Uncommonly, back pain may be a sign of serious disease. It is important for health care providers to consider potential serious underlying issues, which are referred to as "red flags," when assessing the patient who presents for care with back pain. Chiropractors are trained to recognize signs of potential serious conditions and to further evaluate the patient or refer to a different health care provider for additional evaluation and management if appropriate. Some patients with serious disease causing back pain may not be able to receive certain types of chiropractic care, while others may be effectively comanaged with another provider.

Health care providers should also be concerned with identifying the presence of risk factors that are associated with a delay in the normally expected recovery time from low back pain, also known as "yellow flags." Many of the common risk factors associated with back pain chronicity are related to psychosocial factors. These factors include emotional issues, such as anxiety and depression, or can include excessive worrying about the back problem becoming worse with activity, which is called "fear avoidance behavior." Patients with low back pain require an approach that addresses the physical or biological aspects of their problem along with interventions that address the psychosocial dimensions of their problem. An attitude referred to as "fear-avoidance," in which fear of pain leads to avoidance of the activity suspected of inducing pain, can cause a patient to avoid activity and exercise. This leads to deconditioning and decreased back stability, which in turn makes the underlying problem worse. It is important to provide reassurance to patients with noncomplicated low back pain and encourage patients to remain active and avoid prolonged rest.

Spinal Anatomy Overview

The vertebral column, often called the spine, is made up of 26 bones. Twenty-four of these bones are known as vertebrae, divided into three regions. The uppermost region, the cervical spine, contains 7 vertebrae and is commonly referred to as the neck. The middle region, the thoracic spine, contains 12 vertebrae and is commonly referred to as the midback. The low back contains 5 vertebrae and is known as the lumbar spine. The sacrum is a large, triangular-shaped bone directly below the lumbar spine. It is also considered to be part of the pelvic girdle. The sacrum articulates, or forms a joint with, the left and right coxal bone at the sacroiliac joint. The lowest bone in the vertebral column is the coccyx, or tailbone, and it articulates with the sacrum above. The term "low back pain" is often used to describe pain in the lower thoracic spine, the lumbar spine, and in the sacroiliac joint region of the pelvis.

Each vertebra is formed by a central barrel-shaped vertebral body with various processes, or parts of the bone that project from it. One of these processes, the spinous process, projects back from the vertebral body. Two other processes, the transverse processes, project from each side of the vertebral body. These processes are important attachment points for muscles. A potential, but uncommon, cause of low back pain can be fracture of various parts of the vertebrae. Elderly patients and patients who have been exposed to long-term use of steroids have an increased risk of compression fractures of the vertebral body. This type of fracture is usually associated with decreased bone density. The other elements of the spine rarely fracture unless caused by trauma or a pathological process, such as a tumor.

The spine's primary function is to protect the spinal cord. The spinal cord allows the brain and the rest of the body to communicate through the nervous system. Spinal nerves branch off the spinal cord and exit between two adjacent vertebrae through a structure known as the intervertebral foramen. Injury, mechanical conditions, or degenerative processes may directly affect the function of the spinal cord and/or spinal nerves. Patients with low back pain who also show neurological symptoms, such as muscle weakness, altered sensation, or altered muscle strength, will be managed differently than patients with uncomplicated mechanical low back pain. This makes it important for a health care provider to determine if the nervous system is directly being impacted by the condition causing the pain.

When viewed from the side, the spine has four curvatures that give it a shape resembling the letter S. The cervical and lumbar spines both have a concavity that faces the back, known as the cervical lordosis and the lumbar lordosis. The thoracic spine and the sacrum have a convexity that faces the back. These curves allow the spine to have a degree of flexibility needed for normal motion. Changes to the normal sagittal curves in the spine may be associated with abnormal function that leads to pain, including in the low back. Mechanical forces that affect the low back are directly related to the posture of a patient, and changes to the sagittal curves are a common postural deviation seen in the population.

Between all the vertebrae in the cervical, thoracic, and lumbar spine is an intervertebral disc. This small cushion-like structure acts to absorb shock that occurs with normal activities by transmitting that shock to the spongy bone that makes up the central part of the vertebra. The discs also allow the spine the ability to flex, extend, and bend to each side. The tough outer layers of the intervertebral disc are known as the annulus fibrosus. The inner gelatinous portion of the disc is known as the nucleus pulposus. The intervertebral disc is often implicated in patients with low back pain due to its rich innervation. Repetitive motion or traumatic injuries may cause a herniated disc. This condition results from tears to the annulus fibrosus that can sometimes allow protrusion of the nucleus pulposus. If this protrusion puts pressure on the spinal cord or spinal nerves, pain and/or neurological symptoms can result. Protrusion of the nucleus pulposus may also cause an inflammatory reaction that can increase the symptoms of low back pain. Patients with disc pathology often have intermittent recurring episodes of low back pain that may be localized to the low back or may cause low back and leg pain.

Paired joint surfaces exist at the top and bottom of each vertebra. These joint surfaces are known as facets and are covered in hyaline cartilage. These facets form movable joints with the vertebra above and below, allowing for movement. These joints, known as facet joints, zygapophyseal joints, or intervertebral joints, are surrounded by richly innervated soft tissue that forms a capsule containing synovial fluid. The synovial fluid's function is to lubricate and nourish the joint. Some cases of back pain are suspected to be caused by the irritation, either chemical or mechanical, of these richly innervated facet capsules. A substantial number of elderly people experience facet joint pain. Pain in the facet joints may be associated with abnormal motion and is potentially a contributor to patients with low back pain, even in instances when the pain is primarily caused by another tissue.

The spine is also surrounded by various soft tissues, including ligaments, tendons, fascia, and muscles. Support, protection, joint position sense, and movement are provided by this soft tissue, and it can often also be implicated in patients with back pain. Common conditions seen in patients with low back pain related to soft tissue include sprains, strains, muscle spasm, tendonitis, abnormal motion patterns, tissue extensibility disorders, and instability.

A number of ligaments surround the vertebral column and help to stabilize the spine. The anterior longitudinal ligament and the posterior longitudinal ligament run the length of the spinal column and help limit the motions of flexion and extension. Another large ligament, the ligamentum flavum, is elastic in nature and helps protect the spinal cord during certain movements. Additional small ligaments help protect the spine during other motions, such as axial rotation.

The muscle groups surrounding the spine primarily function to stabilize the spine, provide information concerning spinal position, and assist in causing movement in the head and trunk. These muscle groups are frequently implicated as the cause of or a contributor to low back pain. In patients with low back pain, even when not caused by muscles directly, the low back musculature will sometimes react to the pain by shortening and tightening. This causes additional pain and is referred to as the pain-spasm-pain cycle. Abdominal muscles, such as the transversus abdominis, may also be important in stability of the low back. Sedentary lifestyles, injury, or low back pain may contribute to weakness of these stabilization muscles. Without the correct stabilization, the movement in the low back can be altered and may lead to dysfunction. The weakness of stabilization muscles may be a contributing factor to low back pain, both current and potentially in future episodes.

A thin connective tissue known as fascia helps to separate groups of muscles, allows tissues to slide across each other, and may be important in spinal stability. Fascia may also play a role in position sense, as cells that are designed to detect stretch have been found in the tissue of the fascia. Adhesions may form in the fascia of patients who have had an injury or lack appropriate motion in the area, and these adhesions are sometimes considered to be contributors to abnormal function and pain. Fascia may also play a potential positive role related to the low back. The thoraco-lumbar fascia acts much like a brace for the low back by stabilizing the lumbar spine through attachments with the transversus abdominis, the internal obliques, and the latissimus dorsi.

Below the spinal column is the pelvic girdle. The pelvic girdle is formed from two bones known as os coxae, or coxal bones. The two coxal bones articulate (form a joint) with the sacrum at the top and together at the bottom in an area known as the pubic symphysis.

The joint between the sacrum and the coxal bone is known as the sacroiliac joint. The sacroiliac joint is responsible for transmitting the weight of the upper body into the legs and for allowing small amounts of motion necessary for gait. This requires the joint to be stable, and this stability is maintained by both the joint's structure (form closure) and the joint's surrounding tissues (force closure). Problems with either form or force closure can lead to instability of the joint. Instability of the sacroiliac joint as well as limited motion of the joint may lead to mechanical dysfunction and pain. Sacroiliac pain is implicated in some cases of chronic low back pain located below the level of the lumbar spine.

Multiple different types of motion normally occur in the low back. Segmentally, vertebral motion occurs through rotations occurring around three axes. These motions are commonly described as flexion (forward movement), extension (backward movement), left and right rotation (turning to each side), and left and right lateral flexion (bending to each side without turning). Small translations, or sliding motions, are also common in the spine. The thoracic spine allows for more rotation than the lumbar spine. The lumbar spine allows for primarily flexion and extension, with rotation being considerably limited. Motion in the spine is almost always coupled, meaning one motion rarely happens by itself without being accompanied by another motion, even if slight. This coupling of spinal motion is predictable in the upper cervical spine, but in the thoracic and lumbar spine the coupling is not predictable between two people or even within an individual. Normal anatomic asymmetries exist between individuals and even between individual segments within the spine. This large variability in spinal motion complicates the detection of abnormal segmental motion. The sacroiliac joints allow very little motion, approximately two degrees of rotation in flexion and extension. These are very stable joints that allow the upper body weight to be transmitted into each leg. However, the small motion that does occur is important for gait (the motions involved in walking). Limited motion, excessive motion, or instability in the sacroiliac joint may be contributors to low back and pelvic pain.

Back pain is a complicated issue anatomically, in that any tissue in the area, whether ligament, muscle, fascia, joint, or disc, can cause pain because all of these tissues are innervated (have nerves that are sensitive to pain). Distribution of back pain is also not always directly linked to the anatomical site where the pain is actually generated. Back pain can either be local or referred, or a combination of the two. That is, the pain may originate in the location where it is felt (local), or it may originate in an area at some distance from the location where it is felt (referred pain). This makes determining a tissue-specific diagnosis difficult. Radiating, or shooting, pain may also be a symptom of some patients with low back pain.

Evaluation of Low Back Pain

Patients with low back pain should receive a complete and thorough history taking and assessment by a health professional so that serious conditions can be excluded and red flags can be identified. "Red flags" are signs or symptoms that indicate the possibility of serious conditions that would be contraindications for chiropractic care or other manual therapy treatments. Common red flags include history of trauma, age greater than 50 years old, history of cancer, fever, chills, night sweats, unexplained or unexpected weight loss, recent infection, taking medication that suppresses immune function, pain with rest or at night, numbness in the buttocks and perineum, bladder dysfunction, and severe neurological dysfunction in the extremities.[9] Presence of one or more red flag may indicate the presence of serious medical conditions and require further evaluation, including the use of X-ray or other diagnostic imaging techniques.

Some serious diseases can be associated with back pain, with referral of pain to the back or neck because of diseases or dysfunction in visceral organs. Some of the sources of visceral pain that can also have a component of back pain include inflammatory diseases, appendicitis, bowel obstruction, tumors (including benign and malignant lesions), kidney stones, gall bladder disease, endometriosis, prostatitis, chronic pelvic inflammatory disease, pancreatitis, and penetrating ulcer of the stomach. Additional nonmechanical sources of back pain might include malignancy, osteomyelitis, shingles, epidural abscess, and Paget's disease.

"Less is more" may be good advice when evaluating and treating back pain.[10] An initiative of the National Physicians Alliance, the project titled "Promoting Good Stewardship in Clinical Practice," developed a list of the top five activities in primary care for which changes in practice could lead to higher-quality care and better use of limited medical resources.[10] One of these recommendations was to avoid doing diagnostic imaging for low back pain within the first six weeks unless red flags were present. Imaging refers to the use of X-rays and advanced imaging, such as computed tomography and magnetic resonance imaging. These procedures are expensive and often do not change the type of treatment provided; more importantly, they do not ultimately change the outcome. Early use of imaging may even lower the chance of a positive outcome of care in patients with low back pain. If a patient is made aware of a finding, even if an incidental finding, found through imaging, the patient may suffer from psychosocial effects, including fear-avoidance behaviors and catastrophizing.

This should be encouraging for people with back pain, because it means that back pain often gets better, that bed rest should be avoided, and that exercise and movement are actually very good for most people with back pain. Chiropractors can be beneficial in the care of people with back pain as they can screen patients for red flags and encourage return to movement through a combination of passive care and active care interventions.

One cause of back pain that chiropractors frequently encounter is known as segmental dysfunction, subluxation, or vertebral subluxation complex. Within chiropractic practice, a "subluxation" can be defined as a functional entity that consists of an abnormal biomechanical or physiological relationship between adjacent joint structures.[11] This means that the joint does not move or function normally—often, it has restricted movement. Pain related to symptomatic segmental dysfunction may arise from the facet joints, the intervertebral discs, the muscles, or any combination of these. The diagnosis of subluxation is made primarily through a combination of physical examination findings involving pain, asymmetry, range of motion, and soft tissue findings. Various potential mechanisms for the effects of subluxations have been put forward, but it is difficult to ascertain direct evidence of the presence of subluxation. Similar functional pathologies have been described in other health care professions, including osteopathy and physical therapy.

Chiropractic Treatment Overview

Low back or pelvic pain is the most common chief complaint that causes a patient to seek chiropractic care.[11] This pain is most often related to activities of daily living, repetitive stress, motor vehicle accidents, or participation in sports.

Chiropractors treat patients with back pain using a combination of passive and active care interventions. Passive care interventions involve treatment that does not involve the patient actively moving. These treatments are commonly spinal manipulative therapy, various types of massage, heat, cold, electrical stimulation, laser modalities, and passive stretching. Active care interventions include supervised and ongoing home exercises that strengthen the body, especially strengthening core support muscles in the trunk and legs. Chiropractors will often start with mostly passive care modalities when initially seeing a patient who is in pain and then gradually transition to more of a focus on active care as the patient's pain improves. This active rehabilitative approach may lead to less future recurrence, but more research is needed to confirm this theory.

The treatment method most associated with chiropractic care is spinal manipulation, referred to by some chiropractors as the "chiropractic adjustment." The adjustment is a form of spinal manipulation using a low-amplitude, high-velocity dynamic thrust with a controlled velocity, amplitude, and line of drive. These techniques can be either short-leverage (the contact on the patient is close to the targeted joint) or long-leverage (the contact on the patient is not adjacent to the targeted joint and may involve rotation of the patient's thigh or leg). Adjustments of the spine are commonly, but not always, associated with an audible popping sound, known as "cavitation." Cavitation is believed to be from reduced pressure in the joint capsule causing the coalescing of dissolved gasses from synovial fluid. This dissolved gas takes up space in the joint and allows the joint capsule to quickly spring to a new shape to accommodate the increased volume within the capsule. The presence of cavitation is not associated with better or worse outcomes in patient care.

There are a number of subtypes of spinal manipulation therapy techniques commonly used by chiropractors. Some types of spinal manipulation use instruments or devices that deliver a very quick, impulse type of thrust, and this type of manipulation does not typically cause cavitation or popping sounds. Sometimes a chiropractor will use a "drop" or table-assisted manipulation that involves a special table with a spring-loaded section below the patient. Table-assisted and instrument-assisted manipulation may be gentler and more comfortable for some patients. In all cases, spinal manipulation or chiropractic adjustments involve applying loads to the spine and typically include procedures involving an impulse or quick loads to the spine. One goal of spinal manipulation, or the chiropractic adjustment, is to impart small, relative displacements within the affected joints. It is believed that spinal manipulation may also play a role in nervous system function, locally and centrally, which could also explain some of the positive benefits seen in patients with low back pain and other conditions.

The selection of spinal manipulation procedure requires good clinical judgment, including review of patient history and physical and functional assessment. In deciding which procedures to use, the chiropractor should take into account age and size of the patient, muscle mass and weight of the patient, and underlying pathology or prior surgery. The chiropractor will assess a region to determine if functional movement limitations are present and will determine if discomfort is present with provocative movement testing of the symptomatic region.

Spinal manipulation is believed to restore joint motion and function and also produces reflex responses in the adjacent muscles. In many patients, muscle activity decreases immediately following a spinal adjustment. This is evidence that high-velocity, low-amplitude (HVLA) spinal manipulation affects locations remote from the actual treatment site.[12] Spinal manipulation is also theorized to potentially affect central nervous system processing and may influence the autonomic nervous system.

Chiropractic Treatment Methods Used in Addition to Spinal Manipulation

Although spinal manipulation is the primary approach chiropractors use, they usually combine it with other methods to enhance the beneficial effects. Or, if for some reason spinal manipulation is not appropriate, the chiropractor may use only these other methods. Over 97 percent of chiropractors report providing advice on ergonomics and posture, physical fitness and exercise, risky and unhealthy behaviors, nutrition and diet, relaxation and stress reduction, and self-care strategies.[11]

Ergonomic/Postural Advice

The spine is structured in a way to provide a balance of stability and movement when practicing healthy posture. Abnormal posture may challenge muscles, ligaments, and other soft tissues to maintain this balance. Through awareness and active care, chiropractors try to relieve this unnecessary stress to the musculoskeletal system, potentially decreasing or avoiding low back pain.

Physical Fitness/Exercise Promotion

Overall physical fitness is important to overall health. In relation to low back pain, physical fitness and general exercise may help patients avoid stiffness and weakness, decrease severity and duration of low back pain, and potentially decrease the frequency of future episodes of low back pain. Physical fitness will decrease the likelihood of obesity, a known contributor to low back pain.

Lifestyle Modification

Certain behaviors, such as smoking and sedentary lifestyles, are known to increase the chances of experiencing low back pain. Through patient interviews, chiropractors are able to identify these risky behaviors and offer counseling and advice. Lifestyle modification may also be helpful in decreasing obesity-related low back pain and the increased chance of low back pain in patients who smoke.

Nutritional and Dietary Recommendations

Nutritional and dietary recommendations are made by chiropractors for various reasons that may influence low back pain. A balanced, healthy diet is important for overall health, as is a healthy body weight. Obesity is associated with low back pain. This makes weight loss a goal that many chiropractors have for their patients. Through the monitoring of body mass index and dietary intake, a chiropractor has an opportunity to influence this important contributor to low back pain.

Chiropractors also frequently make certain diet recommendations in an effort to decrease inflammation in a patient. Anti-inflammatory diets are often recommended to patients who have inflammation as a contributing factor to their low back pain.

Stress Management

Psychosocial factors are known to contribute to low back pain. Stress is believed to negatively affect patients' perceptions of pain and expected outcomes. A recent study reported patients with chronic low back pain responded more favorably with stress reduction methods added to standard care than with standard care alone.[13]

Self-Care Strategies

Many cases of low back pain will go away in a short amount of time with self-care. Self-care frequently recommended by chiropractors may include activity modification, home exercises or stretches, the use of heat or ice, dietary recommendations, and stress reduction.

Passive Chiropractic Treatment Methods

"Passive" simply means that the doctor does the procedure and the patient does not have to do anything. Most chiropractors report using passive adjunctive procedures, including cryotherapy (ice), trigger point therapy, bracing, electrical stimulation, heat, massage therapy, heel lifts, mobilization therapy, flexion-distraction, and ultrasound.[11]

Cryotherapy

Cryotherapy is the use of cold therapy. Cryotherapy is applied by chiropractors using a variety of methods, including ice packs, gel packs, ice massage, or ice baths. The goal of cryotherapy is to address inflammation and pain, and it is used in the acute phase of treatment of low back pain. Cold decreases blood flow to the area and has an analgesic effect but may also cause shortening of muscles, which can aggravate some patients with low back pain and muscle spasm. In these patients, the use of heat or cycling heat and ice may be recommended.

Trigger Point Therapy

Trigger points are tender points within a muscle that refer pain to a different anatomical site. Trigger points located in the midback, the low back, and the pelvis have been implicated as potential contributors to low back pain. Chiropractors use a wide variety of soft tissue methods to treat trigger points. Trigger point therapy involves strong, deep pressure to an area of pain held for a short period of time and then released. Trigger point therapy is generally considered safe with minimal risk of side effects, but contraindications include infection, fracture, burns, deep vein thrombosis or other vascular problems, and local tumors or malignancy. Precautions should be taken when treating patients who are taking blood-thinning medication.

Bracing

Bracing is used to treat patients with acute low back pain if there appears to be a benefit to providing stability and limiting motion of an area of the spine or pelvis for a short time. The eventual goal of most chiropractors is to allow the patient's body to perform the necessary stabilization on its own. Frequently a patient who initially is recommended bracing will be given stabilization exercises to perform in the office or at home.

Electrical Stimulation

Various forms of electrical stimulation are used by chiropractors, including interferential current therapy, transcutaneous electrical nerve stimulation, and galvanic stimulation. These passive therapies are thought to interfere with pain transmission to the central nervous system and to promote the release of endorphins. Electrical stimulation may also be used to attempt to decrease the tightness of muscles or in some cases to strengthen weakened muscles.

Heat

Chiropractors use heat therapy through the use of heating pads, hydrocollator (moist heat) packs, heated gel packs, and heated wraps. Heat therapy is believed to decrease low back pain through several mechanisms. Blood flow to an area treated with heat increases, and this may speed healing in the area by providing an increased flow of oxygen and nutrients to the area. Heat stimulates the nervous system, which helps to decrease pain perception. Heat also allows soft tissue, such as tight muscles, to lengthen. This lengthening effect may provide relief for certain patients with low back pain.

Massage Therapy

Chiropractors frequently use massage therapy or recommend massage therapy for their patients. Massage therapy is believed to relax tight muscles, improve range of motion, increase circulation of blood and lymph, and increase levels of endorphins. Massage therapy involves the use of the hands or other mechanical devices to manipulate superficial and deep soft tissues. Massage can involve stroking, kneading, percussion, or vibration of soft tissue. Massage is one of the most commonly used interventions among patients with low back pain, and there is some evidence that various types of massage are helpful for these patients. Like trigger point therapy, massage is generally quite safe. Massage should be avoided in patients with infection, fracture, burns, deep vein thrombosis or other vascular problems, and local tumors or malignancy. Precautions should be taken when treating patients who are taking blood-thinning medication.

Heel Lifts and Orthotics

Some patients with low back pain have a leg length difference that may affect standing posture and muscle balance in the pelvis and low back. While functional leg length differences, ones associated with muscular imbalance, are usually addressed with other forms of therapy, a small percentage of patients with low back pain have a true anatomical difference in leg length. In this subset of patients, a heel lift being inserted in their shoe on the short leg side may improve overall body balance and decrease low back pain. Often chiropractors will treat a patient for a period of time prior to use of heel lifts as the apparent initial leg length inequality may be related to the low back pain condition and will improve as muscle tension improves with treatment and return to normal activity and function. Orthotics are also used by chiropractors with some patients, including those with low back pain. Changes in the arches of the foot or the motion of the foot with gait may alter the biomechanics of a patient's lower body, thus affecting the pelvis and low back. Goals of having a patient wear orthotics may include providing stability to the arches, decreasing pronation of the ankle, or improving the motion of the ankle and foot during gait.

Mobilization Therapy

In addition to HVLA spinal manipulation, chiropractors often employ other types of mobilization therapy. Spinal mobilization consists of application of light force to the spinal joints within the passive range of motion but does not involve any thrust movements. Passive range of motion can be used to improve joint mobility, increase circulation, and decrease soft tissue extensibility issues.

Flexion-Distraction

Flexion-distraction is a form of therapy used by some chiropractors that passively puts the patient's lumbar spine into alternating flexion and extension. This passive motion is believed to improve joint motion, decrease soft tissue tightness, and improve the circulation of nutrients within the intervertebral discs of the spine. This method of treatment is often used in patients with low back pain when the intervertebral disc is the suspected pain-generating tissue. In this technique, the patient lies prone (face down) on a special table that is hinged in the middle, which allows the chiropractor to move the table and combine passive, controlled flexion and distraction mobilization to the spine.

Ultrasound

Therapeutic ultrasound is used to treat low back pain during the acute phase. This therapy is believed to deliver heat to deeper structures of the low back than heat packs alone. The goals of ultrasound are similar to heat therapy through decreasing pain perception, improving circulation, speeding healing, and allowing tight tissues to stretch.

Exercise Therapy

Therapeutic Exercise

Many chiropractors use functional muscle testing to determine the quantity, quality, and coordination of muscular contractions during common movements. When a particular problem with muscle contraction is detected, therapeutic exercises targeting a specific muscle or group of muscles may be prescribed to address this movement issue.

Rehabilitation/Stabilization Exercises

The low back does not only require movement; it also requires stability. If a patient has an instability in a joint or region of the low back or lower limbs, other areas of the body react to that instability by attempting to provide stability through an alternate mechanism. This adaptation can lead to altered movement patterns, abnormal muscular balance, and pain. Rehabilitative exercises are often used to attempt to strengthen areas to provide the patient a normal mechanism of stability.

Activities of Daily Living Modifications

Chiropractors are concerned with keeping patients active and maintaining as close to normal activities of daily living as possible. In acute low back pain, modifications to activities of daily living may need to be made to allow the patient to avoid further injury or to allow healing. Addressing inappropriate modifications to the performance of activities of daily living that patients come up with on their own is also an important function of chiropractors.

Evidence of Effectiveness

Spinal manipulation combined with exercise is a common intervention used by chiropractors to treat patients with back pain. A large body of research now exists related to the treatment of back pain.[14] Often chiropractors combine spinal manipulation with other physical modalities and exercise to offer patients the best possible outcomes with respect to pain.

One study found that significantly greater improvement for acute mechanical low back pain (of 16 weeks or less) was achieved with spinal manipulation therapy compared with usual medical care.[15] Patients receiving usual medical care did not have as positive outcomes and were prescribed higher rates of opioid pain medication, for which there is only minimal evidence of effectiveness. Interestingly, patients in the usual medical care group received a high rate (60%) of potentially inappropriate or ineffective treatment, such as bed rest, X-rays, and back support.[15]

Sometimes patients with low back pain are comanaged by chiropractors and medical doctors. One study found that spinal manipulation in conjunction with medical care offers significant advantages for decreasing pain and improving physical function when compared with standard care alone for young adults with low back pain.[16]

In addition to being effective in the alleviation of symptoms related to back pain, chiropractic care has also been shown to be cost-effective. A systematic review of the cost-effectiveness of various care approaches for low back pain demonstrated that spinal manipulation therapy, interdisciplinary rehabilitation, exercise, acupuncture, or cognitive therapy all were cost-effective, while no evidence was found in support of yoga or relaxation techniques.[17] This review also found that care from a general practitioner did not appear to be cost-effective considering that adding spinal manipulation and exercise along with behavioral counseling and education/advice were more cost-effective than usual care from a general practitioner alone.

Another systematic review found "some economic advantage of manual therapy relative to other interventions used for the management of musculoskeletal conditions, indicating that some manual therapy techniques may be more cost-effective than usual general practitioner care, spinal stabilization, general practitioner advice, advice to remain active, or brief pain management for improving low back and shoulder pain/disability."[18]Another review also found that spinal manipulation, either alone or combined with other treatments, was cost-effective.[19] Keeney recently demonstrated that patients with occupational spinal injuries who visited a surgeon first were significantly more likely to receive spinal surgery (42.7%) than those whose first visit was with a musculoskeletal clinician, such as a chiropractor (1.5%).[20] Certainly surgeries are necessary for some patients with spinal injuries, but this study points out the need for accurate triage and diagnosis followed by appropriate care.

Chiropractors are currently not licensed to prescribe drugs in the vast majority of the United States and throughout the world. In the United

States, opioid prescription for low back pain has increased, and opioids are now the most commonly prescribed drug class. More than half of regular opioid users report back pain.[21] Opioid pain medication may have a role in severe back pain, primarily for short-term use, but there is growing concern over the increasing use of opioid pain medication for mechanical back pain. Complications of opioid use include addiction and overdose-related mortality. Use of guidelines-based application of chiropractic care may cut down on the need for patients to use opioids for management of back pain.

The effectiveness of chiropractic care for back pain has been demonstrated in clinical outcomes and cost. Further inclusion of chiropractic care in the future treatment of patients with back pain is likely considering the changing focus of health care reimbursement. As reimbursement models move toward a focus on outcomes, interprofessional collaboration with chiropractors and other health care providers in the treatment of back pain seems inevitable.

Conclusion

Chiropractors have an important role in providing conservative, non-drug interventions in the management of low back pain. Low back pain is a common and costly problem that leads to disability in some patients. Chiropractors offer an array of conservative management strategies that include spinal manipulation therapy or chiropractic adjustments, adjunctive therapies, and exercise and lifestyle recommendations with an emphasis on improvement of movement and function. The use of chiropractic care for low back pain has been demonstrated to be safe and effective.

References

1. Ma VY, Chan L, Carruthers KJ. Incidence, prevalence, costs, and impact on disability of common conditions requiring rehabilitation in the United States: stroke, spinal cord injury, traumatic brain injury, multiple sclerosis, osteoarthritis, rheumatoid arthritis, limb loss, and back pain. *Arch Phys Med Rehabil.* 2014;95(5):986–995 e981.

2. Froud R, Patterson S, Eldridge S, et al. A systematic review and meta-synthesis of the impact of low back pain on people's lives. *BMC Musculoskelet Disord.* 2014;15:50.

3. Dunn KM, Hestbaek L, Cassidy JD. Low back pain across the life course. *Best Prac Res Clin Rheumatol.* 2013;27(5):591–600.

4. Kelly GA, Blake C, Power CK, O'Keeffe D, Fullen BM. The association between chronic low back pain and sleep: a systematic review. *Clin J Pain.* 2011;27(2):169–181.

5. Paulis WD, Silva S, Koes BW, van Middelkoop M. Overweight and obesity are associated with musculoskeletal complaints as early as childhood: a systematic review. *Obes Rev.* 2014;15(1):52–67.

6. Shiri R, Karppinen J, Leino-Arjas P, Solovieva S, Viikari-Juntura E. The association between smoking and low back pain: a meta-analysis. *Am J Med.* 2010;123(1):87 e87–35.

7. Waters TR, Dick RB. Evidence of health risks associated with prolonged standing at work and intervention effectiveness. *Rehabil Nurs.* 2015;40(3):148–165.

8. Shiri R, Karppinen J, Leino-Arjas P, Solovieva S, Viikari-Juntura E. The association between obesity and low back pain: a meta-analysis. *Am J Epidemiol.* 2010;171(2):135–154.

9. Leerar PJ, Boissonnault W, Domholdt E, Roddey T. Documentation of red flags by physical therapists for patients with low back pain. *J Man Manip Ther.* 2007;15(1):42–49.

10. Srinivas SV, Deyo RA, Berger ZD. Application of "less is more" to low back pain. *Arch Intern Med.* 2012;172(13):1016–1020.

11. National Board of Chiropractic Examiners. *Practice Analysis of Chiropractic 2015.* Greeley, CO: National Board of Chiropractic Examiners; 2015.

12. Millan M, Leboeuf-Yde C, Budgell B, Amorim MA. The effect of spinal manipulative therapy on experimentally induced pain: a systematic literature review. *Chiropr Man Therap.* 2012;20(1):26.

13. Cherkin DC, Sherman KJ, Balderson BH, et al. Effect of mindfulness-based stress reduction vs cognitive behavioral therapy or usual care on back pain and functional limitations in adults with chronic low back pain: a randomized clinical trial. *JAMA.* 2016;315(12):1240–1249.

14. Clar C, Tsertsvadze A, Court R, Hundt GL, Clarke A, Sutcliffe P. Clinical effectiveness of manual therapy for the management of musculoskeletal and non-musculoskeletal conditions: systematic review and update of UK evidence report. *Chiropr Man Therap.* 2014;22(1):12.

15. Bishop PB, Quon JA, Fisher CG, Dvorak MF. The Chiropractic Hospital-based Interventions Research Outcomes (CHIRO) study: a randomized controlled trial on the effectiveness of clinical practice guidelines in the medical and chiropractic management of patients with acute mechanical low back pain. *Spine J.* 2010;10(12):1055–1064.

16. Goertz CM, Long CR, Hondras MA, et al. Adding chiropractic manipulative therapy to standard medical care for patients with acute low back pain: results of a pragmatic randomized comparative effectiveness study. *Spine (Phila Pa 1976).* 2013;38(8):627–634.

17. Lin CW, Haas M, Maher CG, Machado LA, van Tulder MW. Cost-effectiveness of guideline-endorsed treatments for low back pain: a systematic review. *Eur Spine J.* 2011;20(7):1024–1038.

18. Tsertsvadze A, Clar C, Court R, Clarke A, Mistry H, Sutcliffe P. Cost-effectiveness of manual therapy for the management of musculoskeletal conditions: a systematic review and narrative synthesis of evidence from randomized controlled trials. *J Manipulative Physiol Ther.* 2014;37(6):343–362.

19. Michaleff ZA, Lin CW, Maher CG, van Tulder MW. Spinal manipulation epidemiology: systematic review of cost effectiveness studies. *J Electromyogr Kinesiol.* 2012;22(5):655–662.

20. Keeney BJ, Fulton-Kehoe D, Turner JA, Wickizer TM, Chan KC, Franklin GM. Early predictors of lumbar spine surgery after occupational back injury: results from a prospective study of workers in Washington State. *Spine (Phila Pa 1976).* 2013;38(11):953–964.

21. Deyo RA, Von Korff M, Duhrkoop D. Opioids for low back pain. *BMJ.* 2015;350:g6380.

CHAPTER EIGHT

The Chiropractic Approach to Neck Conditions, Headaches, and Temporomandibular Joint Conditions

William J. Lauretti, DC

A Chiropractic Approach to Neck Pain

There is good reason that "pain in the neck" is a common phrase for a frustrating problem that just won't go away. Even though most cases of neck pain are not caused by a potentially fatal disease process, many people live with chronic, long-standing pain that can seriously impact their ability to enjoy a productive life. Chronic, long-standing neck pain is a major cause of significant disability worldwide. In the 2010 Global Burden of Disease Study,[1] neck pain ranked fourth highest in terms of disability as measured by years lived with disability, and 21st in terms of the overall disability burden out of all 291 conditions studied.

Neck pain and headache are the second and third most common reason after low back pain for patients to seek care from chiropractors. Millions of chiropractic visits per year are performed for treatment of these complaints. This chapter will discuss the evidence-based chiropractic approach to neck pain and related conditions, such as cervical radiculopathy, headaches, and jaw pain.

Searching for a Cause

In rare cases, neck pain can be a sign of a serious condition, such as a fractured bone, cancer, circulatory disease, or rheumatic disease. Neck pain can even be an initial symptom of a heart attack. The first step for a doctor of chiropractic when seeing a new case of neck pain is to exclude potentially serious causes from the list of possible causes by screening for red flags—indications from the patient's history or exam findings that further follow-up is required to explore possible serious causes. Potential red flags for neck pain patients include a history of a significant trauma, history of osteoporosis, endocrine disease, recent unexplained weight loss or malaise, history of cancer, high fever, nonmechanical pain pattern, loss of consciousness or confusion, or neck pain that is new and unlike any previously experienced (*see Chapter 6*).

The majority of new cases of neck pain seen in the chiropractor's office are not due to an ominous disease process. Instead, the pain is often the result of a mild to moderate injury. Muscular tension, emotional stress, and poor posture are common causes of neck pain in patients without a history of recent injury. Degenerative arthritis of the spinal joints, often identified on cervical spine X-ray, is commonly blamed for causing neck pain in older patients. However, the relationship between degenerative arthritis and chronic neck pain is controversial. Arthritic changes in the spine are an extremely common effect of aging. On the basis of radiologic findings, 90 percent of men older than 50 years and 90 percent of women older than 60 years have evidence of degenerative changes in the cervical spine. While many of these older patients do have neck pain, many with significant arthritic changes visible on X-ray have no pain. In general, the nature and extent of spinal arthritis has a very poor correlation with the presence of spinal pain.

Another commonly cited cause of neck pain is degenerative changes to the discs located between the cervical vertebrae. Like joint degeneration, cervical disc degeneration is also a common effect of aging, sometimes referred to as "the gray hair of the spine." While injuries to the discs, particularly disc herniations, can be a cause of neck pain and cervical radiculopathy, the causal relationship between age-appropriate disc degeneration and chronic pain is unclear.

In the experience of most practicing chiropractors, the majority of patients seen with neck pain have joints in the cervical spine that are stiffer than normal and not able to move freely. Traditionally, chiropractors have referred to these abnormally stiff and misaligned joints as "vertebral subluxations." These stiff joints often cause the muscles that control their movements to be chronically stressed, developing painful, hyperirritable nodules in the muscle fibers called myofascial trigger points. In turn, the tight, sore muscles limit movement in the region, leading to increased joint stiffness and further muscular tightness, eventually setting up a vicious cycle of chronic pain. Chiropractors commonly evaluate for these joint and muscle dysfunctions by performing an assessment using careful manual palpation and functional tests of the spine.

If abnormally stiff joints are found, the preferred treatment includes high-velocity, low-amplitude (HVLA) *spinal manipulation.* In these manipulations, the doctor manually applies a very quick (high-velocity) but very shallow (low-amplitude) movement to a patient's abnormally stiff joints to restore normal pain-free motion. Other techniques may include slower manual mobilization techniques or methods that use a hand-held spring-loaded instrument to move joints with high speed and minimal force in a particular direction. The preferred treatment for the tight muscles often accompanying these stiff joints can be any one of various forms of soft tissue massage, stretching, or exercise. Most patients will also benefit from ergonomic and/or healthy lifestyle advice and a program of home exercise instruction, which are also usually included in the treatment approach taken by most chiropractors.

Regardless of its specific cause, neck pain—particularly pain that is chronic in nature—needs to be viewed in the context of how it affects the life of the patient. Like most other functional musculoskeletal pain conditions, chronic neck pain is a biopsychosocial condition. After the initial pain-generating structural and/or neurophysiological (biological) injury occurs, the nature of the patient's psychological and social response to that pain often has a major role to play in how soon the pain resolves and whether or not it becomes a chronic, long-standing condition. High-quality care for these patients must also consider the psychological issues that can perpetuate chronic pain. These negative beliefs can include a perception that routine physical activities need to be avoided because of a fear they will cause permanent damage, establishing a passive strategy for coping with pain and psychological depression. Social issues should also be addressed, such as encouraging the patient to seek appropriate emotional support from family and friends. The potential for secondary gain from an unresolved painful condition (such as in a case going through litigation) can actually hinder rapid recovery and is an issue that must be recognized and addressed with the patient's best interests at heart.

Neck Pain from Whiplash

One specific source of neck pain that is often considered separately in the research literature is pain that results from *whiplash associated disorders* (WAD). Whiplash is a neck injury due to forceful, rapid, back-and-forth movement of the neck, like the cracking of a whip. These injuries most often result when a stopped or slow-moving vehicle is struck from behind by a faster-moving vehicle. When a stopped vehicle is struck from behind, the stationary vehicle is suddenly accelerated forward while the occupant's head remains still, causing a backward motion of the head relative to the neck and body (hyperextension). The backward hyperextension is limited by the headrest of the car seat and/or the contraction of muscles in the front of the neck, causing the head to suddenly whip forward (hyperflexion). In some cases, this rapid backward and forward motion of the neck can be repeated numerous times. In addition to neck pain and stiffness, WAD often includes symptoms such as headaches, back pain, and jaw pain, and abnormal sensations such as burning, dizziness, or symptoms of concussion.

Effective chiropractic treatment for whiplash is similar to the treatment for neck pain from other causes and can include manipulation, mobilization, massage, and exercise. In addition, the early stages of care should reduce any inflammation by using cold packs and might address any instability by short-term use of braces or neck collars. Long-term use of braces should be discouraged since it has been found to increase the probability of poor recovery.

For many years, conventional belief was that whiplash injuries without any broken bones should resolve completely in four to six weeks, and patients with unresolved symptoms after this time were sometimes accused of engaging in fraud or of being hypochondriac. However, there is evidence that chronic pain after a whiplash injury is a real phenomenon and has an organic basis. Slow-healing whiplash injuries may result from microfractures to the cervical vertebrae, poorly healing ligaments and tendons due to poor blood supply to those tissues, subtle damage to the cervical discs, or chronic myofascial trigger points that develop in the cervical muscles. If painful inputs to the nervous system persist, the body may develop faulty movement patterns and poor coordination of muscular movement, slowing the normal healing process.

Another myth about whiplash is that collisions that occur at a relatively low velocity can't lead to significant injury of the occupants. In reality, there is little evidence that the severity of occupant injury is related to the extent of vehicle damage in low-speed impacts, and even a low-speed impact that results in minimal vehicle damage can transfer a significant amount of energy to the occupants and lead to injury. Most modern passenger vehicles can withstand impacts of up to 8 to 12 mph without sustaining significant property damage, while the risk for injury for many individuals is quite high even below this range.

While chronic pain after a whiplash injury is rarely the result of intentional deception by the patient or the patient's hypochondriasis, the biopsychosocial aspects of the condition need to be considered in an effective treatment plan. A thoughtful, conservative approach is the key to effective management of whiplash injuries. In the absence of red flags in the patient's history and presentation, it is unlikely that further extensive diagnostic testing will yield any clinically useful information. The treating doctor should encourage the patient to remain active, avoiding iatrogenic (doctor-created) disability, clinical depression, and unnecessary work absences. Encouraging the patient to perform specific exercises can increase mobility and give the patient confidence that activity will not cause any catastrophic damage. The best doctors won't invalidate the effect that pain can have on their patient's life, but they also won't make pain and disability the focus of treatment—instead, restoring function and independence should be the goal.

Cervical Radiculopathy

Cervical radiculopathy is any process that causes irritation, compression, or dysfunction of one or more of the cervical nerve roots. A spinal nerve root is the initial segment of one of the spinal nerves as it leaves the spinal cord and travels to the peripheral parts of the body. The eight pairs of cervical nerve roots emerge from the spinal cord and pass between each of the cervical vertebrae.

Cervical radiculopathy is commonly caused by inflammation of the nerve root from an injury. Other common causes include physical compression of the nerve root resulting from bony spurs forming around the vertebrae due to cervical degenerative bony changes or from a herniation of the discs between the cervical vertebrae. Because the cervical discs tend to dry out and become more fibrous with age, cervical herniated discs rarely occur in people beyond middle age.

The major symptoms of cervical radiculopathy, sometimes referred to as a "pinched nerve," include pain and numbness in the upper back, shoulders, arms, or hands, which are the regions innervated by the peripheral nerves that originate from the cervical nerve roots. Signs of more severe nerve damage may include true weakness or true loss of sensation in the hands or arms. Mild to moderate cases can often be successfully treated with nonsurgical, conservative care, but if signs of true nerve damage appear, a surgical approach should be considered.

The first step in chiropractic management of cervical radiculopathy is to determine which nerve is being compressed and where the physical pressure is occurring. Advanced diagnostic imaging, such as magnetic resonance imaging and electrical nerve conduction studies, may be useful in making a specific diagnosis. Since radiculopathy can rarely worsen to the point that permanent nerve damage occurs, the risks and benefits of various treatment options should be discussed

---

Box 8.1

Case Report: Chiropractic Treatment of Cervical Radiculopathy

Nick* was a 37-year-old man with neck pain and stiffness and pain and "tingling" that occasionally radiated into the right upper arm, forearm, and right index finger. An MRI examination of the cervical spine showed a moderate disc protrusion (herniated disc) between the fifth and sixth cervical vertebrae that was pinching the right nerve root.

Nick had previously seen his primary care physician. He was referred to an orthopedic surgeon who recommended cervical spine surgery. Even though his primary care physician agreed with the surgical recommendations, Nick was very opposed to surgery because a family member had had a very poor outcome after having a similar neck surgery. Nick decided to try treatment from a chiropractor before agreeing to spinal surgery.

After a thorough history and examination, the chiropractor discussed his findings with Nick and made him aware of the potential risks and benefits of various treatment options. Nick agreed to the chiropractor's treatment plan, which included heat and electrical stimulation and deep tissue massage to relax the spasms in his neck muscles. The treatment also included judicious high-velocity, low-amplitude manipulation of the cervical spine in the region surrounding the disc herniation. After his first treatment, Nick reported significant improvement in the neck and arm pain. Nick was given home exercises and advised to continue normal activities as much as his pain would allow. After five additional visits over the next two weeks, Nick's pain was completely resolved and he succeeded in avoiding a potentially risky spinal surgery.

*Names and minor details of this case have been changed to protect patient confidentiality.

with the patient, and the patient's informed consent is necessary before beginning care.

One immediate goal of conservative treatment is to manage the patient's pain. This can be done without medications by using electrical therapies such as transcutaneous electrical nerve stimulation (TENS), heat, ice, or topical creams. If the patient is comanaged with a medical physician, it may be appropriate to include nonsteroidal anti-inflammatory drugs, an epidural steroid injection, or, in carefully selected patients, short-term use of narcotics. Effective pain management is an important first step toward gaining patients' confidence and keeping them committed to a nonsurgical approach. Some patients whose pain is not well managed come to believe that surgery will definitely "fix" their problem, but they seldom appreciate the risks involved with cervical spine surgery and how limited the evidence is for its long-term effectiveness in many cases of mild to moderate radiculopathy.

Most cases of radiculopathy will respond well to conservative chiropractic care that includes traction, soft tissue massage, mobilization, and exercise. Carefully applied HVLA manipulation to the involved spinal region is not necessarily contraindicated and is often helpful to restore proper spinal motion. Patients should be closely monitored, and if a patient develops true motor weakness or loss of sensation in the upper extremities or signs of spinal cord pressure, including loss of bowel or bladder control, timely referral for a surgical consultation is necessary to avoid potentially permanent nerve damage.

Evidence Review: Treatments for Neck Pain and Cervical Radiculopathy

Compared to other treatment approaches for musculoskeletal neck pain, the conservative treatments commonly used in chiropractic practice—spinal manipulation, soft tissue massage, exercise, ergonomic advice, and physical modalities—have moderately strong evidence of safety and effectiveness.

The practice of *evidence-based health care* requires integrating individual clinical expertise with the values of the patient and the best available external clinical evidence from systematic research. The least reliable form of evidence is anecdotal. Since there are so many variables from one case to another, a story of one particular patient's success or failure from a particular treatment has very limited usefulness when choosing the most effective treatment for another patient. A more reliable form of evidence is a *randomized controlled trial* (RCT), which seeks to eliminate as many variables as possible to more accurately examine the efficacy of the specific treatment being investigated. The best form of evidence is a *systematic review* of numerous RCTs, in which the quality of the RCTs reviewed are assessed, and the results of numerous RCTs are considered in order to draw conclusions about the evidence basis of a particular treatment option.

The Cochrane Collaboration is one of the most widely respected organizations that perform systematic reviews of clinical treatments. This global, nonprofit, independent network of researchers and health care professionals seeks to gather and summarize the best evidence from research to make better informed choices about treatment possible. Many experts in evidence-based health care consider these *Cochrane Reviews of Evidence* as being among the best and most comprehensive tools for judging the relative effectiveness of clinical treatments in a scientifically sound manner.

One Cochrane review from 2015 compared manipulation and mobilization for neck pain against an inactive control or another active treatment.[2] Among its conclusions was that cervical manipulation for acute or subacute neck pain was more effective than varied combinations of analgesics, muscle relaxants, and nonsteroidal anti-inflammatory drugs for improving pain and function at up to long-term follow-up. However, the review also noted that many studies of neck pain treatments are not of high quality, so choosing the best treatment is still uncertain.

Another Cochrane review from 2011 looked at many types of conservative treatments for whiplash.[3] It concluded that "clearly effective treatments are not supported at this time for the treatment of acute, subacute or chronic symptoms of whiplash associated disorders" due to the lack of high-quality clinical studies, and it was unable to make any specific recommendations due to lack of evidence.

Another Cochrane review examined the effectiveness of patient education for adults with four types of neck pain: pain associated with whiplash, mechanical neck pain, mechanical neck pain with radiculopathy, or cervicogenic headache.[4] The authors concluded that there is no strong evidence for the effectiveness of educational interventions in treating any of these neck disorders.

Still another Cochrane review that looked at the effectiveness of cervical traction for neck pain with and without cervical radiculopathy also had ambiguous finings, concluding that there was no evidence from high-quality randomized controlled trials "that clearly supports or refutes" the use of traction for individuals with chronic neck disorders.[5]

The evidence for the best treatment for cervical radiculopathy is unclear even when considering more invasive and risky treatments. A Cochrane review that looked at surgical treatment for radiculopathy due to spinal degenerative arthritis found some short-term advantage to surgery but little or no difference in the long term.[6] The authors concluded, "It is unclear whether the short-term risks of surgery are offset by long-term benefits."

There is little evidence for the effectiveness of commonly used medications for neck pain. Cochrane has not published a review of this topic, likely due to the dearth of randomized controlled trials. One review performed by the Bone and Joint Decade in 2008 concluded there was "not enough evidence to make a determination" regarding the effectiveness of nonsteroidal anti-inflammatory drugs (NSAIDs) and other commonly used drugs in the treatment of neck pain whether or not it was associated with whiplash, neck pain with radiculopathy, and cervicogenic headache.[7]

Even though nonsteroidal anti-inflammatory drugs are probably the most commonly prescribed medication for neck pain, few studies have been done on their effectiveness for these conditions. One might gain some perspective from the findings of one review of the effectiveness of NSAIDs in the treatment of chronic low back pain, since both conditions are forms of musculoskeletal spinal pain. A Cochrane review found that NSAIDs reduced pain and disability in people with chronic low back pain only very slightly compared to placebo.[8] The differences were extremely small, with NSAIDs improving pain intensity by only 3.3 points on a 100-point scale for pain intensity. They also found no significant difference in effectiveness between different types of NSAID.

In contrast to these unimpressive findings for most commonly used medical treatments for neck conditions, one evidence-based clinical guideline document published in 2014 concluded that moderately strong recommendations could be made for the treatment of acute neck pain using manipulation and mobilization in combination with other modalities, and strong recommendations were made for the treatment of chronic neck pain with manipulation, manual therapy, and exercise in combination with other modalities.[9]

Using Evidence in Practice

Although the desire to practice evidence-based health care is a worthy goal, the reality is that for many conditions the evidence for any of the commonly used treatment options is often incomplete, inconclusive, or even contradictory. This is particularly true of musculoskeletal pain conditions. The good news is that progress is being made. No convincing "winner" has emerged between all the various therapies used to treat neck conditions. Every neck pain patient is unique, and individual responses to therapy are difficult to predict. The "Holy Grail" of spinal care will be the ability to truly individualize care—to predict what specific therapy will work best for each patient. The best hope for doing so seems to lie in being able to identify which specific tissues are generating the pain in a specific patient: Is it the disc, the joints, the muscles, the nerves, or something else? One current trend in the research community is an effort to develop "clinical prediction rules." These are algorithms that, depending on a patient's specific clinical presentation, will lead to a specific treatment plan. While some recent studies suggest we are tantalizingly close to advancing toward the objective of individualized therapy, it is a goal that is clearly still a long way away.[10]

Meanwhile, what should a health care provider do in the face of uncertainty? The best approach is one that is patient centered (not lesion centered or treatment centered), safe, responsible, rational, based on the biopsychosocial model, and based on the best available evidence even if it is not definitive. The typical chiropractic conservative management of neck conditions, which is based on treatments that have been shown to be safe and effective, including manipulation, mobilization, massage, and minimal use of medications, seems to be a good place to start. Combining that low-tech, high-touch care with an approach that empowers patients with positive messages minimizing disability and encouraging rapid return to normal activities is state-of-the-art practice in a field where no one treatment—especially more invasive, expensive, and risky treatments—has been shown to be definitively superior.

A Chiropractic Approach to Headaches

Headaches are among the most common disorders in advanced societies. Worldwide, half to three-quarters of adults aged 18–65 years have had at least one significant headache in the last year and, among those individuals, 30 percent or more have reported migraine. Not only is headache painful, it is also disabling. In the Global Burden of Disease Study, updated in 2013, migraine on its own was found to be the sixth-highest cause worldwide of years lost due to disability.[1] Headache disorders collectively were third highest.

Most surveys show that treatment for headache disorders is among the leading reasons patients visit doctors of chiropractic. There is also a significant amount of evidence that demonstrates chiropractic treatments are effective for a variety of headache disorders.

Types of Headache Disorders

The first challenge facing any clinician caring for a patient with headaches is to determine whether the headache is primary or secondary in nature.[11] *Primary headaches* are benign, recurrent headaches *not caused by underlying disease* or structural problems. Primary headaches are typically not dangerous, even though they may cause significant daily pain and disability. *Secondary headaches* are caused by an underlying disease or structural condition. Secondary headaches can be dangerous if caused by a condition such as an infection, head injury, vascular disorder, brain bleed, or tumor. Or, secondary headaches can be relatively harmless if caused by a benign underlying disorder in structures such as the cervical spine or jaw joint. Certain red flags or warning signs can indicate that a secondary headache may be dangerous. These can be remembered by the acronym "SSNOOP":

- *Systemic symptoms,* such as fever or weight loss
- *Secondary risk factors,* such as HIV or cancer
- *Neurologic symptoms* or signs, such as confusion or impaired alertness
- *Onset:* sudden, abrupt onset of a severe headache can be an ominous sign of an intracranial bleed
- *Older:* the onset of a new type of headache, particularly in a middle-age or older patient, suggests a serious cause, such as a tumor or vascular disorder
- *Previous headache history:* the onset of a new type of headache "unlike any other" in the patient's past experience suggests a serious underlying condition

Primary Headaches

About 90 percent of headaches are primary headaches. The major types of primary headaches doctors of chiropractic are likely to treat include migraine headaches and tension-type headaches.

Migraine headaches

Migraine headaches typically have moderate to severe "throbbing" pain on one side of the head that is severe enough to prohibit normal activities. Migraine headaches are also often accompanied by photophobia (sensitivity to light) and phonophobia (sensitivity to sound). Nausea and/or vomiting are also common during a migraine attack. In one subcategory of migraine called *migraine with aura*, the headache is preceded by visual disturbances (such as seeing flickering lights or experiencing temporary loss of vision) or other unusual sensory disturbances, such as experiencing "tingling" sensations in the head or body.

Tension-type headaches

Tension-type headaches typically have mild to moderate pain on both sides of the head that is often described as "tightening" in nature. The pain may inhibit activity, but often patients can continue normal activities even with the pain. Photophobia, phonophobia, and nausea are rare with tension-type headaches.

The exact cause of most primary headaches remains poorly understood. Formerly, migraines were thought to be caused by abnormal constriction and dilation of the blood vessels in the brain, although that hypothesis is no longer generally accepted. Currently, most specialists think migraines are due to a primary problem with the nerves in the brain. Tension-type headaches are believed to be caused by abnormal activation of the peripheral nerves in the neck and head muscles.

Secondary Headaches

Many types of secondary headaches are caused by a potentially serious health condition and should be referred out of the chiropractor's office to appropriate specialty care. Some secondary headaches are not caused by an ominous condition but rather by underlying conditions that are within the chiropractor's scope of expertise to treat. One example is *cervicogenic headache*. These are headaches caused by referred pain—a structural or functional disorder in the neck is perceived as pain in the head. Diagnosing cervicogenic headache can be challenging and requires a careful history and examination. For example, a past history of neck injury, or the ability to reproduce the headache by manual pressure on tender neck muscles or by certain movements of the cervical spine, suggests a headache of cervicogenic origin. In some cases, cervicogenic headaches share many of the same characteristics as migraine and tension headaches, and making an accurate differential diagnosis between them can be challenging.

Another common type of secondary headache that can be helped by chiropractic treatment is *medication overuse headache*. Ironically, these headaches are commonly caused by the misuse of over-the-counter (OTC) medications taken to manage mild to moderate headaches. Many OTC headache remedies contain an analgesic (such as acetaminophen) or a

---

Box 8.2

The Headache "Spectrum"

For many patients who suffer from chronic headaches, it can be difficult to place their headache type into a single clear category. These patients often have headaches that have some characteristics of several types of headache, or vary on a day-to-day basis. For example, Elizabeth* is a 30-year-old paralegal who gets some type of headache nearly every day. Usually they increase over the course of a workday after cradling the phone between her ear and left shoulder at her job. These headaches tend to be in the back of the head on the left. By the end of the workweek, her headache is nearly constant, and she describes it as "tightening" in nature. About once per month (usually around her menstrual period) she can have one or more severe throbbing headaches that are preceded by her seeing flashing lights and are accompanied by nausea, photophobia, and phonophobia.

Elizabeth has characteristics of cervicogenic headaches (her common, almost daily headache from poor ergonomics), tension headaches (at the end of the workweek), and migraine headaches (around her menstrual period). A chiropractor treated her twice weekly for four weeks with cervical spine manipulation, massage, and stretching exercises and she reported no longer having daily headaches. She still had less severe headaches at the end of each workweek. Advice to use a telephone headset at work and discussing sources of emotional stress reduced these weekly headaches further. She occasionally still had a migraine-type headache with her menstrual period, although these headaches tended to be less frequent and severe. She continued to get chiropractic treatments on an as-needed basis, about one visit every month or two when her headaches began to return.

*Names and minor details of this case have been changed to protect patient confidentiality.

---

nonsteroidal anti-inflammatory (such as ibuprofen) together with caffeine. Besides being a stimulant, caffeine acts as a mild pain reliever and can amplify the analgesic effect of other pain relievers. Many people with chronic headaches frequently take these OTC headache remedies to manage their headaches, but when they stop taking the medications they suffer caffeine withdrawal symptoms—the most common of which is increased headaches. This starts a vicious circle where in effect the patient continues taking the caffeine-containing medication to avoid the headaches that result from discontinuing the caffeine-containing medication.

Daily use of many NSAIDs can also result in headaches. In many cases, chiropractic treatment can effectively treat the primary headache as effectively as the OTC medication, and at the very least the chiropractic emphasis on drug-free treatments can help to break this vicious cycle.

Although patients with headaches are often placed into seemingly distinct categories, the reality in clinical practice is that many patients with chronic headaches have characteristics of various headache types and sometimes defy distinct categorization. In many cases, their headaches have components of the different types of headache during different times. Also, it should be noted that the distinctions between different headaches is somewhat arbitrary and has only limited evidence for its validity. However, the categorization does have some usefulness for determining which treatments will be most effective.

Chiropractic Care for Headaches

After excluding a potentially serious underlying condition, chiropractic care for headache usually focuses on dysfunctions of the muscles and joints of the cervical spine. Chronic muscular tightness can be addressed by soft tissue massage, stretching exercises, electrical therapies, and heat. Restricted mobility in the cervical spine that is a frequent cause of cervicogenic headache often contributes to tension-type headaches and migraines as well and can be treated with spinal manipulation, mobilization, and/or exercises.

There is evidence that chiropractic treatments, including cervical manipulation and soft tissue massage, are most effective for patients who have the characteristics of cervicogenic headaches. Tension-type headache, which is sometimes difficult to differentiate from cervicogenic headache, also often responds well to a chiropractic approach. Migraine headaches can be more challenging to manage conservatively and often are best comanaged with a medical approach. Certain foods and lifestyles are commonly recognized as migraine triggers. These include highly processed foods, foods containing monosodium glutamate (MSG), red wines, smoked cheeses, caffeine, alcohol, tobacco use, and lack of sleep.

Conservative management of headaches should include a comprehensive look at all aspects of a patient's lifestyle, including diet, exercise, and psychosocial factors. Patients with chronic headaches often benefit from interdisciplinary care from a variety of health care professionals. Chiropractors managing patients with tension-type headaches should consider adding stress-reduction therapy and referral to a mental health professional or massage practitioner. Intramuscular injections of short-acting analgesics and/or Botulinum toxin is a common but controversial medical treatment. Chiropractors managing patients with migraine should consider referral to a neurologist for possible medication change (or discontinuation); referral to a nutritionist or acupuncturist may also be helpful.

Evidence Basis of Conservative Treatment of Headaches

Similar to the evidence for neck pain, there is no clearly superior treatment for most types of headache, and the science on the topic continues to evolve. One Cochrane review found multiple sessions of cervical manipulation to be more effective than massage in improving pain and function at short/intermediate-term follow-up.[2]

For chronic tension-type headache, one review found physiotherapy and manual therapy (including massage and mobilization) to be equal in efficacy to prophylactic use of tricyclic antidepressant medication, a commonly prescribed treatment.[12]

Temporomandibular Joint Disorders

Treatment of pain that is associated with the *temporomandibular joint* (TMJ) is a condition most chiropractors treat, although on a somewhat infrequent basis. Many members of the public suffering from jaw disorders usually don't consider a doctor of chiropractic as a primary source of care, but many chiropractors take a special interest in jaw conditions and see a significant number of patients with these problems in their practices.

The TMJ is one of the most active joints in the body, moving over 2,000 times per day in its functions of mastication (chewing), swallowing, respiration, and speech. In many ways, the jaw is functionally part of the neck. A complex biomechanical relationship exists between two of the body's most complicated joint systems—the TMJ and the upper cervical joint complex. Together, these joints and the muscles surrounding them stabilize the cervical spine and the head and brace the region against injuries. A change in cervical spine posture, head posture, or mandibular rest position can create a change in the others. Both of these systems should be evaluated in a patient complaining of chronic head and neck pain, and TMJ dysfunction is often an underlying issue in patients with chronic or poorly responding headache and/or neck pain.

The craniomandibular complex is composed of the temporomandibular joint, the teeth, and the muscles of mastication, which move the jaw joint. Chronic pain in the jaw is often caused by myofascial trigger point activity in the muscles of mastication, bruxism (grinding teeth), temporomandibular joint disorders, or dislocation of the fibrous disc in the joint.

Chiropractic management of TMJ disorders focuses on evaluating the function of the muscles and mobility of the joint. Soft tissue therapies to the muscles controlling the motion of the joint, both intrinsic muscles (that only control the TMJ) and extrinsic muscles (that also control the motions of the neck) has evidence of effectiveness. Abnormalities in the quality of the joint motion can be addressed using low-force mobilizing techniques, precision instruments that apply a fast but low-force impulse to the joint, or by gentle manual manipulation. It is also important to address perpetuating factors, such as diet, posture, sleep habits, and emotional stress. Finally, working in close cooperation with a dental professional to address potential malocclusion of the teeth and other dental issues is often beneficial to the patient.

Evidence Basis of TMJ Treatments

There is little evidence for the effectiveness of any treatment for TMJ disorders, and clinical treatment is often empirical in nature. One randomized controlled trial of 93 patients with chronic TMJ pain found significant improvement in resting, opening, and clenching pain and patient-reported improvement among patients who received chiropractic intraoral myofascial therapies.[13] This improvement lasted even at six months and one-year follow-ups after treatment had ended.

The previously referenced Cochrane review of manipulation and mobilization for neck pain found low evidence that for chronic cervicogenic headache with temporomandibular joint dysfunction, multiple sessions of TMJ manual therapy may be more effective than cervical mobilization alone in improving pain/function at immediate- and intermediate-term follow-up.[2]

A variety of different medications are used to treat pain due to temporomandibular disorders. These include simple analgesics, NSAIDs, and corticosteroids. Muscle relaxant medications, such as benzodiazepines, are sometimes used to reduce tension and spasm in the muscles affected by TMJ disorders. In addition, some antidepressants are used in low doses. One Cochrane review found that there was not enough evidence to decide which medicines are effective in reducing pain due to chronic temporomandibular disorders.[14]

Results from TMJ surgeries are often varied and unpredictable and have a very low evidence basis. At the time of this writing (May 2016) the Cochrane Review of Arthroscopic Surgery for Temporomandibular

Disorders had been withdrawn and is undergoing revision; however, an earlier version found there was no evidence the procedure was more effective than no treatment. Unless there is a clear surgical indication, such as trauma or osseous pathology, patients should be encouraged to pursue all other alternatives before considering TMJ surgery.

Conclusions

This chapter has presented the current evidence for frequently used treatment approaches for a number of common cervical spine–related conditions, such as neck pain, whiplash, cervical radiculopathy, headaches, and temporomandibular disorders. Compared to many more expensive and invasive options, the various conservative treatment options commonly used by doctors of chiropractic for these conditions have a very good track record of effectiveness and safety. *For more in-depth discussion of the relative safety of these treatments, see Chapter 6.*

References

1. Hoy D, March L, Woolf A, et al. The global burden of neck pain: estimates from the Global Burden of Disease 2010 study. *Ann Rheum Dis.* 2014;73:1309–1315.

2. Gross A, Langevin P, Burnie SJ, et al. Manipulation and mobilisation for neck pain contrasted against an inactive control or another active treatment. *Cochrane Database Syst Rev.* 2015;9:CD004249.

3. Verhagen AP, Scholten-Peeters GG, vanWijngaarden S, et al. Conservative treatments for whiplash. *Cochrane Database Syst Rev.* 2007;2:CD003338.

4. Gross A, Forget M, St George K, et al. Patient education for neck pain. *Cochrane Database Syst Rev.* 2012;3:CD005106.

5. Graham N, Gross A, Goldsmith CH, et al. Mechanical traction for neck pain with or without radiculopathy. *Cochrane Database Syst Rev.* 2008;3:CD006408.

6. Nikolaidis I, Fouyas IP, Sandercock PAG, Statham PF. Surgery for cervical radiculopathy or myelopathy. *Cochrane Database Syst Rev.* 2010;1:CD001466.

7. Hurwitz EL, Carragee EJ, van der Velde G, et al. Treatment of neck pain: noninvasive interventions: results of the Bone and Joint Decade 2000–2010 Task Force on Neck Pain and Its Associated Disorders. *Spine.* 2008;33:4Suppl;S123–152.

8. Enthoven WTM, Roelofs PDDM, Deyo RA, et al. Non-steroidal anti-inflammatory drugs for chronic low back pain. *Cochrane Database Syst Rev.* 2016;2:CD012087.

9. Bryans R, Decina P, Descarreaux M, et al. Evidence-based guidelines for the chiropractic treatment of adults with neck pain. *J Manipulative Physiol Ther.* 2014;37:42–63.

10. Murphy D, Hurwitz E. Application of a diagnosis-based clinical decision guide in patients with neck pain. *Chiropr Man Therap.* 2011;19:19.

11. International Headache Society. HIS Classification ICHD-II. http://ihs-classification.org/en/02_klassifikation/. Accessed May 1, 2016.

12. Chaibi A, Russell MB. Manual therapies for primary chronic headaches: a systematic review of randomized controlled trials. *J Headache Pain.* 2014;15:67.

13. Kalamir A, Bonello R, Graham P, et al. Intraoral myofascial therapy for chronic myogenoustemporomandibular disorder: a randomized controlled trial. *J Manipulative Physiol Ther.* 2010;18(3):139–146.

14. Mujakperuo HR, Watson M, Morrison R, Macfarlane TV. Pharmacological interventions for pain in patients with temporomandibular disorders. *Cochrane Database Syst Rev.* 2010;10:CD004715.

CHAPTER NINE

The Chiropractic Approach to the Extremities

Dennis M. J. Homack, DC, MS, CCSP; and Emily Canfield, DC, MS, ATC

Introduction

From the beginning, the founder of chiropractic, D. D. Palmer, recognized the importance of addressing all of the articulations (joints) of the human body. Managing conditions of the spine and limbs is dependent on the clinician's understanding of how forces are transmitted from one body part to the other through what is referred to as the kinetic chain. The "kinetic chain" is the concept that joints that are connected by bones and soft tissue can affect one another as movement takes place. For example, during walking, the joints of the foot, ankle, knee, hip, and low back all affect one another. This concept is most profound in the lower extremity (the leg and foot), as improper biomechanics in one area, such as the foot, can have a dramatic effect throughout the body.

Chiropractors perform treatments to all of the joints of the extremities (arms and legs),[1-4] as complaints ranging from low back pain, neck pain, and even headaches can actually be related to a problem originating in the extremities. Secondly, others will present with primary complaints involving the shoulders, elbows, wrists, hips, knees, ankles, and feet.

Even when the primary complaint may be pain or discomfort in the extremity, the chiropractor will look for the possibility that the primary cause originates in the viscera, muscle, nerves, or joints of the axial skeleton or other soft tissue within the body.[3] In either case, a thorough evaluation beginning with a detailed patient history and investigation as to the precipitating factors of the complaint and continuing with a physical, neurologic, and orthopedic evaluation will help to determine a definitive diagnosis and course of action for management.

This chapter discusses some of the most common conditions of the legs and arms that chiropractors manage. The treatments described represent typical approaches for each condition but may differ in practice in order to meet the individual patient's needs.

The Lower Extremity

The Structure of the Foot

The 26 bones of the foot are divided into three zones:

1. The forefoot contains the majority of the bones. These are the phalanges (toes) and the metatarsal bones (bones connecting to those of the toes).
2. The midfoot includes the navicular cuboid and the medial, intermediate, and lateral cuneiforms (irregularly shaped bones).
3. The hind foot includes the calcaneus (the heel bone) and talus (which sits between the leg and the heel bone).

As with all joints, the bones are held together mostly by ligaments. Muscles connect to bones (and other tissue) through similar tissue called tendons. The function of skeletal structures is very dependent on the health and integrity of these structures. The three zones of the foot need to be able to function independently, sequentially, and in unison. The connection of the leg to the foot (or more precisely, the talus) is the mortise joint, named for its unusual shape. This allows the ankle to move up and down. The joint between the talus and calcaneus is the subtalar joint. It allows the ankle to rock to the inside (inversion) and outside (eversion).

These joints are particularly important in sending information to parts of the brain to let it know its position in space, known as *proprioception*. The ankle sends a large amount of proprioceptive input to the cerebellum and is therefore considered very important for maintaining upright balance and posture.

Arches of the foot

There are three arches of the foot: the medial longitudinal, lateral longitudinal, and the transverse. The medial longitudinal arch is the most important as well as the highest and longest. The bones that make it up are the calcaneus, talus, navicular, medial, and intermediate cuneiforms and first and second metatarsals. While the shape of the talus does help to sustain the arch, it may be more helpful to consider the navicular as the "keystone" of the medial longitudinal arch. Its unique shape and position near the top of the arch create a mechanical wedge that helps to prevent the arch from collapsing.

Reduction of arch height is considered a predisposing risk factor for musculoskeletal injuries.[5] Maintenance of the medial longitudinal arch is highly dependent on the soft tissue structures, including the ligaments and musculature of the foot and ankle. The portion of this arch most likely to yield from overpressure is the joint between the talus and the navicular. This is supported by the plantar calcaneal navicular ligament, otherwise known as the "spring ligament." When pressure is applied, this ligament is quite elastic, giving it the ability to restore itself to its original shape when the disturbing force is removed, as long as the ligament itself is healthy.

The tibialis anterior and the tibialis posterior muscles work synergistically (together) to support the medial longitudinal arch. These two muscles act to help roll the ankle in (invert) and to help support this arch by wrapping their tendon under the arch of the foot. With eversion (rolling the ankle out) ankle sprains, injury to these muscles or tendons can cause dysfunction that may overwhelm the structure of the spring ligament and injure the medial longitudinal arch.

The lateral longitudinal arch (the arch along the bottom of the foot from the heel to the base of the little toe) is lower and flatter than the medial arch. It is made up of the calcaneus (heel bone) and bones along the outside part of the foot. A bone in the middle of that arch, shaped somewhat like an ice cube, called the cuboid, is considered the "keystone" of the arch. When it is out of alignment or doesn't move the way it should, it can cause pain and discomfort in the side of the foot. One muscle on the side of the leg, the peroneus longus (also called fibularis longus), has a tendon that wraps underneath the cuboid to help lift up the lateral longitudinal arch. Another muscle close by, the peroneus (fibularis) brevis, inserts in the fifth metatarsal, the longer bone going to the little toe.

The transverse arch can really be thought of as two arches that combine across the foot from the inside to the outside of the foot. The first of these arches is best visualized at the articulation between the tarsals and metatarsals (between the mid and forefoot). The job of the keystone of this arch is shared between a small bone in the middle of the foot (the middle cuneiform) and the proximal head of the longer bone that reaches out to the toes (second metatarsal).

The second transverse arch, or anterior transverse arch, is across the distal metatarsal heads (often called the "balls of the feet"). This arch can be compromised by tight footwear and by continually walking on flat, rigid surfaces, such as hard floors and sidewalks. The combined transverse arches' functions are to allow the foot to adapt to uneven surfaces and help the other two arches absorb stress and shock.

Plantar vault

The three arches combine to make up the "plantar vault," a dome shape at the bottom of the foot. Evidence of this vault can be seen in most people (with healthy feet) when they walk along the sidewalk barefooted with wet feet, leaving footprints. The middle part of the foot does not usually touch the ground and leaves a dry spot. The plantar vaults can have a significant impact on the kinetic chain. They may affect the musculoskeletal system from the ankle all the way throughout the spine. The association of the kinetic chain is illustrated with the following example of how the loss of the medial longitudinal arch can affect the lower extremity, pelvis, and lumbar spine.

The doctor systematically observes each structure of a barefoot person standing upright, looking straight ahead. He notes that the right foot is turned outward more than the left. The right arch appears much flatter on the inside than the left. Observing from behind the person, the heel and large Achilles tendon (connecting the calf muscles to the heel) of the right foot look bent outward compared to the left. Because the bones of the foot are poorly aligned, the lower leg bones turn slightly inward, causing the leg to appear shorter on that side. Since the lower leg is turned in, the knee is turned in. This torsion (twisting or rotation) of the knee also causes the knee angle to increase in relation to the upper leg (femur). This angle is called the Q-angle and gets its name from the thigh muscle called the quadriceps. These changes cause great stress on the joints, ligaments, muscles, and even bones of the knee.

Thus it can be seen that the fallen arch changes the positioning of the ankle and knee bones. One might ask, how does that affect the rest of the body? For one, the internal rotation of the knee also causes internal rotation of the femur and hip joint. The muscles controlling the hip connect to the pelvis and points along all sides of the lower spine. Uneven tension on the hip muscles results in rotation of the vertebrae. Remember the increased ankle and knee angles? These changes in joint orientation cause the leg to be functionally shorter. That is different than structurally shorter, where a leg bone, for example, is actually a different length than the other side. Functional leg length differences are typically correctable.

The vertebrae have disks between them that hold them together and help protect the spine. On the back of the vertebrae, there are small joints called facets that help guide the motion of the vertebra. When these are injured, they can cause significant pain and discomfort (a "facet syndrome"). This most often happens on the side opposite to the flatter foot. In this way, we can see how pain in the low back on the left can be caused from a flat foot on the right. Of course, these are not the only changes that might occur, but low back pain is one of the more common results of this type of imbalance.

Conditions of the Foot, Ankle, and Toes

Analysis of the foot and ankle begins with a functional assessment done while watching the patient stand and walk, similar to the example previously described. Palpation often reveals tenderness at the point of injury. For many conditions of the lower extremity or, in fact, any condition related to biomechanical problems of the foot, many chiropractors use *orthotics*, specially made inserts for shoes, to help correct the positioning of the foot, combined with manual and other therapies, including corrective exercise.[6]

Understanding custom-made functional orthotics

There are many types and brands of orthotics on the market. An orthotic is a shoe insert that is designed to cushion, protect, or support the feet. Custom-made functional orthotics are superior to off-the-shelf types, as they are specifically designed for the patient's precise anatomy and activities. In general, there are three common methods that are considered accurate measures of the foot, all of which are volumetric (considering three dimensions as opposed to just width and length) in nature. Podiatrists often create a plaster slipper, or cast, with the ankle in a non-weight-bearing position. This is considered optimal for rigid orthotics, which are typically used when there are anatomically abnormal structures of the foot, such as club foot.

Crafting functional orthotics, the usual method among chiropractors, begins with taking precise volumetric measurements of the foot, either using a casting foam box for weight-bearing impressions or an imaging device such as a three-dimensional laser measuring scanner.

The key benefits of functional orthotics over other inserts are that they absorb and return energy in the foot during the gait cycle and that they allow the foot to move and bend in its normal motion during activities. They also prevent the foot from deforming too far, into what is known as the pathologic range. By reducing these stresses and improving function, they can be useful for preventing and managing a number of conditions caused or worsened by dysfunction of the foot.[6,7] It appears that they can improve athletic performance from running to golf as well as helping the patient get the most benefit from chiropractic adjustments and exercise.

Hallux valgus (bunion)

Bunions are characterized by lateral deviation (away from midline) of the big toe, thought to be aggravated by improperly fitting shoes that place stress on the first metatarsophalangeal joint. Other factors that increase this risk include genetic predisposition and stress applied to the toe as a result of long-standing pathologic pronation, joint inflammation related to high levels of uric acid (gout), or spraining of the nine ligaments that surround the first metatarsophalangeal joint, which is known as turf toe. Chiropractic treatment, including manipulation, certain exercises, and orthotics, may be helpful in slowing the progression of bunions and relieving pain. In some individuals, these measures may possibly prevent bunions in the first place.

Turf toe

Turf toe gets its name from injuries caused by playing football on artificial grass. Players often hyperextend the big toe and sprain the ligaments of that joint. Sitting upright with the knees bent less than 90 degrees and ankles crossed can put excessive weight through the big toe and cause similar injuries.

Chiropractic treatment includes reducing the inflammation with ice, cold laser therapy, or ultrasound. Adjusting and mobilizing the joints of the foot and toes can be effective. Splinting or taping the toe can help prevent reinjury. Teaching the patient about how to perform activities is also important.

Plantar fasciitis

Plantar fasciitis is also a common condition of the foot. The plantar fascia is a thick tissue that originates from the bottom of the heel and inserts into the bottom of all of the toes. This structure is very important. When we walk, the normally flexible foot must also provide a rigid base from which to propel ourselves with each step. This occurs as we transfer weight toward the toes and tension builds up in the fascia, causing what is known as the "windlass effect or mechanism." Essentially, plantar fascia tightens up, the arches increase in height, and the various bones of the foot "lock" together to protect the joints as we walk.

With injuries or stress over time, the fascia can become thickened and contracted, and the lack of elasticity can become painful with weight bearing. Symptoms often occur when individuals arise out of bed and take their first few steps, but the sharp pain associated with plantar fascia can continue throughout the day. The plantar fascia can become shortened during the course of the night for people who are tummy sleepers if the feet cannot hang over the edge of the mattress and are forced into a plantar flexed position (toes pointed). The same occurs for individuals who are back sleepers who use heavy blankets over the feet. The feet again are forced into a plantar flexed position and over time result in similar contraction of the plantar fascia.

The calf muscles, notably the gastrocnemius and soleus muscles, are also held in a short position and may resist lengthening upon standing first thing in the morning. Pain and discomfort may be experienced in the Achilles tendon attaching the gastrocnemius-soleus complex (calf muscles) to the calcaneus at the back of the heel.[8]

Addressing the musculature of the lower extremity

Early management of acute plantar fasciitis should begin by reducing the inflammation and controlling pain. Mobilizing and adjusting the joints of the foot helps restore normal motion and function of the three arches of the plantar vault and helps restore elasticity to the plantar fascia. Instrument-assisted soft tissue techniques are commonly used across the bottom of the foot and help break up adhesions that occur between layers of soft tissue.

Along with other stretching exercises, rolling a golf ball or tennis ball under the foot can give temporary relief. Rollers and other products, such as foot wheels, can also be useful. However, a simple, inexpensive home remedy of rolling a frozen bottle of water under the foot can reduce inflammation and be very comforting to most patients. Exercises intended to strengthen the muscles of the foot and restore dexterity can also be useful and may include manipulating small objects with the toes or crinkling newspaper with the foot and performing exercises to restore the arches of the foot.

Proper footwear that provides adequate support and stiffness to avoid overstretching the plantar fascia and the use of custom-made functional orthotics greatly reduce unnecessary stresses. Patient education is warranted as the patient should be aware of postural habits while sleeping and performing other activities that may overstretch the plantar fascia.

Tarsal tunnel syndrome

The tarsal tunnel is an area behind the medial malleolus (the bump on the inside of the leg just above the ankle). This anatomic tunnel, formed of ligaments, contains a nerve that sends branches to different parts of the foot (the posterior tibial nerve). Irritation to this area, such as occurs with ankle sprains or excessive pronation, can injure the ligaments covering the tunnel and put pressure on the nerve.

During evaluation of the patient, a chiropractor will stretch and stress the area and may tap over the region with a reflex hammer or with fingers in order to assess the sensitivity of the neural structures. Upon confirmation of a tarsal tunnel syndrome diagnosis, treatment may include chiropractic adjustments to the osseous structures associated with the foot and ankle, soft tissue treatment including instrument-assisted soft tissue techniques, and restoration of function through exercise and pain control.

An interesting subset of tarsal tunnel syndrome includes the involvement of the medial branch of the posterior tibial nerve. This branch innervates the bottom of the foot and can become irritated, causing numbness and tingling with running or walking. This particular neural entrapment is often termed "joggers foot" and along with other neural entrapments is commonly treated by reducing inflammation, treating the associated soft tissue, improving the biomechanics with adjusting and functional support, and patient education.

Ankle sprain

Manual therapy has been shown to be effective in managing ankle sprains.[1] The chiropractic approach to ankle sprains is generally twofold in nature. The first is management of the acute ankle sprain by reducing pain and inflammation and improving function and range of motion. The second approach is to manage the long-term effects of recovery and rehabilitation while taking steps to prevent reinjury.

The chiropractic approach to sprained ankles is the same as that of any other provider who treats sprains: In the acute stage, it follows "RICE"—rest, ice, compression and stabilization, and elevation. These reduce swelling, inflammation, and pain. Methods of cryotherapy go beyond ice packs, and some may recommend submersion of the injured ankle in a bucket of ice water. Ice water transmits more cold to the limb than ice alone, and the compressive qualities of the hydrostatic pressure of the water will help to push out edema.

The second approach manages the long-term effects of recovery and rehabilitation while taking steps to prevent reinjury. The specific activities the patient participates in and the equipment he or she uses, including shoes, running surfaces, and preparation, should also be investigated, particularly for those participating in athletics. Training regimens, daily walks, and even activities of daily living should be considered when developing a management plan.[9] Appropriate support from properly fitting footwear and the use of orthotics can be very helpful.[6] By understanding the factors that led to the injury, preventive measures can be introduced to reduce the likelihood of new injuries and even improve performance.

Ensuring proper healing of the ligaments can include mild stretching, manual or instrument-assisted soft tissue techniques, chiropractic adjustments, and non-weight-bearing exercises to restore range of motion and minimize deconditioning. Passive motion has been shown to have pain-reducing effects.[10] Chiropractic adjustments can be effective for restoring normal range of motion of the articulations within the ankle. Proper dorsiflexion is critical, for example, if one is to diminish the risk of lower-body and ankle injuries, particularly in at-risk athletes.[11]

Achilles tendon

The Achilles tendon is the largest tendon in the body and connects the powerful gastrocnemius and soleus muscles (calf muscles) to the posterior superior aspect of the calcaneus at the back of the heel. Contraction of the calf muscles causes plantar flexion of the foot and ankle (the foot points down), which is critical for normal gait and balance. It is the same action of the ankle as when people stand on their toes. Although other muscles, such as tibialis posterior and the fibularis brevis, also help to plantar flex the foot, the gastrocnemius-soleus complex performs the majority of this action, particularly during the toe-off phase of gait and when landing on the feet with jumping.

The thick Achilles tendon is most vulnerable approximately 2 to 6 cm from the insertion because of the forces of the powerful calf muscles focusing at that point. Damage to that area is further compounded by the poor blood supply, which results in slow healing. Complete tearing of the Achilles tendon is usually quite obvious, resulting in a dorsiflexed (foot up) position of the ankle when not bearing weight as well as absence of the tendon in the back of the ankle, combined with a muscular mass behind the upper part of the lower leg as the gastrocnemius and soleus muscles contract.

Partial tearing of the Achilles tendon may result in pain in the posterior aspect of the ankle, which needs to be differentiated from posterior ankle sprains or subluxation of the subtalar joint. The examiner will evaluate the tendon from its insertion superiorly in an attempt to find evidence of any scarring or tearing of the tendon or musculature.

As with most injuries, managing tendon injuries will depend on the severity of the injury. In the case of a complete rupture, referral to an orthopedic surgeon is appropriate. Incomplete tears or strains of the tendon can be managed by adding support, such as the use of an ankle orthoses (brace or support), to prevent additional stress. Addressing the musculature can be done with manual or instrument-assisted techniques with the aim of gradually increasing function of the plantar flexors.

Healing may take some time considering the nature of the tissues; however, reducing insult to the area by limiting certain activities and using higher-quality shoes with a stiffer sole and orthotics may also be recommended. Mobilization of the distal tibial fibular joint can increase range of motion of the ankle and can have a positive effect on the associated soft tissue.[12] Adjusting the ankle has been shown to reduce pain and improve function.[2]

Conditions of the Knee

The knee is the largest joint in the human body. The evolutionary development of the knee, allowing people to stand and walk upright, and the fact that it is a weight-bearing structure makes it particularly prone to injury. Although the knee is considered a large hinge joint, the knee also has a natural gliding element and rotational element. The rotational element is most notable at the last 20 degrees of extension as the tibia will externally rotate, allowing the knee to lock in extension, known as the screw home mechanism. This action stabilizes the knee by putting the ligaments of the knee under tension.

Anterior cruciate ligament and posterior cruciate ligament

The anterior cruciate ligament (ACL) and posterior cruciate ligament (PCL) of the knee are responsible for a significant amount of anterior to posterior stabilization and resistance to twisting motion of the tibia on the femur. Common mechanisms of injury to these ligaments involve many sporting activities, particularly contact sports. An impact from the lateral aspect of the knee can tear the ACL, medial collateral ligament (MCL), and medial meniscus. The medial meniscus is one of two structures (the other is the lateral meniscus) that are cartilage parts within the knee joint at the top end of the lower leg. These structures act to absorb stress and help guide motion of the knee.

This collection of tissue damage to the medial meniscus, ACL, and MCL is termed the "unhappy triad" and occurs with impacts from the side while the foot is planted. Rapid directional changes, such as those incurred playing court sports like tennis and basketball, make the ACL particularly prone to injuries. The PCL can be torn or sprained when the proximal lower leg (just below the knee) impacts the dashboard during a motor vehicle collision. Careful examination of the knee can determine the extent of the injuries regarding specific tissues and severity, but some cases may require special imaging, such as MRI. An accurate diagnosis is needed to determine whether chiropractic care can be useful or whether referral to an orthopedic surgeon is warranted.

Patellofemoral pain syndrome/chondromalacia patella

The patella (the knee cap) is a bone that helps protect the tendon of muscles in the front of the thigh (the quadriceps). The forces exerted by these strong muscles push the patella against the end of the femur, and at times the forces can be several times that of a person's entire body weight. The potential for injury is aggravated by postural abnormalities of the knee.

Patellofemoral pain syndrome (PFPS) is part of a condition that includes chondromalacia patella (or simply put, degeneration of the underside of the patella). It affects between 10 and 40 percent of the general population between ages 18 and 45 and is common in athletes, people in the military, and most people suffering obesity. Anterior knee pain, especially when going down stairs, is an extremely common symptom of chondromalacia patella.

Once inflammation is controlled with cold therapy or other treatments, general mobilization of the patella can be quite useful in restoring normal function. Instrument-assisted soft tissue manipulation applied to the structures surrounding the borders of the patella can help to remove areas of adhesion (scar formations).

To help maintain proper alignment of the patella and reduce symptoms, exercises to strengthen the vastus medialis obliquus muscle (the inner part of the front thigh muscles) is recommended to maintain proper alignment of the patella and reduce the level of lateral tracking. It can be found in the literature that the use of foot orthotics is nearly as beneficial as the use of mobilization, exercise, and soft tissue treatment in managing PFPS and chondromalacia patella.[13]

Osteoarthritis of the knee

Because the knee is such a large weight-bearing joint and is affected so significantly by forces of the foot and ankle, it is particularly vulnerable to arthritic changes over time. Common changes in the foot that cause an increase in internal rotation and lateral stress on the knee put a significant amount of stress on a structure called the medial tibial plateau, the widened end of the larger lower leg bone at the knee.

Sports injuries, wearing insufficient or unsupportive footwear, and carrying additional body weight add to the stress and likelihood of osteoarthritis (OA) and damage to the protective cartilaginous structures that line the surfaces of the knee joint. Determination of osteoarthritis can be made initially through observation, orthopedic examination, and palpation, but often X-rays will reveal the level of the degeneration. Addressing the knee early may prevent unnecessary pain and dysfunction later in life. Although total knee arthroplasty (replacement) is increasing in frequency, complications and continued pain are common results after surgery.

Total knee replacement (TKR) has become one of the most commonly performed procedures on people older than 45. Advances in technology and materials are making this a more attractive option for younger populations, but it is still a common procedure among older patients, even into their 90s.[14] While current technology and materials of the artificial knee have continued to improve, revision surgery is still often needed over time, and the life expectancy for a typical TKR is between 8 and 10 years with 15 years currently considered to be optimistic.[14] A better approach to replacing body parts would seem to be preventing the need in the first place.

The conservative approach to management of arthritic disease

The conservative approach initially is to reduce symptoms and improve function and the patient's ability to perform activities of daily living. Even with modest levels of arthritis, patients may experience relief of common symptoms of OA with manipulation of the knee joint as well as exercises designed to restore range of motion and improve function.

More symptomatic or acute phases of OA may require methods of pain control, such as interferential current, micro current, and other ancillary therapies. Many chiropractors will look toward the feet and may recommend the use of functional orthotics in order to improve posture via the mechanism of the kinetic chain. Nutritional supplements are often recommended to improve joint health.

Adhesive capsulitis of the knee

A condition often associated with osteoarthritis is adhesive capsulitis of the knee. The cause of this is the development of fibrous bands that adhere inside the capsule and joint surfaces due to inflammation and the typical disuse one might expect from someone experiencing pain in the knee. This condition presents with limitation of full extension and flexion of the knee and pain with standing and during gait. Examination will reveal the obvious limitations in motion, and the examiner will strive to rule out other conditions that may be limiting the proper function of the joint, such as deterioration of the cartilage, ends of the bone, or menisci.

Chiropractic treatment of adhesive capsulitis usually employs adjustments and mobilization to the knee joint. Initially, the adjustment procedure may be uncomfortable to some degree; however, the effectiveness of restoring proper motion of the joint can have a profound, immediate, and positive effect in function. Subsequent reduction of inflammation and exercises designed to improve range of motion will also be prescribed.

Patients should be reminded that although they may have had a significant improvement initially, they should resist the temptation to overuse the joint during the healing process. Once they feel good, patients often engage in many activities they have not been able to do for some time due to their injury and, of course, do too much. This is a common behavior that will likely delay overall recovery.

Meniscus

The medial and lateral menisci of the knee are disc-shaped structures between the end of the femur and the end of the tibia. These fibrous structures act as shock absorbers between the joint surfaces within the knee joint itself. While commonly associated with injuries such as forced lateral flexion or hyperextension, these tissues may deteriorate over time without outright injuries simply due to overuse and long-term undue stress.

The most common symptoms reported by patients suffering from meniscal tears are pain, popping, clicking, or locking of the knee. Orthopedic exams to identify meniscal tears attempt to reproduce these symptoms.

Conservative treatment of meniscal tears will typically begin with mobilizations designed to restore the meniscus into a flattened position when possible. Once the internal misalignment is minimized, reduction of activities and support from stabilizing knee braces may be prescribed. Care must be given to minimizing the deconditioning of the associated muscles of the knee, and therefore exercises may be prescribed. If symptoms persist or mobilization of the knee is not helpful, referral to an orthopedic surgeon is indicated.

Conditions of the Hip

The hip is a deep ball-and-socket weight-bearing joint. Cartilage covers the head of the femur (thigh bone) and the acetabulum (the socket in the pelvis), and the joint surface is expanded by a fibrous tissue called the labrum, which also serves to absorb some shock with activity. The thick fibrous capsule is made up of a number of ligaments that stabilize this fairly flexible joint. All of the ligaments of the hip restrict extension.

Osteoarthritis of the hip

An estimated 12 million people or more are affected with hip osteoarthritis in the United States, including 10 percent of men and 20 percent of women between the ages of 45 and 65 years. The likelihood increases over time, with as many as 80 percent showing X-ray evidence of OA over the age of 75 years.

Injury or long-term dysfunction and continued excessive stress (such as that produced by obesity) can cause premature degeneration of the hip joint. Conditions such as osteoporosis and other metabolic diseases significantly increase the likelihood of hip OA. Injury to the hip can refer pain to other areas of the body, such as the low back. Not coincidentally, total hip replacements in the United States are the second most common type of musculoskeletal surgical procedures after total knee replacement.

Assessment procedures commonly involve placing the hip in different positions and adding stress or overpressure in an attempt to elicit symptoms. Obtaining X-rays will help confirm the level of degeneration. Once a diagnosis of OA is made, a determination as to whether the patient is a candidate for chiropractic adjustments will be made. For many, the common approach to conservative management of arthritic pain in the hip begins with adjusting and general mobilization and exercises to increase strength and range of motion of the hip. Chiropractic treatment often begins from the ground up, involving the entire lower extremity kinetic chain. Behavior modification and patient education may also be warranted, and proper postural alignment beginning from the feet should also be addressed.

Snapping hip syndrome

Many people, particularly runners, will complain of popping or snapping at the hip. There are several common causes of snapping hip syndrome. Often the involved tissue is located at the location of the snapping. Pain and popping at the lateral hip is most often the result of iliotibial band syndrome. The iliotibial band is a thick, wide ligament-like structure that spans the side of the leg. It originates at the top of the pelvis (the ilium) and covers the muscles of the lateral thigh. It crosses the knee and inserts in a bump on the tibia called Gerdy's tubercle. A small muscle near the top of the iliotibial band (ITB) and inserting into the anterior aspect of it is the tensor fascia lata. This muscle helps to flex the hip and tighten the ITB for stability.

Contracture of the iliotibial band itself or spasm of the tensor fascia lata muscle can cause the band to snap over the greater trochanter of the femur. Treatment of iliotibial band syndrome often includes stretching and manual or instrument-assisted soft tissue techniques to restore the health of the tissue. Aggravating activities must be addressed, including postural faults and possible kinetic chain relationships, necessitating a look at the footwear and consideration of the use of orthotics.

Medial popping or clicking at the hip may be due to degenerative changes to the bone at the upper part of the hip socket (superior acetabular ridge) or other degenerative changes in the hip joint. X-rays and other imaging (such as magnetic resonance imaging) of the hip may be necessary to rule out these changes before considering the more likely cause of medial snapping hip syndrome, the iliopsoas muscle.

Often, due to postural changes or other muscular imbalance syndromes, the tendon of the iliopsoas muscle rubs tightly over the lesser trochanter of the hip, causing a snapping or popping within the hip. This relatively common occurrence is often found on the same side as whichever foot presents with the most severe level of pronation (a condition addressed earlier). This is understandable when considering the idea of the kinetic chain, as the hip itself will be internally rotated, making it more likely that the iliopsoas tendon will get in the way with flexion and extension of the hip during jogging or running gaits, and in some cases, even with walking. When this version of snapping hip syndrome occurs, the patient typically responds quickly to postural corrections and functional support of the feet (to correct the effects of pathologic pronation and asymmetry) in combination with appropriate stretching and strengthening of the iliopsoas muscle.

Another cause of snapping hip occurring on the medial (inside part) of the hip may be due to problems with the labrum of the hip. The labrum is a cartilage-based tissue that serves to protect and expand the hip socket (the acetabulum). In some cases, the labrum may develop a tag or outgrowth, which typically occurs on the inside aspect of the hip socket. With internal rotation flexion and adduction, popping and clicking can be felt by the patient deep within the medial side of the hip. Similar symptoms can also occur if the superior medial aspect of the labrum becomes torn, termed a "Bankart lesion" (which carries the same name as an inferior tear of the glenoid labrum in the shoulder).

The patient may benefit from adjusting the femoro-acetabular (hip) joint as well as performing exercises of the muscles associated with the hip. Although intended to reduce internal rotation for the treatment of chondromalacia and other tracking problems of the patella, a SERF (Stability through External Rotation of the Femur) strap may be useful to reduce the likelihood of continued irritation during the recovery and rehabilitation period.

Although tears of the labrum and growth tags associated with snapping hip syndrome can be managed, the patient may experience reoccurrences with activity and remissions with treatment throughout life. Confirmation of either labral tears or tags may be made using advanced imaging such as MRI, MR arthrography, or CT arthrography to determine the extent of injury. As with other conditions, patients who do not respond favorably to conservative treatment in a reasonable amount of time should be considered for referral to an orthopedic surgeon for consultation.

The Upper Extremity

Conditions of the Shoulder

The shoulder is a complex joint, and people frequently seek chiropractic care for conditions of the shoulder. The most common shoulder conditions are described below.

The rotator cuff

There are four muscles that make up the rotator cuff. These muscles are the supraspinatus, infraspinatus, subscapularis, and teres minor. The primary job of these muscles is to maintain proper alignment of the head of the humerus (arm) with the glenoid fossa of the scapula. The glenoid fossa is a very shallow socket on the scapula that connects the arm to the body. The term "fossa" means "shallow depression" or "hollowed-out region" and is used to describe a number of regions, particularly in different bones throughout the body. The gleno-humeral (shoulder) joint is very flexible, but the flexibility of this large joint makes it very vulnerable to injury. The fossa is covered by a somewhat circular-shaped fibrous structure called the labrum, which serves to cushion the joint and to expand the size of the joint surfaces. Labral injuries will be discussed later. Each of the four muscles have a different role to play but need to work together to ensure alignment.

The secondary actions of the rotator cuff muscles are to assist larger muscles, the primary movers, in initiating motion. While the rotator cuff muscles are always working to some degree, the primary movers take on the majority of the work of moving the arm.

Rotator cuff tears or injuries usually involve the supraspinatus muscle. This muscle sits at the top of the scapula near the top of the shoulder and under the clavicle where that bone attaches to the scapula (the acromio-clavicular, or AC, joint). The supraspinatus attaches to the arm in front of a groove that contains one of the two tendons of the powerful biceps brachii muscle. It is the only rotator cuff muscle to insert in the front of the groove (the other three attach behind the groove). Its position makes it particularly vulnerable to getting pinched, or "impinged" between the acromion of the scapula and a bump on the humerus called the lesser tubercle. The term "tubercle" simply means "bump" or "projection," and there are many in the body. This pinching may create pain when raising the arm, especially with internal rotation (turning the arm inward so the thumb points to the ground). This type of condition is called an "impingement syndrome."

Besides the impingement syndrome, or perhaps because of it, the supraspinatus muscle and tendon may partially or completely tear. Swelling in the space between the AC joint and the rib cage may aggravate symptoms. Posture and overgrowth of tissue can also shrink the limited space the muscle needs to function in. Poor form or improper exercise can put the supraspinatus, and by extension, the entire shoulder, at significant risk for injury.

When evaluating the rotator cuff musculature, the clinician will perform various strength and orthopedic tests to assess function and/or reproduce symptoms. Advanced imaging to visualize the soft tissue structures of the shoulder may be needed to determine the full extent of the injury and whether conservative treatment alone is likely to be helpful.

Adhesive capsulitis (frozen shoulder)

Overuse and inflammation can result in thickening of the shoulder joint capsule and restricted motion. When a type of scar tissue develops and adheres to various tissues (called adhesions), adhesive capsulitis is the result. Adhesive capsulitis tends to be progressive in nature, slowly reducing one's ability to raise the arm or reach to the side, as if the shoulder joint was frozen, hence the term "frozen shoulder."

Examination will reveal the obvious limitations in motion, and the examiner will strive to rule out other conditions that may be limiting the proper function of the joint, such as deterioration of the cartilage, damage to the ends of the bone, or dislocation. X-rays may be used to determine boney changes, and advanced imaging, such as MRI, may be used to determine the extent of the tissue buildup and damage.

Chiropractic treatment of adhesive capsulitis will focus on restoring motion through delivering chiropractic adjustments and mobilization of the gleno-humeral joint (shoulder joint). Initially, the adjustment procedure may be uncomfortable to some degree; however, the effectiveness of restoring proper motion of the joint can have a profound, immediate, and positive effect on function. Mobilizing the scapula on the back will be necessary for overall shoulder function. The surrounding muscles will need to be addressed to ensure they have not atrophied (decreased in size/weakened) from disuse and that they maintain proper function. Subsequent reduction of inflammation will be accomplished by using cold therapy and healing modalities, such as cold laser and ultrasound. Exercises designed to continue to improve range of motion and prevent the return of adhesions within the capsule will also be prescribed.

Bicipital tendinitis

The biceps brachii (biceps) is a muscle of the upper arm that crosses both the elbow joint and the gleno-humeral joint, or shoulder joint. It has three important jobs: it bends the elbow, it helps to raise the arm at the shoulder, and it is a strong supinator of the forearm. "Supination" means to turn the forearm so the palm of the hand is facing up. For example, if a right-handed person is tightening a screw with a screwdriver, the biceps does most of the work. It is also involved in grip strength, as it stabilizes the elbow when the muscles of the forearm going into the fingers (the flexors and extensors) are activated.

The biceps muscle gets its name from the fact that it splits from a combined muscle belly near the elbow into two separate muscle bellies near the shoulder, called the long head and the short head of the biceps. The long head has a long tendon that travels through a groove (the bicipital groove) in the front of the humerus (upper arm bone) and attaches to the top of the shoulder joint socket on the scapula (the glenoid fossa). The short head also attaches to the scapula, but at a projection that comes from the front of the scapula, called the coracoid process.

Traditionally, biceps tendinitis refers to an irritation of the tendon of the long head of biceps as it runs through the bicipital groove. A ligament normally keeps the tendon within the groove, and it can become inflamed or tear. In its early stages, the tendon becomes red and swollen. As tendinitis develops, the tendon sheath, a covering that lubricates and protects the ligament, can thicken. The tendon itself often thickens or grows larger and can even develop calcium deposits similar to bone. Pain is commonly felt in the front and top of the shoulder and is most notable when raising the arm or when lifting. The biceps tendon can rupture, causing pain and discomfort and disfigurement as the muscle contracts in an unusual way.

The biceps tendon crossing the front of the elbow can suffer from tendonitis as well. Pain is typically in the front of the arm into the elbow. This tendonitis may affect any of the various nerves that travel through the arm, sometimes resulting in symptoms that resemble carpal tunnel syndrome. Occasionally, this tendon can rupture, especially if tendonitis is not addressed or the muscle is overloaded. The result can cause the muscle to contract, balling up in the upper part of the arm.

Muscle tests and orthopedic tests are needed to determine the nature of the injury. Advanced imaging, such as MRI, can be very useful in determining the severity of injury in specific tissues involved. If the symptoms include numbness, tingling, pain, or weakness into the forearm and hand, electro diagnosis can be used to determine the damage to the nerves in the area.

Chiropractic care will vary depending on the specific nature and severity of the injury. The goals will be to control inflammation with cold therapy or another modality. Reducing further insult may include temporary immobilization with an arm sling. More often, restoration of function as early as possible is the goal. Adjusting the surrounding joints can help reduce the work the biceps has to do to move the arm. Using manual or instrument-assisted techniques to address the soft tissues will stimulate healing and improve function. Cold laser therapy or ultrasound can encourage nutrient-delivering blood flow and promote cellular regeneration, speeding healing. Rehabilitative exercises will typically start very slowly and increase over time as healing continues. Patients must be educated as to what activities caused the issues in the first place so they can be modified or avoided.

Conditions of the Arm

Although less frequently than for the shoulder, many people also seek chiropractic care for musculoskeletal complaints related to the arm.

Lateral and medial epicondylitis

The deep and superficial extensors of the hand and wrist originate above the elbow at the lateral epicondyle. These are the muscles that straighten the fingers and allow us to raise our hands off of a tabletop. Frequently referred to as "tennis elbow," lateral epicondylitis is a progressive overuse injury that can interfere with normal hand and elbow function. Symptoms become intensified when making a fist or using a power grip of the hand as the extensors of the forearm are engaged to stabilize the wrist.

Assessing the mechanism of injury is particularly helpful when dealing with lateral elbow pain due to the possibility of injury to the radial head, particularly during falls on an outstretched hand. Orthopedic evaluation will include exams designed to stress the proximal muscles and common tendon. Grip strength will be diminished and can be evaluated using a hand grip dynamometer. Any improved strength or decrease in pain when reperforming the grip strength test is a positive finding, indicating lateral epicondylitis.

Medial epicondylitis, also known as "golfer's elbow," is a similar condition involving the tendons of the flexor digitorum superficialis on the medial aspect of the elbow. While the flexor digitorum profundus, a deep intrinsic muscle of the forearm, inserts into the proximal ulna distal to the elbow, flexor digitorum superficialis crosses the joint line to insert into the medial epicondyle. Orthopedic exams designed to confirm medial epicondylitis include resisted flexion of the wrist and elbow. Deep palpation can isolate the specific location of micro tears, as this will elicit localized pain.

There is some evidence that chiropractic treatment for these conditions is helpful in speeding recovery.[3] Treatment of both medial and lateral epicondylitis are treated similarly, targeting the respective involved tissues. Acute phases may include cryotherapy, such as ice, and rest, perhaps with additional bracing until the patient can tolerate treatment. Once the level of pain and inflammation have been sufficiently controlled, the practitioner may use manual soft tissue techniques, such as cross friction or deep tissue massage, or instrument-assisted soft tissue techniques directed at the muscles and tendons to encourage healing. Ancillary modalities, such as cold laser therapy or ultrasound, may also be used to encourage the healing process.

Using a strap orthosis (a type of brace) just below the elbow joint can be very effective by creating a temporary insertion of the tendons on the forearm. The use of this device may be recommended during the healing phase and may also be recommended for use during activities that provoke the conditions, such as playing golf or tennis. Osseous adjustments and mobilization to the elbow and wrist have also been shown to be useful.[3] Rehabilitative exercises are designed to strengthen the extensors and flexors with both concentric and eccentric contractions. Ergonomic considerations, particularly for the use of computer keyboards, can also help to reduce some of the stress of the elbow.

Besides adjustive procedures and soft tissue treatments, associated musculature and fascial inflammation can be addressed and controlled with ancillary methods, such as cryotherapy, ultrasound, and/or cold laser therapy. Nutritional support and dietary recommendations are frequently also recommended as part of a comprehensive treatment plan and protocol designed to prevent further injury.

Conditions of the Hand, Wrist, and Fingers

Each hand has 27 bones. The five phalanges (fingers) have a total of 14 bones (the thumb has one less than the rest). Connecting the five fingers to the wrist are the longer bones called metacarpals. There are eight small, irregularly shaped bones of the wrist called carpal bones. The carpal bones and their attachments to the end of the forearm are connected by a complex group of tissue mostly made of a network of ligaments

Carpal tunnel syndrome

Carpal tunnel syndrome (CTS) is the most commonly diagnosed repetitive stress injury in the human body. Repetitive stress occurs when a person does the same type of movement repeatedly over an extended period of time, usually as part of his or her job, such as typing at a computer. Symptoms of CTS include pain, numbness, and tingling from the palm of the hand into the thumb, index, and middle fingers and may extend to the lateral aspect of the ring finger. Symptoms can increase while sleeping, and the patient will often shake out the hand in an attempt to diminish the discomfort.

The effectiveness of treatments for carpal tunnel most certainly depends on the severity and progression of the condition. Surgery for carpal tunnel syndrome is among the most rapidly growing surgeries performed in the United States. While it is beyond the scope of this discussion to talk about the outcomes of surgical procedures in general, it is worth mentioning that, as with all surgeries, risks of complications, including continued carpal tunnel symptoms, are somewhat common. Recommendation for surgery is often made for those with more severe or complicated cases. Outcomes after surgery can be improved by cotreating the patient with chiropractic care to maximize function and encourage proper healing during recovery.

"Ergonomics" refers to how people interact in the environment and is closely related to posture and the use of tools and how we do things. Simply, improperly performing our usual activities of daily living and violating basic ergonomic principles can contribute to the repetitive stress associated with CTS. Using computer keyboards can put the wrist at angles that increase the pressure on the median nerve that travels through the carpal tunnel. Resting the wrists on a keyboard or computer desk can add to the compression. Using gripping tools and opening jars are similar activities. Cold temperatures, vibration, and long periods of repeated stress are all aggravating factors. In most cases, ergonomic changes during the performance of activities such as keyboarding or using gripping tools along with nocturnal use of wrist braces designed to hold the wrist in a neutral, slightly extended position have been shown to be very beneficial. To reduce the pressure exerted upon the median nerve, manual stretching or instrument-assisted soft tissue work can be applied to the transverse carpal ligament and the wrist retinaculum. The retinaculum is a tough ligament-like structure that wraps around some joints, such as the ankle, knee, elbow, and, of course, the wrist. Its thick, fairly inflexible nature helps stabilize the joint, but in certain conditions, most notably CTS, it can contribute pressure to the underlying structures.

Proper diet can help reduce body fat that encloses entrapment sites, and improved nutrition may help to restore neural structures' ability to resist injury and encourage healing. Again, ancillary procedures, such as ultrasound and cold laser therapy, may be used to reduce inflammation and speed healing. Cryotherapy, ranging from ice packs to ice bath submersion, will also reduce inflammation and pain transmission and allow the patient to better perform rehabilitative exercises in a pain-free environment. Stretching of the muscles of the forearm and both wrist and finger extensors and flexors can also be useful. Using soft tissue techniques may be helpful in some cases.[3] Patient education is paramount, as most treatments will have little effect if patients continue to perform the same activities that caused a problem in the first place. If patients do not respond well to conservative care, surgical consideration is appropriate.

Trigger finger

Thickening or a nodular growth on the flexor tendons in or near the digits may cause pain and locking of the fingers during flexion and extension. This snapping action is referred to as trigger finger and may affect any of the fingers in the hand but occurs most often in the fourth digit or ring finger.

Direct physical injury can create scar tissue, and long-term repetitive stress, such as the action of gripping or using a digit to pull a trigger (the origination of the term), is a primary cause, but this condition is also frequently found in individuals diagnosed with early stages of diabetes or prediabetes. This thickening will glide under the small strips of the ligamentous tissue called the retinaculum, which hold the tendons near boney structures of the hand. While the diagnosis of trigger finger is usually easy due to the very obvious physical signs, the clinician will typically look for systemic causes, such as diabetes and nutritional deficiencies. Daily activities and ergonomics must also be considered.

Chiropractic management will involve soft tissue techniques, such as instrument-assisted work focusing on releasing the tension on the retinaculum fibers and any deformity developing within the tendon itself. Focusing a tool and rubbing in precise directions will help break down scar tissue and encourage healthy tissue to take its place. Modalities such as ultrasound or cold laser therapy can help reduce inflammation and stimulate healing. Chiropractic adjustments to the joints of the hand, wrist, and fingers can ensure proper motion that requires less force from the muscles that move them. Attention to strengthening, stretching, and improving function of the muscles of the hand and forearm will also take stress off of the tendon at the point of the trigger-finger lesion.

References

1. Southerst D, Yu H, Randhawa K, et al. The effectiveness of manual therapy for the management of musculoskeletal disorders of the upper and lower extremities: a systematic review by the Ontario Protocol for Traffic Injury Management (OPTIMa) Collaboration. *Chiropr Man Therap.* 2015;23:30.

2. Brantingham JW, Bonnefin D, Perle SM, et al. Manipulative therapy for lower extremity conditions: update of a literature review. *J Manipulative Physiol Ther.* 2012;35(2):127–166.

3. Brantingham JW, Cassa TK, Bonnefin D, et al. Manipulative and multimodal therapy for upper extremity and temporomandibular disorders: a systematic review. *J Manipulative Physiol Ther.* 2013;36(3):143–201.

4. Clar C, Tsertsvadze A, Court R, Hundt GL, Clarke A, Sutcliffe P. Clinical effectiveness of manual therapy for the management of musculoskeletal and non-musculoskeletal conditions: systematic review and update of UK evidence report. *Chiropr Man Therap.* 2014;22(1):12.

5. Wilken J, Rao S, Saltzman C, Yack HJ. The effect of arch height on kinematic coupling during walking. *Clin Biomech (Bristol, Avon).* 2011; 26(3):318–323.

6. Williams AE, Hill LA, Nester CJ. Foot orthoses for the management of low back pain: a qualitative approach capturing the patient's perspective. *J Foot Ankle Res.* 2013;6:17.

7. Berbrayer D, Fredericson M. Update on evidence-based treatments for plantar fasciopathy. *PM R.* 2014;6(2):159–169.

8. Rosenbaum AJ, DiPreta JA, Misener D. Plantar heel pain. *Med Clin North Am.* 2014;98(2):339–352.

9. Verhagen EA, Bay K. Optimising ankle sprain prevention: a critical review and practical appraisal of the literature. *Br J Sports Med.* 2010;44(15):1082–1088.

10. Yeo HK, Wright A. Hypoalgesic effect of a passive accessory mobilisation technique in patients with lateral ankle pain. *Man Ther.* 2011;16(4):373–377.

11. Bell DR, Oates DC, Clark MA, Padua DA. Two- and 3-dimensional knee valgus are reduced after an exercise intervention in young adults with demonstrable valgus during squatting. *J Athl Training.* 2013;48(4):442–449.

12. Fujii M, Suzuki D, Uchiyama E, et al. Does distal tibiofibular joint mobilization decrease limitation of ankle dorsiflexion? *Man Ther.* 2010;15(1):117–121.

13. Brantingham JW, Globe G, Pollard H, Hicks M, Korporaal C, Hoskins W. Manipulative therapy for lower extremity conditions: expansion of literature review. *J Manipulative Physiol Ther.* 2009;32(1):53–71.

14. Karuppiah SV, Banaszkiewicz PA, Ledingham WM. The mortality, morbidity and cost benefits of elective total knee arthroplasty in the nonagenarian population. *Int Orthop.* 2008;32(3):339–343.

CHAPTER TEN

The Chiropractic Approach to Other Musculoskeletal Conditions

Clinton Daniels, DC, MS, DAAPM

Introduction

The purpose of this chapter is to focus on musculoskeletal conditions that complicate syndromes of the spine and extremities. Tendinitis and tendinopathy, osteoarthritis, myofascial pain syndrome, and fibromyalgia are maladies that affect millions of individuals worldwide. They may present as primary pain generators or contribute to other neuromusculoskeletal disorders.

Tendinitis and Tendinopathy

Chiropractors frequently manage tendon injuries and can provide a number of conservative treatment options. A tendon is a tough band of fibrous connective tissue that connects muscle to bone. "Tendinitis" and "tendinopathy" are terms that have long been used to describe tendon injuries. "Tendinitis" has devolved into an archaic term over the previous couple of decades. The designation "tendinitis" implies a presence of inflammation within the injured tendon. However, research studies have failed to confirm the presence of inflammation in chronically injured tendons.[1] As a result of these studies, "tendinopathy" and "tendinosis" have become more readily accepted labels. "Tendinopathy" simply refers to disease of a tendon without reference to cause, and "tendinosis" is chronic tendon injury with damage present at the cellular level.

The anatomy of healthy tendons consists of a firm, dense, parallel-fibered, collagenous connective tissue containing an organized fibrillar matrix of a white, glistening nature.

The presence of tendinopathy causes specific modifications to the tendon, making it appear gray or yellow-brown and morphing it to be soft, crumbly, fragile, and thin. Under light microscopy, tendinopathy looks like disrupted collagen fibers that are thinner than normal. The chemical composition of the tendon changes in such a way that more cells die than normal, accompanied by neovascularization (new blood vessels) associated with tendon repair.[2] The cellular changes noted under the microscope indicate tissue remodeling due to repetitive insult.

Tendinopathy injuries tend to be caused by chronic overuse, also known as cumulative trauma disorders, through job- or sport-related activities. Chronic disability from tendinopathies is associated with a substantially higher health care costs and costs to society. One study reported that the most frequent upper limb diagnosis submitted to workers' compensation boards is tendonitis and that people suffer with tendonitis for an average of eight months before filing a claim. A substantial portion of workers with cumulative trauma disorders, such as tendinopathies, had additional injury-related absences after their initial return to work.[3] In sports medicine, tendon injuries account for 30 to 50 percent of all injuries.

Biomechanical risk factors for tendinopathies have been studied exhaustively. Tendons are designed to sustain great tensile (stretching capability) loads. Tendon changes in tendinopathy are consistent with adaptive responses to shear or compression forces. Repetition and forceful exertion, typical of work and sport activities, are implicated in the development of tendinopathies. When mechanical loads exceed the strength of the tendon, it can become progressively damaged. This results in the breakdown of collagen fibers and induces progressive internal tendon degeneration, partial tears, and even ruptures. Tendon injuries typically progress slowly with no obvious mechanism of injury. Pain often follows a history of recent increased activity and is described as a localized "sharp" or "stabbing" sensation. In early phases, the symptoms commonly diminish after a warm-up period and later the patient may feel a "dull" or "achy" type of pain after activity or even at rest.

Increased age and obesity may increase personal risk of developing tendinopathy. The aging tendon has a lower metabolic rate, progressive decrease in elasticity and tensile strength, and a decreasing tendon blood flow. Disability due to tendinopathy is complex and multifactorial. Psychosomatic problems, previous injury, and depression are all risk factors for tendon injuries.

Common upper extremity tendinopathies include rotator cuff impingement, lateral epicondylitis (tennis elbow), medial epicondylitis (golfer's elbow), and De Quervain's tenosynovitis (wrist). Common tendinopathies of the lower extremity include Achilles and patellar tendinosis. Some less common injuries include tendinopathy of the iliopsoas (hip), quadratus femoris (thigh), popliteus (back of knee), pes anserine (medial—inner side—knee), and longus colli (neck).

Tendinopathy Evaluation and Diagnosis

Evaluation and diagnosis of tendinopathies relies heavily on physical examination. Manual palpation of the tendon along the area where it attaches to the bone tends to reproduce symptoms in a well-localized pattern. Various orthopedic tests that place stress on the tendon of interest are done to re-create the patient's pain, which helps support the diagnosis. The basis for many of these tests includes either the doctor stretching the involved tissue or resisting as the patient attempts a movement involving the tendon. Any test that reproduces the chief complaint without weakness is considered to support the diagnosis of tendinopathy. In cases of muscle weakness, more testing is needed to investigate the possibility of a muscle tear or nerve injury.

Use of diagnostic imaging has relatively little utility to diagnose tendinopathy. Plain film radiography (X-rays) are generally not helpful since they only image bone. Although they are not very useful for visualizing tendons, X-rays can be helpful to show congenital joint malformations and signs of chronic injury, such as bone spurring and arthritis. In some cases, the patient may have acute deposition of calcium within tendons that can be visualized on X-ray. Diagnostic ultrasound (US) and magnetic resonance imaging (MRI) are more capable of imaging muscle and other soft tissues, but they often do not correlate with patient symptoms. False positives are frequent, and the treating physician should make an effort to associate imaging findings with patient symptoms. Due to a high rate of false positives and expense, US and MRI are typically reserved for cases that do not respond well to conservative treatment.

Clinical Management

The chiropractic physician scope of practice allows treatment of tendinopathy using a variety of interventions, including joint manipulation, cryotherapy (ice), bracing/orthotics, massage, electrical stimulation, therapeutic exercise, and acupuncture (depending on local jurisdictional law). The Council on Chiropractic Guidelines and Practice Parameters (CCGPP) reviewed the most common treatments for tendinopathy and determined that there is good evidence that ultrasound therapy provides clinically important improvement in the treatment of calcific tendonitis and fair evidence to support the use of eccentric exercise in the treatment of tendinopathy.[4] Eccentric exercise is the motion of contracting a muscle while lengthening it; an example would be slowly lowering down from a pull-up position. There is limited evidence to support the use of manipulation, mobilization, friction massage, acupuncture, surgery, and topical nonsteroidal anti-inflammatories (NSAIDs). According to the CCGPP, there was insufficient evidence to recommend extracorporeal shock wave therapy, corticosteroid injections, laser therapy, use of bracing/orthotics, and cryotherapy. It is important to note that the most common medical strategies for tendinopathy fare no better than those used by chiropractors.

Brosseau et al. reviewed treatment with friction massage for tendonitis. They found deep tissue massage with other physiotherapy modalities did not show consistent benefit in control of pain.[5] Woodley et al. reviewed effectiveness of eccentric exercise in treatment of chronic tendinopathy. They concluded there is limited evidence that eccentric training has a positive effect on clinical outcomes, such as pain, function, and patient satisfaction or return to work.[6] Another study concluded that eccentric exercise may reduce pain and improve strength in lower extremity tendinopathy, but there is uncertainty over whether eccentric exercise is more effective than other forms of exercise.[7]

In complicated cases of tendinopathy that do not respond to a conservative trial of chiropractic care, referral to a medical provider may be warranted. Arroll and Goodyear-Smith studied subacromial injections of corticosteroids and found them to be effective for rotator cuff tendinopathy up to a nine-month period and likely more effective than oral NSAIDs.[8] Treatments like cortisone injections have a greater risk of side effects than manual treatments. These include decreased tendon strength and risk of rupture several weeks after the injection. Extracorporeal shock wave therapy has been suggested as an intermediate treatment modality after failure of conservative care but before surgical intervention. This treatment involves using high-amplitude pulses of energy, similar to sound waves, to treat calcium deposits within a muscle or tendon. Evidence supports the use of ESWT for treatment of calcific tendinopathy but not in cases of chronic noncalcific tendon injury. This is likely because the shock wave is able to break up the calcium deposits. Medical and surgical interventions recommended by the CCGPP in treatment of elbow disorders include acetaminophen and aspirin, topical NSAIDs, oral NSAIDs, and surgery after at least six months of conservative treatment with failure to show signs of improvement. Surgical intervention should be reserved as a last-case scenario due to both the greater risks associated with surgery as well as the greater cost.

Osteoarthritis

Osteoarthritis (OA), also known as degenerative arthritis, is a painful joint condition that involves the breakdown of cartilage and failure of supporting bone structure and commonly results in the formation of osteophytes or bone spurs. OA is considered as a noninflammatory arthritis and is the most prevalent of all forms of arthritis. A major cause of disability in individuals aged 65 and older, OA has been projected to affect 60 million people in the United States by 2020. Osteoarthritis can occur in any joints and commonly occurs asymmetrically—that is, affecting just one side. It can occur in multiple joints or just at a single overused joint. The incidence and prevalence of OA vary by whether a clinical or radiographic (X-ray) definition is used. The number of individuals with arthritis diagnosed by X-ray is considerably higher than for those with a clinical diagnosis. This means that not everyone with X-ray evidence of arthritis has pain or other symptoms. For example, 6 percent of adults over 30 have symptomatic knee OA, and 10–15 percent of adults over 60 have symptoms, but at least 33 percent (some studies report 68 percent) of adults over 55 have X-ray evidence of knee OA. Other studies show that 30 percent of adults over 30 years old have evidence of hand OA, while only 10–15 percent of the elderly show hand OA symptoms, and an estimated 1–4 percent of adults have symptomatic hip OA.

Osteoarthritis develops when a healthy synovial joint structure is damaged. To understand the OA disease process, it is first necessary to understand the normal anatomy and physiology of a healthy joint. Synovial joints consist of subchondral (under cartilage) bone, articular (joint) cartilage, synovial membrane, synovial fluid, and the joint capsule. Joints may additionally be supported by labral tissue, interosseous ligaments, menisci, and fat pads.[11] Normal healthy cartilage consists of three layers: surface, middle, and deep. The surface layer has a very high collagen content, which runs parallel to the joint surface. The middle layer has collagen fibers running in multiple directions, and a high proteoglycan (protein core with sugar chains) content. In the deep layer, the collagen fibers run perpendicular to the joint surface and attach to subchondral bone. Articular cartilage reduces friction, provides shock absorption, and transmits weight loads to underlying bone.

Articular cartilage is made up of an extracellular matrix and chondrocytes. Extracellular matrix is comprised of water, collagen, and proteoglycans. Proteoglycans have a protein core and one or more glycosaminoglycan side chains, such as hyaluronic acid, chondroitin sulfate, and keratin sulfate. Chondrocytes function to produce and maintain cartilage matrix—collagen and proteoglycans.

Subchondral bone plays a role in joint protection and can attenuate about 30 percent of loads through the joint. Articular cartilage only absorbs 1–3 percent of the load. Subchondral bone is porous and contains bone marrow, trabecular bone, end arteries, and veins. The porous nature allows for the arrival of nutrients and removal of metabolic waste.

Synovial membrane is another protective joint layer. It consists of a thin layer of tissue that forms synovial fluid and produces hyluronate. Synovial fluid has a consistency similar to egg white. It is involved in shock absorption, reducing joint friction, protecting against inflammatory debris, and shielding nerve receptors from inflammatory mediators. Normal loads on articular cartilage include forces caused by the action of muscles as well as the force of body weight transmitted through the joint. The forces from muscle contraction and body weight can be tremendous. Although articular cartilage is an excellent shock absorber, the protection it can provide a joint is limited because it is only 3–6 mm thick. The surrounding muscles play a substantial role in helping synovial fluid, subchondral bone, and articular cartilage absorb shock. Therefore, adequate muscle bulk, strength, and neuromuscular responses are necessary to protect the joint.

Osteoarthritis is classically associated with wearing down and loss of articular cartilage, thickening and remodeling of subchondral bone, formation of osteophytes (bone spurs), and ultimately loss of joint space. Typically, OA involves many or all of the tissues that form the synovial joint, including articular cartilage, subchondral bone, synovial tissue, ligament, joint capsule, and muscles surrounding the joint. In the early stages of OA, irregularities of the articular cartilage develop with clefts and fissures present in the deepest layers. In later stages, the cartilage may wear away completely, exposing bone. As OA progresses, signs of bone involvement include formation of new extra bone, known as subchondral sclerosis, formation of cyst bone cavities, and development of osteophytes (bone spurs). Osteophytes typically occur around the periphery of the joint but may also occur along insertions of joint capsule or protrude from degenerative tissues. Microfractures can occur within the subchondral bone due to excessive loading. These microfractures heal with callous formation and remodeling. The remodeled bone may be stiffer than the original tissue, leading to reduced capacity to absorb shock and furthering the cycle of microfracture in the presence of persistent overloading. On a cellular level, OA is thought to represent an imbalance between the destructive and reparative processes of the articular cartilage. Early cellular signs of OA include elevated levels of water content accompanied by loss of extracellular matrix. Initially, chondrocyte cells multiply and increase activity, producing increased quantities of collagen and proteoglycans. As disease progresses, the proteoglycan concentration decreases to 50 percent or less, and the new cartilage formation is thinner and more disorganized than healthy cartilage. Failure of the body's ability to restore and maintain cartilage tissue leads to loss of articular cartilage accompanied or preceded by a decline in chondrocytic response. Chondrocyte deterioration is thought to be the result of chronic oxidative stress, specifically exposure to anabolic cytokines. Once inflamed, the synovium directly produces cartilage-degrading enzymes and indirectly contributes to release of prostaglandin E2. Enzymatic degradation further contributes to decreased cartilage thickness and volume.

Investigation into the causes of OA have shown that the disease is multifactorial and can be broken up into systemic and local factors. Systemic factors are thought to influence the whole person and include such factors as ethnicity, age, gender, hormonal status, genetic factors, bone density, and nutritional factors. Local factors include obesity, altered joint mechanics (i.e., ligamentous laxity, misalignment, impaired proprioception, muscle weakness), prior joint injuries, occupational injuries, and sports activities. Ethnicity may be related to genetics as well as many other underlying variables and habits that affect lifestyle, leading to disparities between populations. For example, hip OA and anatomic deformities that are common in the United States are rare in China, whereas knee OA is far more common in China. In this case, the primary difference in OA location is thought to be due to varying patterns in squatting between the two cultures. The prevalence and incidence of OA at all joint sites increases with age. The increase of OA with age is thought to be due to biological changes with aging. As we age, a number of events occur that inhibit cartilage repair—chondrocytes are less responsive to growth factors and glycation end products accumulate in cartilage. In addition to cellular changes, aging causes decreased strength, slower reflex responses, thinning cartilage, and increased shear stress in joints.

The relationship between bone density and OA is unclear. Studies have shown that in the presence of generalized OA there is an increased bone mineral density in the lumbar spine. However, it has been hypothesized that the increase in bone density is linked to osteophyte formation with cartilage loss, and the increased bone mineral density may in fact be a sign of damage. In theory, a diet high in antioxidants could have a protective role in preventing formation of OA. High dietary and blood serum levels of vitamin C and D may be protective against both the incidence and progression of hip OA.

Local risk factors for osteoarthritis are those biomechanical factors that increase stress and load through an individual joint. These are the factors that are most commonly of interest to chiropractic physicians, because they seem to have the highest potential for modification. From a local standpoint, any major injuries that alter joint alignment and/or function may predispose an individual to cartilage loss and arthritis changes. Irregularity in the cartilage surface can lead to increased joint friction, which further perpetuates degeneration and formation of OA. A high body mass (obesity) increases the prevalence of OA and has been shown to precede arthritis development. Fortunately, a relatively small reduction in weight—as little as 11 pounds—can result in a dramatic clinical reduction in pain. Obesity has been linked to increased levels of OA even in non-weight-bearing joints, leading researchers to suspect an inflammatory or metabolic component to osteoarthritis as well.

Repetitive-use injuries through work, sport, and/or physical activity are all associated with an increased risk of OA. Occupational activities, such as repetitive grasping, squatting, and bending, are often linked to injuries of specific joint groups. Jobs with a large physical demand, such as miners, dockworkers, concrete workers, and carpenters, are also associated with a higher degree of OA when compared with desk and office staff. OA associated with sports seems linked to torsional loading, or high-intensity, acute, direct joint impact as a result of contact with players or equipment. Early diagnosis and treatment of sports-related injuries may decrease the risk and prevent the development of OA.

Evaluation and Diagnosis

OA is diagnosed on the basis of detailed history, physical examination, and radiographic examination. Diagnostic criteria established by the American College of Rheumatology include the presence of joint pain, osteophytes on X-ray, and one or more associated symptoms, including stiffness, crepitus, point tenderness, enlargement or deformity, and narrowing joint space on X-ray. There is often a disconnect between clinical signs and symptoms and X-ray evidence of OA. When present, pain can be either unilateral or symmetrical and commonly develops slowly, gets worse with activity—particularly weight bearing—and is relieved by rest. Patients frequently report stiffness after prolonged periods of rest, such as awaking in the morning and getting up from a seated position. Movement of the involved joints frequently mitigates this stiffness, and it generally resolves in 20 to 30 minutes. Swelling of the joint, also known as effusion, is often present in early stages of OA. Crepitus is a crackling, grinding sound often reported by patients with OA that can be heard with range of motion and felt with palpation. Crepitus develops as the joint degenerates and irregular cartilage and bone surfaces rub together.[9]

Physical examination should evaluate range of motion, muscle strength, ligament stability of affected joints, and tenderness present at the joint line and identify the presence of joint deformities and many movement/mechanical sensitivities. Neuropathic pain may also be present if there is an impingement on surrounding nerves.

Plain film X-rays are the gold standard for confirming clinical findings of OA and ruling out other conditions. Radiographic findings consistent with OA include asymmetrical joint space narrowing, presence of osteophytes, bony cysts, and subchondral sclerosis. Disease progression is difficult to determine by X-rays due to slow advancement of the disease. The American College of Rheumatology has guidelines available for the diagnosis of hand, hip, and knee OA. For OA, computed tomography (CT) scans and magnetic resonance imaging (MRI) demonstrate little clinical advantage over X-ray, and lab studies have limited value.

Clinical Management

Management of mild to moderate OA should be individualized to the patient with a focus on functional levels, maintaining joint mobility, improving muscular stability, providing pain relief, and enhancing quality of life. Initially, this care should be focused on educating the patient in self-management strategies rather than on passive therapies delivered by providers. When heeded, education on the importance of lifestyle changes involving exercise, pacing regular activities, and weight reduction can have a dramatic impact on progression and suffering related to OA. Patient-driven programs that have shown success include the Arthritis Self-Management Program (ASMP)/Arthritis Self-Health Program and the

Chronic Disease Self-Management Program. All three of these programs focus on physical activity and weight management among their recommendations.

Rest can be beneficial when joint pain occurs after long exposures to activity. However, prolonged rest can lead to loss of joint motion and disability. Patients with OA should be encouraged to establish a regular routine of aerobic, muscle-strengthening, and range-of-motion exercises. Regular exercise is associated with maintaining joint health, increasing range of motion and strength, and improving mood and outlook. Deconditioned and/or sedentary patients may need to begin with water exercises or flexibility training before beginning land-based training. The use of braces, splints, patellar taping, proper footwear, and wedged insoles may be beneficial in aiding patients pursuing a more active lifestyle.[10]

OA patients should be counseled on healthy diet and, when appropriate, on weight loss. Even modest weight loss can lead to improvement in pain and function. According to the Arthritis Foundation, as low as a 10 percent reduction in weight can reduce joint pain by as much as 50 percent. Individuals with OA commonly pursue nutritional supplementation to aid joint support. Vitamin D, glucosamine, and chondroitin are the most commonly considered supplements. Dietary intake of vitamin D is well understood to play a role in increasing bone density; individuals with lower bone density are at a higher risk for developing OA. Despite a scarcity of published evidence, it is logical that vitamin D supplementation would be beneficial for patients at risk of developing OA. Treatment with glucosamine and/or chondroitin sulfate may provide symptomatic relief for OA. Glucosamine and glycosaminoglycan chondroitin sulfate are both naturally occurring building blocks of cartilage proteoglycans. A trial of three to six months is generally recommended to test patient response to these supplements.

Manipulation and manual therapy have been shown to be beneficial for patients with knee and hip OA.[11] The effect of a manual therapy program on hip function has been shown to be superior to exercise therapy in patients with OA. The recommended manual therapy consists of stretching shortened musculature (hamstrings, psoas, piriformis, etc.) followed by traction mobilization and manipulation of the hip. In addition, chiropractic manipulative therapy may contribute added benefit when performed on the full kinetic chain: lumbar spine, pelvis, knee, ankle, and foot.[12] Clinician-directed home exercise programs can improve muscle length and strength, joint mobility, pain relief, and walking ability.

Severe and/or progressive OA cases may be appropriate for comanagement or referral to a medical provider. Medications such as acetaminophen (up to 4g/day) may be helpful with initial pain relief in mild to moderate OA pain. NSAIDs may be beneficial; however, they carry significant risk for the gastrointestinal and cardiovascular systems. When used, they should be taken at the lowest possible effective dose, and long-term use should be avoided.[13] Topical NSAIDs and capsaicin can be effective alternatives to oral anti-inflammatories and pain relievers. Opioids and narcotics may be considered when pain does not respond to other medications and conservative therapies. An appropriate medical specialist can perform procedures such as intra-articular injections of corticosteroids or hyaluronate and a myriad of surgical strategies, including total joint replacement.[13]

Myofascial Pain Syndrome

"Myofascial pain syndrome" refers to the presence of myofascial trigger points (MTrP) and their associated clinical symptoms of sensory, motor, and autonomic dysfunction. Janet Travell and David Simons famously recognized that each muscle has its own specific trigger point pain pattern, which they subsequently identified, classified, and mapped.[14,15] Within the chiropractic profession, Ray Nimmo is most well known for describing the management strategies for MTrP.

Myofascial trigger points are recognized to be one of the most common causes of musculoskeletal pain and dysfunction and possibly a precursor to other conditions, such as osteoarthritis and tendinopathies. Several studies have attempted to quantify the presence of MTrPs. They found them to be present in more than half of asymptomatic individuals and in the majority of painful musculoskeletal disorders.[16] It is exceedingly difficult to establish if trigger points precede degenerative conditions or if the trigger points are the result of such disorders. A MTrP is a tender point within a taut band of skeletal muscle but not including the whole muscle. The tender points are accompanied by a predictable pattern of pain referral, pain on sustained compression, and a local twitch response within the muscle on a plucking type of palpation. The presence of pain referral is important as it distinguishes trigger points from tender points, which are only painful with palpation. Trigger points can be further subclassified into active versus latent trigger points. An active trigger point (ATrP) is a tender point that produces spontaneous pain with a referred pain pattern. Latent trigger points (LTrP) are points that do not cause pain while at rest but may restrict muscle movement and cause local pain with direct pressure on the point. It is believed that latent trigger points, though possibly contributory, are not the primary pain generator in musculoskeletal syndromes.

Myofascial trigger points are principally located at the center of the muscle in its motor endplate zone. This zone is where the motor nerve, on entering a muscle, divides into a number of branches with each of these having a terminal point embedded in the surface of a muscle fiber. These terminal branches consist of a neuromuscular bundle made up of motor nerve endings and sensory nerve fibers specifically related to pain. Microdialysis studies have been used to examine the biochemistry of MTrPs. In the presence of ATrPs, they have identified significantly elevated concentrations of certain inflammatory agents: protons, bradykinins, calcitonin gene-related peptide, substance P, tumor necrosis factor, interleukin-I beta, serotonin, and noradrenaline. Interestingly, if the microdialysis needle was manipulated to stimulate a local twitch response, there was a decrease in concentration of a number of inflammatory mediators.

Many factors are believed to be contributory to the development of MTrPs. The most common explanation is the development of painful sensory activity following either direct sudden muscle injury or recurrent overloading leading to repetitive strain injury. In addition, anxiety, muscle wasting, muscle ischemia, visceral pain referral, radiculopathy, and climate changes have all been linked to trigger point formation.

Evaluation and Diagnosis

Patients with trigger points commonly present with pain described as deep, aching, and poorly localized. The pain is typically regional, aggravated with activity, and often appears with decreased range of motion. Myofascial TrP pain is reproducible but does not follow dermatomal (nerve root) distributions. In the head and neck, TrPs can manifest as tension headaches, tinnitus, dizziness, orofacial dysfunction, neck pain, and torticollis. The head and neck muscles most commonly involved are masticatory (mouth closing) muscles, sternocleidomastoid, scalenes, and craniocervical paraspinals, upper trapezius, and levator scapula. Upper extremity TrPs can lead to complaints of shoulder, elbow, and wrist pain mimicking tendonitis, bursitis, and cardiac symptoms. Most commonly involved muscles of the upper extremity include pectoralis major/minor, subscapularis, middle trapezius, supraspinatus, infraspinatus, and forearm extensors. In the lower extremities, trigger points may limit knee and ankle movements; cause hip, knee, leg, and foot pain; and mimic sciatica symptoms. Myofascial TrP hypersensitivity in the gluteus maximus, gluteus medius, and quadratus lumborum (all low back and hip muscles) have all been implicated as potential sources of lower back pain.

Evaluation for trigger points involves palpation of a nodule of muscle fiber that is harder than normal consistency. Identification of a trigger point is based on the clinician's subjective sense of feel and assisted by the patient's recognition of pain referral and palpable observation of a local twitch response.[14] This palpation elicits pain over the palpated muscle and/or causes radiation of pain in a predictable pattern in addition to a twitch response. To assess for a local twitch response, the palpating finger is snapped across the taut band of an active MTrP and often there is a detectable contraction. When a tender point is localized, the practitioner should ask the patient if it is his or her usual pain while applying pressure to the trigger point and further ask the patient to indicate the pattern of pain produced. Thanks to the predictable pattern of pain referral outlined by Travell and Simons, it is frequently possible to narrow down the trigger point search of involved muscles by history alone.

For the evaluation of trigger points, several procedures have been explored, including microdialysis, biopsy, imaging techniques, and electromyography. Unfortunately, none of these has risen above the others to become the definitive standard of diagnosis. Two studies investigated the reliability of agreement between examiners on palpation of the location of latent trigger points. Both found a large degree of discrepancy of agreement, which makes it very difficult for practitioners to accurately use precision-based therapies, such as dry needling and injections. No studies have reported on the reliability of identifying the exact location of active trigger points or the reliability of detecting all diagnostic criteria simultaneously. The presence of tenderness and pain reproduction achieve satisfactory reliability; however, they are not specific to trigger points. Physical examination of firm palpation and patient feedback remains the only means to establish diagnosis.

Recent advances in ultrasound technology may lead to a more accurate visualization and eventually a better characterization of myofascial trigger points. Diagnostic ultrasound may also be used to distinguish active from latent trigger points. Research has shown sonoelastography may be used to classify trigger points by area. Further study is warranted in this area, as physical examination alone cannot be recommended as a reliable diagnosis for myofascial trigger points.

Clinical Management

Chiropractic physicians have a long history of treating myofascial pain syndromes and trigger points. According to the CCGPP, there is moderate evidence in support of spinal manipulation and ischemic pressure for immediate pain relief. However, there is only limited evidence for long-term effects. Clinical research additionally supports treatment of myofascial trigger points with laser therapy, transcutaneous electrical nerve stimulation, acupuncture, and magnet therapy. Several studies have investigated the effects of chiropractic manipulation and manual therapy on paraspinal musculature. Consistently, spinal manipulation has been shown to immediately increase pressure pain thresholds. Manual therapy, with a variety of different techniques, is believed effective at relieving pain from trigger points. Ischemic compression involves direct digital pressure applied on a trigger point to a tolerable level of pain for a few seconds, followed by pressure release, and then repetition with a gradual increase in pressure as discomfort subsides. Vascular congestion within trigger points is thought to adversely affect cellular metabolism, causing a shortage of oxygen and glucose and ultimately resulting in a painful situation. Ischemic compression is believed to flush out the congested blood and allow for recirculation with fresh blood supply.

Post-isometric relaxation (PIR) is a muscle relaxation technique that can treat trigger points. PIR first involves taking up the slack in a specific muscle by stretching it to its barrier (maximum length). From this position, the patient is instructed to resist with a minimum amount of force, breathe in, and to hold this resistance for 5 to 10 seconds, after which the patient is told to let go and slowly breathe out. The practitioner slowly guides the muscle toward a new barrier, which may take 10 to 30 seconds. This procedure is repeated until the muscle is relaxed and the trigger point is resolved. Wherever possible, breathing should be used to assist the muscle relaxation effects of PIR. The effect of PIR is believed to be due to the fact that minimal force is used and the only muscle fibers that contract are those with a low stimulus threshold (such as trigger points). In cases where PIR is ineffective, more aggressive myofascial therapies may be warranted.

Myofascial release is another manual system of treatment that can address muscle shortening, trigger points, fascial restriction, and myofascial pain. It involves palpating involved musculature for a taut band or hypertonic tissue and tenderness. Once tissue restriction or trigger point has been identified, the practitioner then positions the muscle into its most shortened posture. While applying a deep digital tension at the area of tenderness, the muscle is either passively or actively lengthened. This is performed repeatedly until there is a decrease in symptoms or improved tissue flexibility. The goal of myofascial release is to stretch and loosen muscle and surrounding connective tissue, allowing the tissues to glide freely over each other.

There is strong evidence to support *laser therapy* treatment of trigger points. Laser therapy is essentially a type of light therapy in which a specific area is targeted. A number of studies have shown that in the short term, laser therapy is superior to placebo in the management of trigger points.[17] A wide variety of type, dose, and frequency of laser have been investigated with none clearly outperforming others. One study compared laser therapy to dry needling and found laser therapy to be more effective.[18]

In recent years, chiropractic has seen a growth of interest in *dry needling* to manage myofascial pain. Dry needling is the application of an acupuncture needle deep into a trigger point. Once inserted, the needle is manipulated in an attempt to stimulate a local twitch response of the muscle, followed by a reduction of local inflammatory mediators, which is believed necessary for effective treatment. Medical physicians commonly inject anesthetics into trigger points; however, this practice has not been shown superior to dry needling. A recent interdisciplinary evidence and expert-based recommendation proposed that myofascial pain should first be managed with the least invasive modality and progressed with more aggressive therapies as needed. Lisi et al. advocated beginning with patient education and progressing from self-stretching and massage, to over-the-counter topicals, passive application of manual and myofascial therapies, dry needling, and finally Botox injections as indicated.[19] A 30 percent reduction in pain is recommended as adequate to continue care at any given step.

Fibromyalgia

Fibromyalgia syndrome (FMS) is a common and perplexing syndrome of unknown origin and is commonly described as a diagnosis of exclusion. Frequent complaints of people with this diagnosis are widespread chronic pain, fatigue, sleep disturbance, and cognitive difficulties. Clinically there is a tremendous amount of confusion surrounding fibromyalgia because the hallmark symptoms may also be associated with symptoms of latent pathology, metabolic syndromes, or chronic musculoskeletal disorders.[20] Before chiropractors can even begin to consider treatment options, they must first rule out a large laundry list of different conditions. Widespread pain and fatigue are also primary symptoms of hypothyroidism, anemia, diabetes, Lyme disease, rheumatoid arthritis, undiagnosed cancer, and other conditions.

Fibromyalgia is the second most common "rheumatic condition," following only osteoarthritis. The prevalence of fibromyalgia is estimated between 2 percent and 8 percent of the population, with the difference based largely on which diagnostic criteria is used.[21] The gender ratio is similar to other chronic pain conditions, 2:1 female to male. Studies of twins suggest that approximately 50 percent of the risk of developing fibromyalgia is genetic and 50 percent is environmental. Environmental factors likely to trigger fibromyalgia include certain types of infections (Epstein-Barr virus, Lyme disease, Q fever, viral hepatitis), trauma, or deployment to war.[21] Obesity and weight-control problems often occur in FMS patients and are related to worsening quality of life in terms of higher pain, fatigue, worsened sleep quality, and higher incidence of mood disorders.[22] Nonceliac gluten sensitivity is increasingly recognized as a frequent condition with similar manifestations that overlap with FMS.[22]

Psychological, behavioral, and social issues certainly contribute to the development of fibromyalgia and grossly complicate its treatment. Individuals with FMS are much more likely to exhibit psychiatric symptoms, including depression, anxiety, obsessive-compulsive disorder, and post-traumatic stress disorder (PTSD). It has been hypothesized that this may result from common triggers for these psychiatric conditions and fibromyalgia, such as early-life stress or trauma.[21] Potentially modifiable risk factors for developing FMS include poor sleep quality, obesity, physical inactivity, poor nutrition, and poor job or life satisfaction. Insomnia is a common complaint with FMS and has been reported by as much as 75 percent of patients.

The American College of Rheumatology first described fibromyalgia in 1990. The term "fibromyalgia" refers to pain spreading from fibrous soft tissue and/or muscles. However, investigations into fibromyalgia have failed to provide any evidence that there is injury to these structures. Contrary to its name, studies with functional MRI support the notion that fibromyalgia is in fact a disorder of pain processing within the central nervous system (brain and spinal cord) and not a condition of the peripheral tissues. Fibromyalgia is frequently misdiagnosed because the diagnosis is not based on any laboratory or diagnostic tests. According to the most recent ACR diagnostic criteria, fibromyalgia diagnosis relies on composite scores of self-reported symptoms using the widespread pain index (WPI) questionnaire and a symptom severity (SS) scale.[23]

The WPI is a list of 19 different body regions that is used to record the number of painful regions, and the SS scale consists of categorical scales for cognitive symptoms, unrefreshed sleep, fatigue, and the number of somatic symptoms.[20] Fibromyalgia is classically associated with extreme tenderness to touch. This extreme level of tenderness is known as allodynia and can result in pain from even minor stimuli, such as wearing clothing or light touch. The presence of allodynia typically implies a disorder of pain-stimulation pathways within the central nervous system and not an abnormality of peripheral tissues themselves.

Fibromyalgia Evaluation and Diagnosis

When presented with a patient suffering from chronic widespread pain, chiropractors must first ensure the absence of a myriad of other health conditions before entertaining the diagnosis of fibromyalgia. They should establish if the patient truly has chronic widespread pain or if she or he has a regional pain that may be explained by another musculoskeletal or visceral origin. The ACR defined "chronic widespread pain" as pain above the waist, pain below the waist, pain on both sides of the body, and pain involving the axial skeleton, and they defined "chronic" as meaning present for at least three months. If patients have true widespread pain, they should be investigated for signs of joint swelling. In the presence of joint swelling, specialized laboratory studies to rule out types of arthritis, such as Lyme disease, rheumatic arthritis, lupus, gout, and ankylosing spondylitis would be in order. If those tests are negative or there is an absence of joint swelling, then a full medical history, physical examination, and routine blood/urine test should be run. These tools are appropriate to determine if the patient shows signs of classic fibromyalgia: widespread allodynia, significant sleep disorder, history of significant anxiety/depression/PTSD, and fatigue.

In 2010, the ACR updated their diagnostic criteria for fibromyalgia.[23] They updated prior guidelines by eliminating the physical examination portion of the diagnosis and instead substituted inclusion of the WPI and SS scales. The WPI is a 0–19 count of the number of body regions reported as painful by the patient. The SS scale looks at a series of symptoms characteristic of fibromyalgia and rates their severity from 0 to 3. The symptoms assessed include fatigue, nonrefreshed sleep, cognitive problems such as memory loss, and the extent of somatic symptom reporting. The two scales can be combined to tabulate a score of 0–31, with a higher score indicating a higher likelihood of a fibromyalgia diagnosis.

Clinical Management

Presently, there is no one treatment or intervention that is considered curative. Fibromyalgia is a syndrome that is complex and may be the result of a number of different causes, thus requiring a number of treatments.

Future studies seem to be geared toward identifying subgroups of FMS patients that are more likely to respond to one treatment or another. The most up-to-date evidence-based approach to FMS syndrome consists of prescription low-dose antidepressants, cognitive behavioral therapy, and mild aerobic exercise. The American Pain Society recommends tricyclic antidepressants, selective serotonin reuptake inhibitors, anxiolytics, and pain medications for improving sleep, reducing anxiety/depression, and decreasing pain. NSAIDs, corticosteroids, and opioid medications are not recommended as primary medications for FMS.

Cognitive behavioral therapy (CBT) should be provided by a trained mental health professional. CBT is geared toward reduction of pain and psychological disability by enhancing self-efficacy, self-management, and skills for coping with pain. Chiropractors can assist CBT by avoiding catastrophizing symptoms, reenforcing skills of active coping (such as exercise and nutrition), preventing patient dependence on chiropractic manipulation, helping to identify and modify pain behaviors, and promoting healthy sleep hygiene.

Physical exercise has been demonstrated to minimize pain, improve sleep quality, enhance self-efficacy, and increase positive mood. A number of different exercise recommendations have been made for FMS, including aquatic exercise, aerobic training, resistance training, Pilates, yoga, and tai chi. Adding chiropractic manipulation to exercise training has been shown to increase patient adherence to training programs and facilitate greater improvements in functionality. The American Pain Society guidelines suggest that clinicians offer their patients complementary therapies, such as acupuncture, biofeedback, chiropractic manipulation, hypnosis, spa therapy, and massage. It is important that these patients be approached with team-based integrative care to incorporate two or more strategies to decrease pain and improve function. Additionally, it is crucial that an emphasis be placed on sleep hygiene as part of the treatment plan, using both medication and nonmedication techniques as needed.

When chiropractic manipulation is used for FMS patients, low-force techniques may have added value. Conversely, high-velocity, low-amplitude manipulation may aggravate symptoms in some patients. Examples of low-force chiropractic techniques that may be appropriate for FMS include Activator methods, flexion-distraction, and a myriad of soft tissue techniques. *See Chapter 4 for more information about different types of chiropractic manipulative techniques.* Physical modalities, such as ultrasound and laser heat therapy, are within most chiropractic scopes of practice and may be beneficial in reducing the impact of FMS.

Establishing a regular exercise routine can dramatically impact the quality of life of patients with fibromyalgia. Regular incorporation of physical fitness leads to a multitude of body adaptations, such as decreased mental stress, improved cognition and mental clarity, increased energy, increased strength, increased lean body mass, and decreased body fat percentage. There are many methods of exercise that have been shown to help improve function and quality of life, including aquatic therapy, yoga, and low to moderate aerobic and resistance training. The chronic fatigue and allodynia associated with FMS are the primary limiting factors to implementing a training program. Ideally, aspects of all the aforementioned exercise styles would be used; however, finding an enjoyable and endurable source of physical fitness is more important for the long haul of symptom management and recovery. Within a controlled environment, a physician or trainer can monitor resting fatigue levels by measuring resting heart rate and blood pressure while performing a 1.5-mile walk test to calculate VO2 max. (VO2 max is the maximum amount of oxygen one can use during intense exercise and is related to aerobic endurance,) These tests can be administered at regular intervals to track progression of improvement.

A comprehensive 12-week exercise and recreational protocol for FMS was recently proposed. The authors recommended beginning exercise with a baseline of intensity at week one limited to 40 percent of maximum heart rate. As the patient progresses through the weeks, they propose a gradual increase in intensity of exercise by 5–10 percent each week until the patient peaks at 80 percent of maximum heart rate. In week one, the patient will complete five sessions of general aerobic training (walking, cycling, elliptical) and two sessions of yoga with an emphasis in diaphragm breathing, stretching, and meditation. In week two, they suggest adding aquatic therapy, and in week three light resistance training with TheraBands, body weight, and/or free weights. By week seven, the patient should be using all the listed forms of physical exercise plus participating in recreational activities that aim to decrease stress, such as meditation, art therapy, and/or music therapy.

An important part of helping individuals with FMS is motivating them to adapt lifestyle habits to help them cope with their pain and symptoms. Sleep hygiene comprises a variety of different practices aimed at facilitating normal, quality nighttime sleep and refreshed wakefulness. The primary goal of sleep hygiene is to establish a seven-days-a-week routine for wake and sleep patterns. Sleep hygiene is important for everyone but particularly so for individuals suffering from FMS. The most telling signs of poor sleep hygiene are daytime sleepiness and nighttime sleep disturbance.

To address sleep hygiene, the National Sleep Foundation recommends a variety of simple strategies. Avoid napping during the day because it can disturb the pattern of sleep and wakefulness. Avoid stimulants, such as caffeine, nicotine, and alcohol close to bedtime. Alcohol close to bedtime may speed the onset of sleep, but as the alcohol metabolizes it can cause arousal from sleep. Exercise vigorously in the morning or late afternoon. Relaxing exercise such as tai chi done before bed may help initiate restful sleep. Avoid large meals, spicy foods, and chocolate in the evening as these may disturb sleep. Ensure adequate exposure to natural light. Light exposure helps regulate a healthy sleep-wake cycle as well as helping the body to synthesize vitamin D. Establish a regular relaxing bedtime routine and try to associate bed with sleep. It is not a good idea to watch TV, listen to the radio, or read in bed. Lastly, make sure the sleep environment is pleasant and relaxing.

References

1. Khan KM, Cook JL, Kannus P, Maffull N, Bonar SF. Time to abandon the "tendinitis" myth. *BMJ.* 2002;324:626–627.

2. Kaux JF, Forthomme B, LeGroff C, Crielaard JM, Croisier JL. Current opinions on tendinopathy. *J Sports Sci Med.* 2011;10:238–253.

3. Baldwin ML, Butler RJ. Upper extremity disorders in the workplace: costs and outcomes beyond the first return to work. *J Occup Rehabil.* 2006;16:303–323.

4. Pfefer MT, Cooper SR, Uhl NL. Chiropractic management of tendinopathy: a literature synthesis. *J Manipulative Physiol Ther.* 2009;32:41–52.

5. Brosseau L, Casimiro L, Milne S, et al. Deep transverse friction massage for treating tendonitis (review). *Cochrane Database Syst Rev.* 2002;4:CD003258.

6. Woodley BL, Newsham-West RJ, Baxter GD. Chronic tendinopathy: effectiveness of eccentric exercise. *Br J Sports Med.* 2007;41:188–198.

7. Wasielewski NJ, Kotsko KM. Does eccentric exercise reduce pain and improve strength in physically active adults with symptomatic lower extremity tendinosis? a systematic review. *J Athl Train.* 2007;42:409–421.

8. Arroll B, Goodyear-Smith F. Corticosteroid injections for painful shoulder: a meta-analysis. *Br J Gen Pract.* 2005;55:224–228.

9. Sinusas K. Osteoarthritis: diagnosis and treatment. *Am Fam Physician.* 2012;85(1):49–56.

10. Kalunian KC. Nonpharmacologic therapy of osteoarthritis. In: Rose BD, ed. *UpToDate.* Waltham, MA: Wolters Kluwer; 2012.

11. Brantingham JW, Bonnefin D, Perle SM, et al. Manipulative therapy for lower extremity conditions: update of a literature review. *J Manipulative Physiol Ther.* 2012;35:127–166.

12. Brantingham JW, Parkin-Smith G, Cassa TK, et al. Full kinetic chain manual and manipulative therapy plus exercise compared with targeted manual and manipulative therapy plus exercise for symptomatic osteoarthritis of the hip: a randomized controlled trial. *Arch Phys Med Rehabil.* 2012;93:259–267.

13. Zhang W, Moskowitz RW, Nuki G, et al. OARSI recommendations for the management of hip and knee osteoarthritis, Part II: OARSI evidence-based, expert consensus guidelines. *Osteoarthr Cartilage.* 2008;16:137–162.

14. Travell JG, Simons DG. *Myofascial Pain and Dysfunction. The Trigger Point Manual. The Upper Extremities.* 1st ed. Vol. 1. Baltimore, MD: Williams & Wilkins; 1983.

15. Travell JG, Simons DG. *Myofascial Pain and Dysfunction. The Trigger Point Manual. The Lower Extremities.* 1st ed. Vol. 1. Baltimore, MD: Williams & Wilkins; 1983.

16. Schiffman EL, Fricton JR, Haley DP, Shapiro BL. The prevalence and treatment needs of subjects with temporomandibular disorders. *J Am Dent Assoc.* 1990;120:295–303.

17. Vernon H, Schneider M. Chiropractic management of myofascial trigger points and myofascial pain syndrome: a systematic review of the literature. *J Manipulative Physiol Ther.* 2009;32:14–24.

18. Illbuldu E, Cakmak A, Disci R, Aydin R. Comparison of laser, dry needling and placebo laser treatments in myofascial pain syndrome. *Photomed Laser Surg.* 2004;22(4):306–311.

19. Lisi AJ, Breuer P, Gallagher RM, et al. Deconstructing chronic low back pain in the older adult—step by step evidence and expert-based recommendations for evaluation and treatment: Part II: Myofascial Pain. *Pain Med.* 2015. [epub ahead of print]

20. Schneider MJ. Clinical brief: challenges with the differential diagnosis of fibromyalgia. *Top Integr Health Care.* 2011;2(3):ID:2.3007.

21. Clauw DJ. Fibromyalgia: a clinical review. *JAMA.* 2014;311(15):1547–1555.

22. Rossi A, DiLollo AC, Guzzo MP, et al. Fibromyalgia and nutrition: what news? *Clin Exp Rheumatol.* 2015;33(1 Suppl 88):S1117–1125.

23. Wolfe F, Clauw D, Fitzcharles M, et al. The American College of Rheumatology preliminary diagnostic criteria for fibromyalgia and measurement of symptom severity. *Arthritis Care Res.* 2010;62(5):600–610.

CHAPTER ELEVEN

The Chiropractic Approach to Nonmusculoskeletal Conditions

Cheryl Hawk, DC, PhD, CHES

Introduction

As discussed in previous chapters, chiropractic care, especially spinal manipulation, has a substantial amount of evidence for its effectiveness for patients with many musculoskeletal conditions.[1] The evidence is much less plentiful with respect to nonmusculoskeletal conditions.[1] Before proceeding to present this evidence, it is first necessary to clarify what the term "nonmusculoskeletal" means. This is really a catch-all term that refers to anything that is not *directly* related to the muscles, bones, and tissue that connects them (ligaments and tendons). Thus, nonmusculoskeletal conditions might be what has in the past been referred to as "visceral" conditions. The term "viscera" refers to the organ systems of the body, such as digestive, respiratory (lungs), cardiovascular, and reproductive. However, the category of "nonmusculoskeletal conditions" is more encompassing than only visceral. It also includes neurological conditions (e.g., multiple sclerosis, Parkinson's disease), immune system disorders (e.g., allergies, cancer), and psychological conditions (e.g., depression, anxiety, posttraumatic stress disorder).

With such a mixed bag of conditions, it is not surprising that the evidence base for chiropractic care is somewhat sparse. Research is expensive, and resources to date have primarily been directed toward conditions frequently seen by chiropractors: those associated with musculoskeletal pain. However, some speculate that research findings may (and probably *should*) shape practice, rather than the other way around. That is, if the majority of research is conducted to investigate the effectiveness of chiropractic care for low back pain, then patients will tend to use chiropractic for low back pain.

Whichever may be the case, only a small minority of patients go to chiropractors with a primary complaint that is nonmusculoskeletal. One study found that only about 1 percent of patients did so, compared to about 34 percent of patients seeing a naturopathic doctor.[2] However, many patients who see chiropractors for a musculoskeletal complaint like back pain also have nonmusculoskeletal conditions and sometimes are surprised to find that these complaints also improve with a course of chiropractic care.[3] This type of evidence is termed "anecdotal" when it is simply an unsystematic clinical observation. Unfortunately, it is difficult to fund research looking more intensively into secondary complaints that seem to have fortuitously improved.

The purpose of this chapter is to summarize the clinical research related to chiropractic care for nonmusculoskeletal conditions. "Clinical research" refers to research done with human patients. Therefore, basic science research, which is usually conducted in a laboratory and often with animals rather than humans, cannot explain many aspects of effects that occur in clinical practice. However, basic science research is very important for learning more about possible mechanisms for how spinal manipulation or other aspects of chiropractic might affect nonmusculoskeletal conditions.[4]

The reader should keep in mind that physiological effects of spinal manipulation and other types of manual therapies are only one component of the entire clinical encounter. It is difficult, and sometimes impossible, to determine exactly which part of the entire doctor-patient encounter produces a treatment effect. In fact, this may vary greatly depending on the individual patient and doctor. Factors such as the general emotional and physiological effects of human touch, psychological factors like belief and expectation, and other actions the doctor may take, such as providing nutritional, exercise, and lifestyle advice, all contribute to treatment effects, inseparable from spinal manipulation. In fact, the placebo effect, once discounted as being produced by a combination of expectation and belief colored by aspects of the clinical encounter, is now recognized to be an important part of clinical practice that should be maximized, not discounted.[5] In fact, the treatment/healing effects that result from the clinical encounter are now referred to as "contextual healing."[6] It is likely that contextual effects a patient experiences when visiting a medical physician, a chiropractor, an Oriental medicine practitioner, or a massage therapist may be quite different.

It should also be kept in mind that many nonmusculoskeletal health problems, including hypertension, asthma, depression, and insomnia, are made worse by stress and its physical correlate, muscle tension. Any type of therapy that helps with relaxation of muscles can thus have an effect, even if indirectly, on such conditions. Chiropractic manipulation often has a relaxing effect on the muscles. Furthermore, there is some basic scientific research that suggests that spinal manipulation may help regulate the autonomic nervous system, although this is not definitive.[4] Because stress reactions are directly related to the action of the sympathetic nervous system (the part of the autonomic nervous system responsible for the stress reaction of "flight, fight, or fright"), this is also a possible avenue through which spinal manipulation may be helpful.

It should also be kept in mind that chiropractic care is not simply spinal manipulation. Chiropractors use a variety of approaches and procedures, as has been discussed in other chapters. These may include other manual therapies, like soft tissue techniques, as well as nutrition, exercise, dietary supplements, herbs, and general lifestyle counseling. Many chiropractors are trained in additional therapies, such as acupuncture. Therefore, it is a good idea for patients to discuss their chiropractor's approach to their particular health problems to see if it makes sense and has worked for other patients with similar issues. Of course, this applies to any type of health issue, not only nonmusculoskeletal ones.

Summary of Clinical Research Related to Chiropractic Care for Nonmusculoskeletal Conditions

Clinical research generally does not attempt to determine *how* a treatment effect was produced. Instead, it attempts to measure *how much of an effect* was produced, among *which group of patients*, using *which types of interventions*. The rest of this chapter will summarize current clinical research related to chiropractic care for common nonmusculoskeletal conditions. The reader must keep in mind the caveat that evidence from clinical research, the highest level of which is considered randomized controlled trials, is limited in that it looks at large groups of people receiving a very carefully restricted protocol of interventions. This is necessary in order to attempt to isolate the "active" ingredient, which in chiropractic research is almost always spinal manipulation. However, in real life, real patients generally want, and get, an individualized intervention that includes an array of therapies plus the doctor-patient interaction itself, which adds to the effect of the intervention.

It is unquestionably important to consider whether the spinal manipulation portion of the clinical encounter has a unique effect. Readers just need to keep in mind that their own experience might entail a greater or lesser impact, depending on individual factors of both the patient and the doctor. It is always important for both patients and doctors to remember that the focus of the clinical encounter is a *patient* who has a particular set of symptoms we call a "condition." The doctor is treating a patient, not a condition! And so the treatment should always be individualized to the patient's needs.

The most recent and thorough evaluation of the effect of manual therapies on nonmusculoskeletal conditions is the updated U.K. Report published in 2014 by Clar et al. This is a group commissioned by the U.K. to do an independent and nonbiased assessment of the research on manual therapies, both on musculoskeletal and nonmusculoskeletal conditions.[1] In this report, "manual therapies" included massage, manipulation, mobilization, and soft tissue techniques. It did not matter what type of practitioner performed the procedure. It could have been an osteopathic or chiropractic physician, a physical therapist, a massage therapist, or other type of manual therapist (sometimes physical medicine medical physicians do manual therapies). However, often the type of manipulative therapy is specified in the study as being "osteopathic manipulative therapy" or "chiropractic manipulative therapy." This is because there are various manipulative techniques used more commonly by osteopathic physicians and others used more commonly by DCs. In most cases, the techniques themselves could be performed by any trained and qualified manual therapist. Thus, all these manual therapy techniques listed in the table could theoretically be done by a DC, if he or she had training in them, even when they are labeled "osteopathic"—and, of course, vice versa.

The reader should also note that this chapter includes information about conditions common among adults; Chapter 13 covers conditions common among children.

The conditions discussed in this chapter are those with positive or negative evidence for spinal manipulation or mobilization from at least one systematic review and at least one comparative clinical study. A *systematic review* is an exhaustive and carefully structured literature review in which the quality of the research studies is factored in when assessing the strength of the evidence. A *comparative study*, usually but not always a randomized controlled trial, is one that compares the treatment of interest to an established treatment or a placebo in terms of patient

Table 11.1 Evidence for Effects of Spinal Manipulation on Patients with Nonmusculoskeletal Conditions[1]

Condition	Type of Manipulation	Type of Evidence*
Cardiovascular/ Circulation		
Hypertension	Spinal manipulation, high-velocity, low-amplitude	Negative
	Upper cervical spinal manipulation	Favorable
Intermittent claudication	Osteopathic manipulation	Favorable
Digestive System		
Irritable bowel syndrome	Osteopathic manipulation	Favorable
Neurological (Nervous System)		
Cervicogenic vertigo (dizziness)	Spinal manipulation and mobilization	Positive
Parkinson's disease	Osteopathic spinal manipulation	Favorable
Reproductive and Urinary Systems		
Dysmenorrhea	Spinal manipulation	Negative
Urinary incontinence in women	Osteopathic spinal manipulation	Favorable
Chronic prostatitis in men	Osteopathic spinal manipulation	Favorable
Respiratory Systems		
Asthma	Osteopathic spinal manipulation	Favorable
Chronic ob3structive pulmonary disease (COPD) or pneumonia, in elderly people	Osteopathic spinal manipulation	Favorable

*For the type of evidence, "Favorable" means the evidence is inconclusive, due to not enough high-quality research studies on the topic, but suggests a beneficial effect. "Positive" means there is enough evidence to say that the treatment has a beneficial effect on the symptoms of the condition listed. "Negative," in this context, means that there is enough evidence to say that the treatment has no effect on symptoms of the condition.

outcomes—that is, whether or not the patient's condition improved. A note about evidence: "positive" evidence means that the treatment improved the patient's condition-related symptoms. "Negative" evidence indicates that the treatment either did not help the condition or actually made it worse. "Inconclusive" evidence means that there is simply not enough research to be sure one way or the other. However, sometimes there is enough research to say that the evidence is "inconclusive but favorable" or "inconclusive but unfavorable." This chapter will list the conditions with positive, negative, or inconclusive favorable or inconclusive unfavorable evidence. Of course, many conditions are not listed—why not? Those conditions not listed simply indicate that there is not enough research to make a judgment one way or the other. It does *not* mean that chiropractic could not help; we simply don't know for sure.

Cardiovascular or Circulatory Conditions

Hypertension

Hypertension, or high blood pressure, is extremely common and is a risk factor for heart attacks and stroke. It is defined as having blood pressure that is equal to or greater than 140/90 mm Hg. Prehypertension is now defined as having systolic pressure (the top number) of 120–139 and diastolic pressure (the bottom number) of 80–90 mm Hg.

Although genetics play a part in developing hypertension, it is well known that lifestyle-related factors, such as obesity, poor diet, smoking, alcohol use, and lack of physical activity are important contributing factors. However, small research studies and personal experiences (again, we return to anecdotal evidence) have historically suggested that spinal manipulation might help normalize blood pressure through its effect on the autonomic nervous system. Cumulative research now indicates that traditional chiropractic manipulation, which is the type that causes the familiar cracking or popping sound in the joint (termed "high-velocity, low-amplitude manipulation") does not appear to affect blood pressure significantly, although it is certainly not harmful.[1] Interestingly, a different type of chiropractic technique, which uses a very small amount of force and is applied only to the upper neck vertebrae, has some evidence of having a beneficial effect in normalizing high blood pressure.[1,7] In general, patients who want to actively address their hypertension through natural methods—in conjunction with medical management as appropriate—should rely first on well-documented lifestyle interventions, such as improved diet, increased exercise, and stress reduction such as through mindfulness-based techniques or progressive muscle relaxation.[8] Certainly, chiropractic care involving spinal adjustments and soft tissue techniques may promote relaxation and better resilience to stress, and most DCs also advise patients on healthy lifestyle. At most, spinal manipulation should only be considered a component of a comprehensive lifestyle approach to management of hypertension, which may or may not include medications, depending on the individual case and the patient's physician's recommendations.

Intermittent Claudication and Peripheral Artery Disease

"Intermittent claudication" refers to cramping pain in the legs that comes on with exercise and then subsides. It is an indication of peripheral artery disease, which means that the blood vessels in the "periphery"— that is, the parts of the body furthest from the center—are constricted, mainly by the presence of atherosclerosis ("hardening of the arteries"). Although the evidence was only considered inconclusive, it suggested that osteopathic manipulation had an effect on improving patients' circulation so that they could walk farther without pain.[1] The techniques used included not only spinal manipulation of the high-velocity, low amplitude type but also soft tissue techniques and craniosacral manipulation.[9] It is also important to note that people with peripheral artery disease should make the lifestyle modifications that help improve circulation and prevent atherosclerosis: quit smoking, improve the diet, and increase moderate physical activity, particularly walking. In fact, simply getting on a regular walking program may improve symptoms of intermittent claudication because the body actually develops what is called "collateral circulation" in response to gradually increasing exercise.

Digestive System

Irritable Bowel Syndrome

Irritable bowel syndrome (IBS) is a common condition in which the person has bouts of diarrhea and constipation with accompanying abdominal discomfort and bloating. As with the other conditions discussed so far in this chapter, there are self-care actions people can take to help themselves, including avoiding "trigger" foods and taking probiotics.[10] A DC who has training in nutrition, particularly functional medicine, could advise a patient with IBS on which probiotic supplements and dietary changes would be most helpful. There is some inconclusive but favorable evidence that osteopathic spinal manipulation may also be helpful in restoring normal function of the large intestine.[1]

Neurological

Cervicogenic Vertigo (Dizziness)

"Cervicogenic" means that the dizziness is caused by a problem with the nerves in the neck. Most people do not realize that the nerves connected to the cervical (neck) vertebrae have an important effect on balance. This is an effect separate from the role of the inner ear, with which people are more familiar. Determining whether dizziness is cervicogenic or not can be difficult, and it is often a "diagnosis by exclusion." That is, if other causes are ruled out, then it is assumed that the cause is cervicogenic. However, when the dizziness is accompanied by neck pain, restricted neck movement (stiffness), or seems to increase or decrease depending on the position of the neck, a cervicogenic cause may be suspected. It may be complicated by the presence of problems with the inner ear as well.

There is moderate positive evidence that spinal manipulation of the neck is helpful in cases of cervicogenic dizziness.[1] Chiropractors are also taught, at most chiropractic training institutions, to do the Epley maneuver, which is a set of exercises with the neck, done either by the DC or at home by the patient, that help dizziness originating in the inner ear. The combination of gentle neck manipulation and the Epley exercises can be helpful for many patients suffering from cervicogenic vertigo.

Parkinson's Disease

In this neurological condition, the person's ability to move becomes progressively more limited, and he or she also has pronounced tremors. Although there is no treatment that will cure it, there is some inconclusive but favorable evidence that osteopathic spinal manipulation and also rehabilitation programs in which joint mobility is improved may help allay the symptoms.[1]

Reproductive and Urinary Systems

Dysmenorrhea

Painful menstruation is thought to be largely due to fluctuations in hormones. There has been a fair amount of research done on spinal manipulation for dysmenorrhea, and it appears that it is not, in general, helpful for relieving the symptoms or correcting the condition, although spinal manipulation certainly does not aggravate the condition or cause harm.[1] A chiropractor who is trained in nutrition, diet, and exercise might be able to advise individual patients on dietary and activity regimens that may help with dysmenorrhea.

Urinary Incontinence in Women and Chronic Prostatitis in Men

Unlike dysmenorrhea, which is greatly influenced by hormone balance, these two conditions of the female and male genitourinary tract do seem to respond in some cases to spinal manipulation.[1]

"Urinary incontinence" simply means urinating when one doesn't want to; that is, involuntary leakage of urine. It is much more common in women than men, probably because pregnancy, childbirth, and menopause are all factors that may contribute to developing incontinence. Weak muscles of the bladder and pelvic floor are common contributors to incontinence. Some evidence shows that osteopathic manipulation may be helpful. However, it should be noted that manipulation, although helpful, was not shown to be better than pelvic floor muscle training, usually known as Kegel exercises, which women can do on their own.[1]

Chronic prostatitis in men is also fairly common, mainly among older men. Incontinence may be an associated symptom. Even more commonly associated is an inability to urinate readily. Some evidence was found that osteopathic spinal manipulation and also myofascial therapy—a type of manual therapy many chiropractors, osteopathic physicians, and physical therapists may use—may be helpful.[1]

Respiratory

Asthma

Asthma is a complex condition involving the respiratory and immune systems. Osteopathic manipulation that includes soft tissue techniques has inconclusive but favorable evidence for its effect on symptoms of asthma. It cannot be claimed that it cures the condition, but it helps manage the symptoms. It should also be noted that osteopathic, chiropractic, or massage techniques that focus on relaxing the muscles in general, and the accessory muscles of respiration in particular (the muscles in the top of the shoulders and neck, which are brought into play when someone is having difficulty breathing), can be very helpful for asthmatics. Even though these treatments do not "cure" asthma, they can make the person much more comfortable.

Chronic Obstructive Pulmonary Disease or Pneumonia in Elderly People

Pneumonia is often a serious complication of an initial upper respiratory infection in older adults. Influenza is one of the most important precursors to pneumonia, which is why influenza vaccination is recommended so strongly for older adults. Once an elderly person has pneumonia, he or she may not realize it because symptoms are somewhat less severe at first than they are in younger people. Once symptoms become severe, the person must be hospitalized and treated with intravenous antibiotics, and fatalities are not uncommon. Promising research on spinal manipulation—specifically osteopathic manipulation—suggests that it may reduce the symptoms and decrease patients' need for medication as well as the number of days they need to be in the hospital.

Conclusion

Clearly there is not a great deal of research in the area of spinal manipulation or chiropractic care for patients with nonmusculoskeletal conditions. This is not only due to the scarcity of funding for clinical research on so many different conditions; it is also because nonmusculoskeletal conditions are so often complex and multifactorial, with lifestyle factors playing a very large part in the course the illness follows. Thus, people who are interested in exploring comanagement with a combination of medical care, chiropractic care, and possibly other approaches, for any nonmusculoskeletal condition, should seek a DC who is not only skilled in spinal manipulation but also in soft tissue techniques, nutrition, and lifestyle counseling.

People who are already seeing a chiropractor for a back problem or other musculoskeletal condition might mention any other nonmusculoskeletal conditions they also suffer from to their DC. The DC will note it in her or his records (although it is probably already there from the history the doctor took at the first visit). Then the DC can offer treatments and lifestyle advice that might help and be sure to check spinal or soft tissue structures that might have a relationship to the problem. Since research into the effects of spinal manipulation is still in its infancy, a therapeutic trial—that is, a course of treatment to explore whether it will help the problem—may be useful. This is something that a patient should discuss with the chiropractor and come to an agreement with no promises of a "cure" but assurance that no harm will be done.

References

1. Clar C, Tsertsvadze A, Court R, Hundt GL, Clarke A, Sutcliffe P. Clinical effectiveness of manual therapy for the management of musculoskeletal and non-musculoskeletal conditions: systematic review and update of UK evidence report. *Chiropr Man Therap.* 2014;22(1):12.

2. Hawk C, Ndetan H, Evans MW, Jr. Potential role of complementary and alternative health care providers in chronic disease prevention and health promotion: an analysis of National Health Interview Survey data. *Prev Med.* 2012;54(1):18–22.

3. Leboeuf-Yde C, Pedersen EN, Bryner P, et al. Self-reported nonmusculoskeletal responses to chiropractic intervention: a multination survey. *J Manipulative Physiol Ther.* 2005;28(5):294–302.

4. Bolton PS, Budgell B. Visceral responses to spinal manipulation. *J Electromyogr Kinesiol.* 2012;22(5):777–784.

5. Kaptchuk TJ, Miller FG. Placebo effects in medicine. *N Engl J Med.* 2015;373(1):8–9.

6. Miller FG, Kaptchuk TJ. The power of context: reconceptualizing the placebo effect. *J R Soc Med.* 2008;101(5):222–225.

7. Bakris G, Dickholtz M, Sr., Meyer PM, et al. Atlas vertebra realignment and achievement of arterial pressure goal in hypertensive patients: a pilot study. *J Hum Hypertens.* 2007;21(5):347–352.

8. Hughes JW, Fresco DM, Myerscough R, van Dulmen MH, Carlson LE, Josephson R. Randomized controlled trial of mindfulness-based stress reduction for prehypertension. *Psychosom Med.* 2013;75(8):721–728.

9. Lombardini R, Marchesi S, Collebrusco L, et al. The use of osteopathic manipulative treatment as adjuvant therapy in patients with peripheral arterial disease. *Man Ther.* 2009;14(4):439–443.

10. Aragon G, Graham DB, Borum M, Doman DB. Probiotic therapy for irritable bowel syndrome. *Gastroenterol Hepatol (N Y).* 2010;6(1):39–44.

CHAPTER TWELVE

Health Promotion and Wellness

Marion W. Evans Jr., DC, PhD, MCHES

"Wellness" as an Operational Term

"Wellness" has enjoyed many definitions over the years; today, the meaning of the word is vague, and consumers and patients hear it applied to a host of applications. In some cities, a wellness program may be a yoga studio where one can purchase whole-food smoothies at the end of a session. Perhaps it is a visit to the massage therapist, acupuncturist, or herbalist. It may be a chiropractic office that uses the term in the name on the sign. Physical therapy offices, medical offices, naturopathic offices, and even medical marijuana clinics in the Pacific Northwest sometimes have the word on their signs as well. In other areas, it may simply be a fitness center or outpatient hospital clinic that specializes in hospital-based care for heart attack, rehabilitation, or restoring health after a sickness. For others, it clearly represents what some might term "chronic disease management."

Groups like the American Heart Association encourage citizens to "know their numbers," which means tracking their cholesterol values, A1C, or other vital health indicators, such as blood pressure, as a means of determining how well one is at a given time. However, if these numbers are managed by medications, is a person really well? If we reach a point where regular medical care is required, how well are we?

It seems that some question remains about what really constitutes wellness. At times, the sensibility of clinics and services that offer what is labeled as "wellness" can be confusing for the consumer and the health care providers that deliver it. The term "wellness" is certainly popular in current branding efforts by many groups of business and health care providers. From a chronic disease perspective, if we "meet people where they are," a common phrase used in wellness and health promotion, then at times we must work within a chronic disease management model. We may have to start with restoration of health after a portion of health has been lost. For so many Americans, as well as people in other developed nations, that is simply where they are in their quest for health and well-being. The term "behavioral health" has been associated with substance abuse treatment programs and addictive disease management, adding to the confusion when it comes to addressing needed health behavior changes that are such an essential part of any wellness paradigm.

The National Wellness Institute (NWI) is one of the oldest organizations in America dedicated to wellness. This organization is also very open to most legitimate provider groups who want to learn more about wellness from the science-based sense of the term. They have a paradigm that offers six unique dimensions of wellness. In this paradigm, wellness is considered to be a process to achieve full potential in a manner that is conscious, self-directed, and always evolving. It is not only holistic but also includes aspects of lifestyle as well as mental, spiritual, and environmental well-being. Further, NWI contends that the experience should be positive and affirming. In order to better define where wellness can occur, the NWI lists the six dimensions of wellness separately (see Box 12.1).

Box 12.1

The Six Dimensions of Wellness

1. Occupational
2. Physical
3. Social
4. Intellectual
5. Spiritual
6. Emotional

Source: National Wellness Institute

According to NWI, the model best defining wellness takes into account how a person will contribute to the environment and community and how better living spaces and social networks create opportunities for wellness, how we enrich our lives through work and play, how our belief systems and world view can shape our lives for the better, and how personal self-esteem, self-control, and self-confidence foster a better life. Engaging in mentally stimulating, creative endeavors and sharing gifts and talents with others creates a strong sense of social wellness. These ideals should help a person achieve a sense of full personal potential and affirm positive qualities and strengths.

It is easy to see that we can be well in one environment and perhaps lacking wellness in another. The workplace is a good example. If one does everything right at home but has to sit all day in a cheap, unsupported chair, over time, that person is likely to have negative health consequences. The same is true if work brings added stress, as many jobs do today. But if the employer recognizes this, sets standards for better seating, encourages moving around, and teaches stress-management strategies at work, then this area is addressed for the workers whether they select wellness at home or not. It is from this more comprehensive view of wellness that this chapter is framed. In addition, the chapter will also discuss what people should expect to find in a legitimate wellness-based clinical practice when seeing a chiropractic physician, or any other physician for that matter.

Levels of Prevention

All health care providers should endeavor to help their patients prevent disease, and an active approach for preventing disease is to strive to be well. To be certain, everyone will eventually suffer from "mortality." The death rate is still, at some point, 100 percent. However, if health care providers aim to help patients live as many well years as possible—with the cooperation of the patient, of course—they should understand a few levels of intervention. Leavell and Clark described three levels of prevention:[1]

1. *Primary prevention* means keeping healthy people on course and helping them stay healthy for as many years as possible. New cases of disease are prevented from occurring.
2. *Secondary prevention* means helping a patient reestablish better health after some health risk has become evident. This is a reversal of misfortune related to health. Many Americans see the doctor when there is a need for intervention at the secondary or tertiary level. An example of secondary prevention

might be that an unhealthy diet has led to higher cholesterol levels in between visits to the doctor. If so, and if no harm has been done overall, reversal of that high cholesterol reduces risks for that patient and restores his or her health to a better baseline level of wellness. Theoretically, this could be accomplished with diet and exercise.

3. *Tertiary prevention* is essentially damage control. For example, a person has a disease or condition that has manifested in some way, and there is no getting back to a baseline level of being truly well. That is, some damage has been done. This could be a person who has had unhealthy habits for many years and within the last few months has started to experience chest pain. After a visit to the doctor, it turns out that the person had a mild heart attack and an artery to the heart is partially blocked. While surgically placing a stent in the artery to help it stay open is an everyday procedure, there is often not a lot that can be done to reverse all of the damage the heart attack may have caused. There are studies that show some damage can be reversed with major lifestyle changes, but for the most part, once some health damage has occurred, it is difficult to reverse it completely. Therefore, tertiary prevention becomes damage control or preventing the condition from becoming worse.

Being well means embracing primary prevention when possible. This is what we should strive for in our patient population, but we acknowledge that secondary prevention may be where most health care providers find themselves in their day-to-day dealings with their patient population.

Every provider should work with patients to help restore health and establish a better state of wellness where they can within the six dimensions. While not all conditions will be discovered at the point at which complete reversal can be accomplished, reducing risk is still a preventive measure. However, not every aspect of a patient's life is under the control of the health care provider. Often, achieving a better state of wellness comes down to behavior change. This must occur in a partnership with the patient. After all, no one can or should be forced to change.

World Health Organization Definition of Health

In order to more clearly define "wellness," it's helpful to have a good working definition of "health." For decades, the World Health Organization (WHO) has offered this definition: "Health is a state of complete physical, mental and social well-being and not merely the absence of disease or infirmity."[2]

With this definition, health is achieved in many of the same areas as described by the NWI's six dimensions, and as such, "wellness" becomes the personal, and often social, steps or measures one takes in order to achieve this level of health. The person, the surroundings, and the behaviors are all involved in the triad of wellness, and this has been described for decades in several health behavior models. Some of them will be described in this chapter.

Health Promotion

What does the term "health promotion" bring to mind? Many people have some intuitive knowledge of what they think the term means, but, unfortunately, many people have no idea what it is or, further, that there are professions built on its concepts! While "health promotion" is a term that is often used in both clinical practices and in community health, hospital, or school health programs, it will help to offer an accepted, working definition. By definition, health promotion combines efforts to educate people about health and wellness with opportunities to advocate or arrange for changes in policies or laws in order to create a place where wellness can occur.[3] Health promotion stems from the field of health education, which in turn was a spin-off of early physical education models but directed more at school health. Health education is what most people think it is: it is about offering education to the public on choices they should make to be healthy or to improve health. However, models of health promotion are often "ecological" in nature, taking into account not only the personal attributes needed to make behavior changes that facilitate wellness, such as knowledge, but the social dynamics or cultural norms of a region that may be in need of change. The best ecological model that has been described is by McLeroy and colleagues.[4] Their model (Table 12.1) states that health promotion efforts must often look at the intrapersonal or individual issues, such as knowledge and beliefs; interpersonal issues or relationship-based issues involved in ties with family and friends; community issues; institutional or organizational issues, including norms and rules; and public policy factors.

The ecological system surrounding the patient influences choices, and health care providers should take that into account when offering interventions. The ecological health model takes into account the personal knowledge, attitudes, and beliefs of a patient, which can be largely attributed to education; social interactions with friends, family, and significant others; and even the social norms of the region. It may even take into account how people in a particular culture tend to eat or exercise. Most people can think of a time peer pressure or family habits had some effect on their health choices, whether positive or negative. Along with taking into account laws and policies that may either enable healthy choices or

Table 12.1   Ecological Model of Health Promotion

Ecological Construct	Application of the Model in Clinical Environment
Intrapersonal	Knowledge, attitude, and beliefs about a behavior or a risk factor; belief about wanting to, or thinking they can, make a change factors in to action
Interpersonal	Family members' thoughts, other health care providers' thoughts, friends, peers, social support for needed changes (or perception of this support)
Community Level Institutional	Rules; regulations at work; policy at the local, county, state level; formal and informal rules that enable or reinforce certain behaviors
Basic Community Factors	Social networks, community norms, infrastructure, attitude toward community availability of resources, support agencies
Public Policy Issues	Support for healthy policies and laws to protect the public, policy for health screenings and preventive services in the community or state, state government attitude toward federal support

Sources: National Cancer Institute: *Theory at a Glance a Guide for Health Promotion Practice.* US Dept of HHS, NIH 2005:1–52.

McLeroy KR, Bibeau D, Steckler A, Glanz K. An ecological perspective on health promotion programs. *Health Educ Q.* 1988;15:351–377.

hinder them, the model is a comprehensive example of health promotion that has been studied for decades and shown to be very predictive of influences in health behavior. It may also involve what a community thinks about or is willing to spend on infrastructure, such as bike lanes or sidewalks and other external examples of the "built environment." At times, even what family doctors, dentists, or chiropractors think about health themselves can have a bearing on choices patients make. For example, if health care providers do not emphasize anything more than a "know your numbers" plan in their office, they operationalize wellness only at a secondary or tertiary level. If this has undue influence on patients (make no mistake; it can), they may feel that taking a pill every day or getting an adjustment at the chiropractor once a month is all they need to do to be well. This should not be all that is done to help a person reach a state of wellness, and frankly, it will not likely lead to an overall state of wellness. After all, a person is only in a doctor's office a few times a year, and that encounter cannot reestablish wellness in most cases. Most medicines alleviate pain or symptoms, but, even if we lower a single health risk indicator such as high bad cholesterol, they do not address the total risk to the patient. Wellness is an active process, and in most cases, the patient has to take on new behaviors and make personal changes on a daily basis to achieve wellness. It is truly about overall lifestyle changes for most people. There are few quick fixes or magic bullets for restoration of overall health.

Wellness as Applied to Clinical Practice

Clinical practice provides opportunities to influence patients to make healthier choices or adopt healthier attitudes and practices that may extend their life expectancy. While *life-span*, which suggests an average number of years a person in a given population is likely to live, is determined by large, epidemiological studies, *life expectancy* is how long we will likely live based on environment, choices, or genetic makeup. Our healthy or unhealthy social interactions, described in the ecological model of health promotion above, have a direct impact on outcomes in this area. We can even predict health status based on zip codes today.

Wellness should be a central theme at clinical practices, but often that is not the case. For instance, there are many studies that suggest the primary care physician is not likely to advise the patient on disease prevention or how to become and remain healthy. The National Ambulatory Medical Care survey, which asks physicians what they did with a patient on a given day, found that physicians often identified risk behaviors but missed opportunities to address them even when they filled out a form asking them if they provided such advice.[5] The physicians reported engaging patients on a health education topic in fewer than 40 percent of encounters on a given day. Unfortunately, other provider groups, including doctors of chiropractic, also do not do as much as they could in this area. Providers of all kinds tend to be more reactive than proactive and do not act from a preventive mind-set. However, there are studies that show that health care providers are the people most likely to influence healthy behavior changes in their patients. In addition, short, systematic, regular messages about positive behavior change can indeed have a cumulative effect on a patient's desire to make changes. The health care provider should engage the patient, know what to recommend to aid in disease prevention and promotion of wellness, and know what not to say that could demotivate a person who wants to make a change in behavior. They also need to make sure resources are available to the patient, instead of simply saying, "You need to lose 15 pounds this month," followed by, "See you next visit."

For example, it is not helpful to remind people who know they are overweight of this fact and then leave them to try to lose weight with no support. It is probably unfair to address the issue with the patient if the doctor has no plan to offer support. For practitioners to have an opportunity to advise patients on health and wellness, first they must have made this a part of their practice. When seeing health care providers, it may be prudent to ask them how they feel about working with someone who wants to try lifestyle changes in place of medicine or hands-on treatment. In some cases, insurance companies may reimburse providers for wellness and preventive care. In the case of the Affordable Care Act, this is certain for some screenings. Providers may receive compensation for the time spent talking to patients about a variety of things, from smoking or tobacco cessation to healthy weight, stress levels, and sleep levels. That means more providers should be willing to discuss wellness with patients and provide a pathway for prevention if patients want it. There are billing codes for preventive services and health education that is delivered in the practice setting. Practitioners may think they don't have the time or the knowledge to advise patients on these topics. If that is the case, it might be a good idea to find another provider. These issues need to be resolved.

However, there are many resources available for clinical providers to update their knowledge of wellness issues and healthy behavior change. Behavior change is often needed in the doctor's case as well! To reiterate, it is critical to have a mind-set that is ready to attempt a behavior or lifestyle change if the process is going to be effective. We are all in various stages of readiness to make changes, and some times of year or points in one's life can be better than others. But when we are ready as a patient to make a change, any provider who is interested in prevention and wellness should also be ready and willing to assist in this process. That is another hallmark of a wellness-based doctor.

Wellness in Chiropractic Practice

There are several reasons why a chiropractic office is the perfect place to promote health and wellness to patients. First, some studies indicate that patients tend to perceive chiropractic physicians as wellness oriented. This is probably due, in part, to the fact that chiropractic doctors emphasize a check-up style of practice more similar to dentistry than to traditional medicine. Satisfied patients tend to go to the doctor of chiropractic to prevent recurrences of the types of pain that brought them there in the first place. When patients come in periodically to have their joints checked for improper function or mobility and then have those areas adjusted before they cause pain, chiropractors have the opportunity to engage them on lifestyle changes that can lead to a better state of health. Patients miss out when doctors fail to discuss preventive measures and lifestyle changes that can improve longevity. Furthermore, patients may miss an opportunity to make a behavior change when they are ready to do it, which would be very unfortunate. Chiropractic physicians with an interest in wellness and prevention should offer more than once-a-month chiropractic adjustments. Prospective patients must keep this in mind as they consider providers.

In a typical condition-specific treatment plan, patients do not come in once for a prescription; rather, they tend to come in several times over the course of a few weeks for manual or hands-on care (adjustment). This provides multiple points of interaction and opportunities for dialogue with patients about wellness or better health. In clinical care circles, this is referred to as "dose response"; that is, the more often a concept (or treatment, for that matter) is described, the more likely the patient is to hear it and potentially act on it and have it do some good. These "doses" of health advice tend to have a cumulative effect. Similar to talking a pill for wellness several times rather than once or twice a year, dose response suggests that the more times the doctor engages the patient, the better the chance a message will stick. Studies have shown that short, focused messages have led to measurable behavior changes in patients over time. Therefore, patients who have health risks that can be improved through lifestyle modification should receive ongoing information and support from their doctor.

Valid Approaches to Wellness in Clinical Chiropractic Practice

Because the term "wellness" has been used in so many different settings in so many different ways, it is important to establish what actually constitutes a valid approach to wellness. To better understand what makes up a valid approach, let's first consider what is not a valid approach to wellness in clinical chiropractic practice. For many years in the early part of the chiropractic profession, many providers would help resolve patients' painful spine problems only to tell them that they now needed to come in once a week (or once a month) for the rest of their lives as a preventive measure. While this may have made the doctors' wallets well, it may or may not have promoted wellness in the patient.

Consider the example of a person who has a minor problem with the spine from a long day running or playing softball and no other major health problems. If all this patient needs is a few chiropractic treatments, then this is what he should get, and then he should be released. There may not be a real need for continued care. Now, if that person feels better and his softball swing improves and so he wants to come in periodically for a chiropractic checkup, there is nothing wrong with that. Patient experience and preference is also a part of evidence-based health care. Doctors should always take into account what the patient wants out of the experience of a visit. However, prescribing a regular schedule of care at the same rate for every single person is not wellness oriented and is simply an invalid practice; especially if all the patient gets is a spinal adjustment. After all, there are opportunities to talk about diet, exercise levels, tobacco use, sleep patterns, seat-belt use, and all sorts of positive behavior changes that could be guided by the doctor on that visit and subsequent visits.[6] This is what one should expect from a true wellness-based chiropractic visit.

There are times when a person with a chronic condition may need to receive regular chiropractic care. This is no different than diabetics who need regular care from their medical physician to manage the condition. However, if all the medical physician were to do on subsequent visits is refill a prescription and never talk about diet and daily exercise, would that be a valid wellness practice for the patient? Probably not. As long as health care providers can justify that a patient can benefit from some schedule of regular care and talks about preventive measures that can be taken within the six dimensions of wellness, there is a valid opportunity for wellness care to occur in that office.

Some wellness measures that can, and indeed should, be taken in the chiropractic office, or any health care office for that matter, are vital signs. Blood pressure is easy to check, and it has been called the "silent killer" because a person can have elevated blood pressure and not know it. However, making some simple lifestyle changes can often lower blood pressure and reduce the risk of stroke and heart attack. Dietary changes, regular exercise, and reductions in salt intake are all valid lifestyle changes to make if one has a higher than normal blood pressure reading. This should be recommended by the doctor. Good wellness practitioners will offer this advice regardless of what discipline of health care they practice. Imagine the health and wellness benefits that could come from monitoring the blood pressure of every patient as a part of regular medical and chiropractic practice.

Health care providers should also measure height and weight to determine body mass index (BMI). A high BMI, indicating that the patient is overweight or obese, can indicate a higher risk of diseases. BMI is not a useful measurement for all people (e.g., a body builder could have a high BMI but not be overweight), it can be valuable for most subgroups of people. A high BMI measurement can serve as a reminder to the clinician to advise the patient to get more physical activity and improve dietary habits. If this is not happening in a provider's office, there may be a problem.

Other vital signs are temperature and pulse rate; these can be simply evaluated on every new patient visit or follow-up visit as needed. Indicators of basic overall health are a starting point in the assessment of how well a patient is. These should be a routine part of any clinical practice. There are also those who will contend that tobacco use is so important that it should be considered a vital sign as well.[7] Whether one smokes or uses other forms of tobacco, or has used tobacco in the past and for how long, is very important to know. Risks factors for cardiovascular disease diminish with time once someone stops using tobacco, but risks for some forms of cancer, such as lung cancer, never go back to the baseline level. Many other cancers are more common in tobacco users as well. This information is needed in not only the assessment of a patient but in identifying other potential causes of chronic pain. For example, smokers tend to recover less rapidly and completely from chronic spinal pain than nonsmokers.[8] Only by asking the right question on a patient intake form or in a discussion with the patient in a review of their various systems and history will one actually know what risks a patient carries with him or her on a daily basis. A good patient assessment and diagnostic workup is always the start of a wellness-based practice. Questions about lifestyle should be asked in the intake and exam. If they are not, the provider is not focused on wellness and prevention.

What if every health care provider on every checkup visit asked the patient about the following six things: diet, exercise levels, tobacco use, alcohol use, sleep levels, and stress levels? And if the patient exhibited a risk in one of those areas, what if the health care provider was willing and able to offer him or her resources to improve each of those risk factors? Do you think people would improve their overall health and wellness levels? The answer is yes. Studies have shown that changes in diet to more of a Mediterranean diet, exercising between 150 and 300 minutes a week,[9] and getting enough sleep all help patients to become or continue to be well. We have known for decades about the risk of tobacco use for the cardiovascular system, and we now know that although a drink or two a day is probably okay, excessive use is not. These are simple questions that one can ask to assess basic health risks.

It is not difficult to gather resources that can be offered to patients who want to make lifestyle changes—including information about other groups in the community, such as gyms and yoga studios; lists of healthy foods and health food stores; and resources from various agencies and philanthropies—and make all these available in the health care clinic. However, some providers either don't see this as part of their role or are simply unwilling to take the time to set up these valuable resources. A good wellness-based provider will know what resources are already available in the community and point them out to patients.

Signs of a Wellness Practice

If a health care provider is truly focused on wellness and preventive care, there should be signs of this in the office. First, wellness-oriented practices are often attached to a fitness center or CrossFit gym. More of these are popping up today, and they can be legitimate practices with much to offer. In addition, a nutritionist or dietician may be on staff. Doctors and dieticians, naturopaths, nurse practitioners, and chiropractors are increasingly working together to develop highly specialized dietary recommendations for those with chronic conditions, in what is called "functional medicine." Led by the Institute for Functional Medicine, these providers take an even more detailed history of diet and lifestyle and often provide more nutrition-based care than traditional medical care.

Wellness practices will also ask more detailed questions about diet and health habits, particularly exercise and physical activity, on intake forms. They may ask specific questions about sleep patterns, stressors, and other features of daily life that can indicate a need for behavior change. In addition, they may encourage the use of supplements in place of medications, but not as a substitute for lifestyle changes necessary for better health.

An exam in a wellness doctor's office will include a check of vital signs. Specific importance will be placed on height and weight to calculate BMI, as well as potentially the waist-to-hip ratio, which is a means of assessing belly fat. Increased belly fat is an indicator for cardiovascular risks but varies between men and women (and between pre- and postmenopausal women). The doctor or nurse can explain these differences so that patients understand what the risks are, if any, for their body type. Blood work may be done, as well as urine testing. These will give the provider some information about things like cholesterol, A1C, and inflammatory biomarkers that have been found to indicate risks of everything from arthritis to heart disease.

In the report of findings, wellness doctors may talk about changes that need to be made to diet, exercise levels, sleep patterns, and other behaviors. They may offer a recheck later in the year after patients have adopted a healthier lifestyle plan. The idea here is that patients will stick with this plan and try to make those changes prior to a subsequent reevaluation. Of course, they will address the patient's chief complaint as well. The report should give the patient's levels of cholesterol, low-density and high-density cholesterol, A1C, and inflammatory indicators, and it should indicate some things that can be done to reverse any unhealthy trends. The provider should help the patient to set some goals, making very specific suggestions regarding supplements or exercise levels and offering resources to help reach the goal.

Treatment in a chiropractic office can be manual care or it could mean advice on how to make a dietary change, supplement use, physical activity in general, exercise, and sleep suggestions or stress-reduction activities. This may involve several visits, but a good provider will set up a reasonable number, such as two or three times a week for a week or two. The provider will see how the patient responds and adjust the schedule accordingly. Chiropractic care is more akin to physical therapy visits than to seeing a medical physician for a prescription. The use of supplements, exercise, or other home-care methods is meant to speed recovery and help patients get into a habit of taking better care of themselves for the rest of their life.

In contrast, some chiropractic physicians may offer a long treatment period for a single condition with very little follow-up. This is not considered good practice if the patient's pain levels, ability to function, or state of health do not dictate it. If recommendations seem unreasonable, they may be. Other chiropractic physicians may make a very accurate diagnosis of the patient's specific condition and set up very reasonable treatment plans that will be reevaluated in two or three weeks. However, the difference is that in a wellness practice, they will do more than address the specific condition. The intake and examination will look and feel different. The questions related to current lifestyle will go into more depth and will include aspects of life that could be changed if needed, in most cases. It is not uncommon for a doctor to focus very specifically on the main problem that brought the patient to the office; however, to truly address better health and wellness, more is needed, and this is very evident from the current assessment of physical well-being in the general population, particularly in the United States. While the United States spends by far the most money on medical care, prescriptions, and other "health" care, it lags behind most developed nations in well-being! This is at least in part due to clinical health care providers focusing exclusively on their patients' primary complaint and not taking a more holistic view of health. No provider group is doing a great job here. There is room for improvement from all providers, and that is why it is increasingly important to think about what a wellness provider looks like.

Changes That Can Be Seen Today

Today, patients have more choices related to wellness than ever before. For example, the new functional medicine movement, which relies heavily on diet, lifestyle, and conservative care, is moving along rapidly. The famous Cleveland Clinic, a functional medicine clinic, was established in 2013, and the program has since doubled. This movement addresses inflammation, causes of food sensitivity, and other chronic conditions in a way that traditional health care has often overlooked. They also stress the importance of the microbiome or healthy bacteria of the gut. Exciting new information supports the notion that these healthy bacteria also play an important role in inflammation and immunity, and supplements and diet can have positive effects on these bacteria. Antibiotics have a very negative effect, obviously. At this time, an increasing number of chiropractors are getting postgraduate training in functional medicine.

Culinary medicine is another emerging field in which medical colleges, such as Tulane University School of Medicine's Goldring Center,[10] will now teach future physicians how to prepare healthy meals so that they can teach their patients how to eat healthy and thereby avoid premature chronic disease. This effort is one of a few programs based on the idea that most of the chronic health conditions in this country are related to either poor dietary choices or other bad habits that can be changed or avoided. Since the health care provider is among the most powerful people to cue others to take action about their health, this is considered a fantastic step in the right direction. In fact, "food as medicine" and "exercise as medicine" are two common phrases that, if embraced by all health care providers in the United States, could lead to a reversal of bad fortune for many Americans, should they make an effort to work with those health care providers to change their health behaviors.

The emerging field of epigenetics is also adding to our understanding of nutrition. We now know that long-term, or sometimes even short-term, changes in diet can have an effect on genetically modified signals that either enhance health or diminish it.

As more options become available for patients to make healthier choices, it is important to make sure patients know to keep their doctors and other health care providers informed. For instance, some diets and supplements can interfere with drug absorption, and some drugs can react poorly with certain foods and other substances. It is a good idea to have everyone on the same page, and that means informing the primary care provider of choice. Patients should let their primary care doctor know about the other providers that care for them as well as the results they are getting. That way, each one can respect what the other brings and perhaps they can all work together to keep patients healthy and not simply treat condition after condition.

Closing Thoughts and Take-Away

At the end of the day, the biggest threats to premature disease and premature mortality are mostly related to lifestyle and health behavior. While these may be influenced by friends, family, and surroundings, when people choose positive health behavior, they tend to live longer and more productive lives. Genetics may play a role, so some factors can't be changed by choice. However, nutritional epigenetics is changing some of the perceptions on this front, and we will learn more about this in the next decade than ever before. Still, the majority of risk for premature morbidity and mortality is related to four things: tobacco use, excessive use of alcohol, bad dietary choices, and lack of recreational physical activity. Sleep levels may be the next indicator to make the list. People in most developed countries have become considerably less active since the 1970s, and fast food has become more readily available since then. We now know what kind of exercise is needed and even what type of diet, in most cases. The information and resources are available to support positive changes. While no one is suggesting taking away everything that makes life enjoyable, almost everyone needs more physical activity or movement and a healthier diet. Tobacco use is declining, but many people still use it; their health care providers should help them quit. Many Americans drink too much as well.

If all health care providers addressed those four issues in practice as a key part of what they talked about every day, health care practices would have a major impact on the health outcomes in their communities. They would grow as well. Patients need someone to advocate for change, and they need resources and guidance that is not typically provided in the family medical clinic environment. Chiropractic professionals are filling that void in many cases, but patients interested in assistance with their wellness process must take a little time to find the right doctor. Ask a friend who uses a chiropractic physician about his or her experience. Think of the ideas noted above and ask questions about what the provider offers in the way of prevention. Is it once-a-month care with nothing but chiropractic adjustments, or is there more? It is also possible to "interview" doctors and call for a simple consultation to find out what they truly offer and believe as a paradigm for better health. Don't be afraid to do this.

Chiropractic physicians are in a unique situation in that they see patients with some frequency, their patients have a tendency to choose preventive adjustments for spinal conditions, and they are often thought of as having a preventive mind-set by health care consumers. If most doctors of chiropractic would learn the basics about wellness, advising and applying health promotion in their offices, major changes would be seen, and over time, the brand of health care focused on wellness and prevention would be more associated with the profession than perhaps any other health care discipline. This is true of all providers; a change is desperately needed. Patients need to know how to choose better health care providers. More choices are available today than ever, and people must seek out opportunities to connect with a better healer for the sake of their health and that of their family. Our culture needs health care providers that will lead them down a path to better health outcomes instead of only treating symptoms and relieving aches and pains.

References

1. Leavell HR, Clark EG. *Preventive Medicine for the Doctor in His Community.* 3rd ed. New York: McGraw-Hill; 1965.

2. World Health Organization. WHO definition of health. http://www.who.int/about/definition/en/print.html. Accessed April 10, 2016.

3. Glanz K, Rimer BK, Viswanath K, eds. *Health Behavior and Health Education.* San Francisco: Josey-Bass; 2008:11.

4. McLeroy KR, Bibeau D, Steckler A, Glanz K. An ecological perspective on health promotion programs. *Health Educ Q.* 1988;15:351–377.

5. Evans MW, Ndetan H, Singh KP. Primary prevention: what are we missing in primary care? *Am J Heal Stud.* 2012;27(2):82–96.

6. Hawk C, Schneider M, Evans MW, Jr., Redwood D. Consensus process to develop a best-practice document on the role of chiropractic care in health promotion, disease prevention, and wellness. *J Manipulative Physiol Ther.* 2012;35(7): 556–567.

7. Ahluwalia JS, Gibson CA, Kenney E, Wallace DD, Resnicow K. Smoking status as a vital sign. *J Gen Intern Med.* 1999;14:402–408.

8. Rechtine GR, Rechtine JC, Bolesta MJ. Smoking cessation in the spine surgeon's office: a review. *J Spinal Discord.* 1999;12(6):477–481.

9. U. S. Department of Health and Human Services. *Physical Activity Guidelines for Americans: Be Active, Healthy, and Happy!* www.health.gov/paguidelines. Accessed April 10, 2016.

10. The Goldring Center for Culinary Medicine. Tulane University School of Medicine. http://tmedweb.tulane.edu/mu/teachingkitchen/. Accessed April 10, 2016.

CHAPTER THIRTEEN

Chiropractic Care for Special Populations: Pregnant Women, Children, and Older Adults

Sharon Vallone, DC, FICCP; Cheryl Hawk, DC, PhD, CHES; and Lisa Zaynab Killinger, DC

This chapter describes the chiropractic approach to care of special populations commonly seen by chiropractors: pregnant women, children, and older adults.

Pregnant Women

Conception and the development of life in the womb is affected by a woman's emotional and physical state of well-being. Her nutrition, her body mechanics, her sleep and exercise habits, her stress levels and state of mind have all been shown to have a potential effect on her ability to conceive and the health and well-being of her child. If any of these are less than optimal, it can result in anything from a woman's inability to conceive to the later development of adult health disorders in her child.

Pregnancy, to rephrase a popular saying, is a journey *and* a destination. The destination, delivering the baby, is profoundly affected by the journey. Where does the chiropractor play a role on this momentous journey?

The miracle of having a child can be supported by chiropractic in a number of ways. Chiropractors can be invaluable members of the pregnant woman's support team on the journey toward bringing a healthy baby into the world.

When a woman plans to become pregnant, her healthy lifestyle is of paramount importance, and preparing the body for this journey will prevent many problems along the way. Chiropractors will counsel their pregnant patients to eat a healthy, organically clean diet; reduce their stress; sleep enough hours to recharge their body regularly; drink plenty of clean water; and exercise appropriately. This can help set the stage for the important timing of events required to successfully conceive and have a healthy pregnancy. Chiropractic manual care can be helpful in maintaining proper body biomechanics with the changes in a woman's body that occur through pregnancy as well as relieving stress on the musculoskeletal system.

Safety

The first concern of pregnant women and their doctors is that the treatment is safe for the pregnant woman and her unborn baby. Fortunately, evidence is beginning to accumulate related to the safety of chiropractic care, specifically spinal manipulation, for pregnancy. A 2012 systematic review of adverse events among pregnant and postpartum women receiving spinal manipulation stated, "There are only a few reported cases of adverse events following spinal manipulation during pregnancy and the postpartum period identified in the literature. While improved reporting of such events is required in the future, it may be that such injuries are relatively rare."[1] In none of the cases were there any adverse effects on the pregnancy, delivery, or baby.

Chiropractic education includes training and supervised clinical experience on how to modify manipulative techniques and patient positioning for pregnant women. These modifications increase patient comfort and minimize the risk of adverse effects. Students are also taught to recognize situations in which manipulation is not appropriate. Because X-rays cannot be used during pregnancy to rule out some conditions that might be contraindications to traditional high-force spinal manipulation, it is essential that chiropractors are skilled in modified manipulative techniques. Also, due to the relaxing of the ligaments from hormonal changes preparing the woman's body for delivery, lower-force techniques are likely to be not only more comfortable but just as effective. The chiropractor will be careful in positioning the patient to avoid pressure on the abdomen by using side-lying or supine (lying face up) positions.[2]

Low Back Pain during Pregnancy

Chapter 7 discussed the chiropractic approach to low back pain among adults in general. This is perhaps the best-researched topic related to chiropractic care, with ample evidence that chiropractic care and specifically spinal manipulation are beneficial for acute and chronic low back pain.[3]

Low back pain is very common among pregnant women, due to the change in posture from the pregnancy and the relaxing of ligaments that occurs in preparation for childbirth. Although the evidence is not yet strong due to the relatively small number of studies, it indicates that spinal manipulation is beneficial to pregnant women with low back pain.[3] Chiropractors also have training in therapeutic exercise and can suggest safe and effective physical activity and exercises for pregnant women.

Pain during Labor and Delivery

Compared to the evidence for chiropractic care for low back pain during pregnancy, research related to the effect of chiropractic manipulation, or spinal manipulation in general, on reducing back pain during labor is sparse.[3] There is some preliminary research investigating the effect of spinal manipulation that is provided as a regular part of prenatal care that suggests a possible positive effect.[4]

Breech Presentation Correction

Babies in a breech position (head under the rib cage and buttocks presenting at the cervix—head up/bottom down) are usually delivered by Caesarean section (C-section). Mothers and their doctors who would prefer a vaginal birth might consider seeing a chiropractor to structurally assess the movement of the joints of the spine and pelvis that could present a restriction to the fetus moving freely enough in the womb to present head down for delivery. Many chiropractors are also trained in a particular manipulative technique, the Webster technique. Practitioners of this technique believe that imbalances in the biomechanics of the lumbar spine and pelvis may affect the uterus in such a way that a breech position occurs. The purpose this technique is to correct these imbalances. It does not involve an attempt to move the fetus in the mother's abdomen. The chiropractor may use a variety of different chiropractic techniques modified for pregnancy to manipulate the sacrum (the triangular bone at the base of the spine that makes up the back of the pelvis) and then a very light application of pressure (three to six ounces, approximately) to the round ligament (palpated halfway between the belly button and the boney point on the front of the pelvis), a ligament that helps to suspend and support the position of the uterus in the lower abdomen.[5] No adverse effects were noted by chiropractors trained in this technique who used it for pregnant women with diagnosed breech presentation.[5]

Children

Parents frequently seek chiropractic care for their children in both the United States and internationally. In fact, chiropractic is the complementary and integrative medicine profession used most often by children in the United States.[6] Usually, parents take their children and teens to a chiropractor for the treatment of musculoskeletal conditions.

A 2010 survey collected demographic data of pediatric patients presenting to a chiropractic teaching clinic in Great Britain, of which 20.5 percent were pediatric patients between two days and 15 years old. The most common presenting complaint was musculoskeletal (35%). Excess crying (30%) was the most common complaint in the largest presenting age group, which was under 12 weeks of age (62.3%). All children had previously presented for medical care for the same condition. Most (83%) of the infant patients under 12 weeks of age were referred for care by a medical practitioner.[7]

For infants, colic is one of the more common reasons for parents to seek chiropractic care.[8,9] It is also fairly common in the United States for parents to take their children to a chiropractor for "wellness care." This is a sort of check-up in which the chiropractor checks the child's spine, muscular system, and often diet and exercise habits in order to prevent problems from arising later.

Safety

There is a great deal of scientific evidence for chiropractic care for many health problems, primarily musculoskeletal, suffered by adults. However, at this time, the amount of research done specifically on chiropractic care for children is relatively modest but growing.[10] The most important concern of any parent when considering chiropractic care is, of course, safety. It is fortunate that a substantial amount of effort has gone into establishing the safety of chiropractic care for children. *Chapter 6 discusses safety issues in detail.* Here the focus is on the evidence related specifically to the safety of chiropractic care for children. A 2015 systematic review evaluating the safety of chiropractic care for children found that serious adverse effects related to chiropractic care are rare, and no deaths have been reported in the literature. For the few reported cases of serious adverse effects, in most cases the child had some type of preexisting condition—for example, a malformation of a bone, joint, or nerve structure. This makes it extremely important that the chiropractor does a careful history and examination before using any manual therapy.[11]

Best Practice Recommendations for Chiropractic Care for Children

The profession has now published a set of practice guidelines for "best practices" for chiropractic care of children.[12] These recommendations were updated, accompanied by a systematic review to inform the consensus process, in 2016.[13] Below are some of the key points that this set of recommendations makes:

- Children's musculoskeletal and nervous systems are different from adults' and also differ according to children's developmental stage. Chiropractic treatment must be tailored to the individual child's developmental stage and individual characteristics. There is not a "one size fits all" chiropractic treatment, especially for children.

- The chiropractor should explain everything he or she recommends being done, as well as the diagnosis, in clear and simple terms, to both the child and his or her accompanying adult. The child and parent should have all their questions answered to their satisfaction so that they can make an informed decision about their choice of care.

- Chiropractors treating children, just as any other chiropractor, should adhere to the principles of evidence-based practice. These are to make clinical judgments based on the best available scientific evidence combined with the patient's preferences and values and the clinician's experience.

- Children who see a chiropractor are likely to also be under the care of their primary care physician or other types of health care professionals. If so, the chiropractor should communicate with these professionals appropriately in order to best serve the patient's needs. The chiropractor is also expected to know when it is appropriate to refer the child to another type of provider for care. This might be the case when a child is not showing clinical improvement after the first trial of chiropractic care (which might be several treatments over a one- or two-week period).

- The chiropractor should make an immediate referral to the child's primary care physician or a specialist if the examination or history shows any "red flags"—findings that suggest a serious problem. Delay of appropriate care, which is one cause of some reported adverse effects, will then be prevented.

- The history and examination should be tailored to the child's developmental stage.
- Concerning X-rays (diagnostic imaging): these should not be used routinely or repeatedly for children. They should only be used when there are clear clinical reasons for doing so, such as a recent severe injury.

Especially important to most parents who are new to chiropractic will be considerations for treating children with manual procedures. In using manual procedures, chiropractors consider the patient's size, developmental stage, joint flexibility, and the patient's and parents' preferences. The child's needs and comfort are of the greatest importance.

Another important consideration is the concept of "well child" visits. Just as in medical care, well child visits may be used as opportunities for health promotion counseling and catching risk factors before they cause ill health. Chiropractors should talk to children and parents about physical activity, nutrition, injury prevention, and a healthy lifestyle.

Any tests or procedures used for public screenings must be based on recognized evidence of their benefit for disease prevention and health promotion.

Chiropractic Care for Children with Specific Conditions

The 2016 best practices recommendations cited above found that only a few conditions had published research evidence to support their treatment with chiropractic care.[13] These were almost all for nonmusculoskeletal conditions: asthma, colic, and bedwetting (nocturnal enuresis). Only one musculoskeletal condition has research support: headaches. However, it is important to be aware that "no research evidence" does not mean that the treatment doesn't work. It simply means that there hasn't been enough research done yet to be sure one way or the other. Clinical research is extremely expensive, and research investigators who are experts in chiropractic are scarce, and that has a great deal of bearing on why there is not more research in this area.

Therefore, we will describe a number of conditions common among various age groups of children, which, in the authors' experience, often benefit from a chiropractic approach.

Infants

Nothing affects parents as deeply as the cry of their newborn child who cannot be comforted. A paper published by a professor of the

Anglo-European Chiropractic College states, "With 21% of parents taking their excessively crying infant to a healthcare professional, chiropractors are often selected to treat these infants. The personal, family and social costs of this crying syndrome are high, yet there is no agreed treatment protocol. A large number of studies have been aimed at providing useful interventions, but no 'cure' has been demonstrated. With some evidential backing, chiropractors are well-placed to provide therapy for this syndrome."[14]

Since chiropractic care for infants has been shown to be safe, particularly when guidelines are followed for best practices and the chiropractor has training in pediatrics,[13,15] a variety of challenges infants face may be worth a reasonable trial of chiropractic care, such as difficulty sleeping, excessive crying or colic, feeding difficulties, muscle restriction (wry neck or torticollis), and flattening of the head (plagiocephaly) to name just a few.

Infantile Colic

A recent systematic review[16] done by the prestigious Cochrane Collaboration found some support for manipulative therapy such as is done by chiropractors for reducing crying time in infants with colic. Colic is when an otherwise healthy infant cries more than three hours a day, three days a week, for three weeks or longer. Nothing a parent can do appears to help the baby during these episodes. Infantile colic is a distressing problem characterized by excessive crying, and excessive crying is the most common complaint seen by physicians in the first 16 weeks of a child's life.[14] It is usually considered a benign disorder because the symptoms generally disappear by the age of five or six months. However, questions have been raised about the longer-lasting effects on the child. Chiropractors may provide treatment to infants to attempt to first rule out any underlying musculoskeletal disorder that could be the cause of the infant's distress and then to ameliorate the symptoms if possible. A review of six randomized trials involving 325 infants were of insufficient "quality" to confidently conclude that chiropractic or osteopathic therapies were useful in the treatment of colic, but rigorous research requires providing treatment to one group of children while denying it to another and the ethics of denying treatment presents a challenge to setting up a large-scale study.

Besides taking a careful history and evaluating the infant for musculoskeletal dysfunction, a chiropractor might review lifestyle (overstimulation or other environmental stressors, overzealous siblings, parental fears, or other parental issues like postpartum depression) and nutrition (underfeeding, overfeeding, poor oral motor function resulting in swallowing air or slow motility, or breastfed vs. formula-fed infants and potential gastrointestinal sensitivities, for example) and evaluate whether the infant is developing a healthy microbiome (natural bacterial flora in the gut), which is often disturbed by the intervention of antibiotics at birth. All of these could contribute to excessive crying in an infant, and symptoms improve (and general family demeanor improves) when the offending problem is recognized and averted.[16]

Nursing Dysfunction

Although little formal research has been done, a literature review of chiropractic and breastfeeding dysfunction published in 2014 revealed a number of case reports and case series as well as a clinical trial conducted at a university that indicated that chiropractic care may be helpful for certain infants with nursing dysfunction resulting from musculoskeletal issues.[17]

These issues can include a baby who won't root (turn) to the breast or suckle (absence of normal infant reflexes), problems opening the mouth (temporomandibular joint problems) or moving the head into positions that make it possible to breastfeed (poor mobility of the head and neck), or other joint misalignment that may make it painful for the baby to be held in the breastfeeding position.

The chiropractor would perform a careful evaluation, and treatment would consist of specific chiropractic techniques modified for the age and size of the infant patient. Treatment usually consists of two to six treatments over a two- to three-week period when there are no other problems that need to be addressed (e.g., a tongue tie or incidental injury like a fracture of the clavicle in an infant whose shoulder was lodged behind the pubic bone during birth). In these cases, the compensatory musculoskeletal issues may require support beyond the initial two- to three-week period.

For uncomplicated cases, the specific outcome desired is to achieve exclusive breastfeeding. In one study, it was found that of 114 infants who presented to the chiropractor due to feeding difficulties, all infants showed some improvement, with 78 percent being able to exclusively breastfeed at the end of two weeks.[17]

Plagiocephaly and Torticollis

Deformational plagiocephaly, also known as positional plagiocephaly, describes changes in the shape of the infant skull. How an infant is repeatedly positioned after birth can play a role in the development of this condition. Tremendous growth of the brain and skull occurs during the first weeks of life, yet infants cannot actively reposition themselves. If the child is placed in the same position for sleep, favors a certain side (as in the case of torticollis), or looks at a mobile while only in a certain position, this can result in a flattening of the area of the skull that carries the weight of the resting head. This often develops gradually over the first few months of life.

Torticollis involves the rotation and lateral flexion of the head and neck due to contracted musculature. It can be caused by a wide range of things, from lack of room in the womb to injury during the birth process. The infant may be born with it or it may develop over the first few months of life.

Regardless of the cause, the contracted musculature restricts range of motion, keeping the head in one position, which results in a flattening of the head. The contracture may also contribute to changes in the face and to the shape of the ear. In this case, parents are often advised to perform neck exercises on the infant at home to increase mobility and allow repositioning of the head to prevent plagiocephaly.

Once believed to be only a cosmetic problem, studies are now linking deformational plagiocephaly to developmental delays, including hearing and vision disorders and uneven development of bones of the skull, such as the jaw. "Watching and waiting," frequently changing an infant's head position, physical therapy, cranial remodeling using a cranial helmet, and, in the rare case, surgical procedures are traditional treatments. Due to the possibility of long-term problems, early intervention and a proactive approach would appear advisable.

Chiropractors present another treatment option for this condition. An Australian study of 25 infants diagnosed with positional plagiocephaly suggested full resolution of the condition after receiving three to four months of chiropractic care.[18] In another report, evidence-based recommendations concluded that it was "appropriate to propose a course of pediatric chiropractic manual therapy along with advice and recommendations regarding active counter-positioning, 'tummy time,' and appropriate infant placement."[19] Parents should also be well educated about the use of car-seat carriers, bouncers, and swings, as well as the risk factors for SIDS, with a thorough explanation concerning chiropractic care as a treatment option.[18]

What Does Chiropractic Care of the Infant Look Like?

As parents tentatively place their infant into the hands of a chiropractor, their own experience, or lack of experience, with a chiropractor may generate questions and concerns. Chiropractic techniques are modified according to the age and specific stage of bone and muscle development of the child,[13] whether performed manually (by hand) or with an instrument (a hand-held tool that can be set to administer a very low force for infants). When done by hand, the adjustment or manipulation is a controlled low-force (or non-force as in a technique where the joint is contacted with a fingertip, pressed and held until movement is restored by the infant moving against the finger) short ranges of motion (little movement) with a specific contact and understanding of the specific architecture of the joint.

Infants have a higher percentage of cartilage that will convert to hard bone as they mature and muscles that can become tight or strained during the birth process or in compensation for another problem and can require gentle soft tissue techniques like massage or myofascial release to prepare the area before adjusting. The chiropractic treatment may begin with some mild evidence of discomfort as tender muscles are palpated and released, but by the end of the treatment, the infant is often so relaxed he or she falls asleep.

The course of treatment depends on the problems the individual child presents with, but the chiropractor will assess progress after a number of treatments to recommend whether further treatment would be advantageous or whether it is more appropriate to collaborate with another health care provider.

Children (Ages 1–12) and Adolescents

As children become weight bearing and begin to develop their motor skills and cognitive function, chiropractors can play an important role in observing and proactively supporting their development with "well visits" to be sure that milestones are being appropriately reached and to prevent any compensations or roadblocks from impeding their progress. "Well child visits" are an opportunity for parents and children to ask questions about their health and lifestyle as well as for the chiropractor to assess the child and detect any early signs of problems that may not yet have symptoms (like an alteration in a normal walking pattern or a lateral curvature of the spine, called a scoliosis).

As children enter school and become more actively involved in both cognitive pursuits and athletics, a chiropractor can monitor their musculoskeletal health and general well-being. Chiropractors should counsel children and their parents in healthy behavior and lifestyle, including but not limited to the following topics: adequate age-appropriate physical activity and decreased screen time, such as TV, electronic games, and computer use; healthy diet; adequate sleep; injury prevention; and substance use (e.g., caffeinated beverages, alcohol, tobacco, steroids, and other drugs). The chiropractor can also be another attentive adult that children can talk to as they begin to face performance and social stresses.[13]

Some of the nonmusculoskeletal complaints that the older child presents with to the chiropractor are described below.

Otitis Media

Ear infections, both acute and chronic, are the bane of parents who sit with a crying child who cannot be soothed in the middle of the night, rocking the child back and forth and holding the child's ears. Children with restricted cranial or cervical movement and blocked lymphatic channels that empty the head and neck are supported with chiropractic treatment to mobilize the joints and help release the lymphatic flow by relaxing and releasing the associated soft tissues. Although the published evidence for the effectiveness of manipulation for otitis media is not sufficient to draw a conclusion, the evidence does indicate that there are no adverse effects.[3]

Constipation

Constipation can occur at any age and can be caused by beginning solid foods too early, dehydration, food sensitivities, or lack of healthy bowel flora and yeast overgrowth. It may also occur because of musculoskeletal dysfunction, and normal bowel function is often restored if this is the root of the problem and is addressed with appropriately provided chiropractic treatment, sometimes supported by a change in diet or addition of a probiotic to the child's diet. As is the case with most of the research on chiropractic care for children, there is insufficient evidence at this time to draw firm conclusions.

Enuresis

Bedwetting past the age of toilet training can be a problem for a number of reasons, including the child losing self-esteem or being unable to participate in certain social functions. Like constipation, bedwetting has been linked to food sensitivities in some cases; it can also be caused by slow development or poor neurologic control of the bladder or reduced feedback to the nervous system that the bladder is full but needs to be controlled until the appropriate time to empty, which may be associated with joint dysfunction and can be helped by a chiropractic treatment. The research evidence for the effectiveness of spinal manipulation on enuresis in children is favorable but inconclusive, due to the small number of studies.[3]

Asthma

Although the evidence is inconclusive due to a shortage of high-quality studies,[3] one 2001 clinical study pointed out an interesting finding: children treated with chiropractic care for their asthma used their bronchodilators less and rated their symptoms and quality of life to be improved, even though their lung function tests did not change.[20] Reducing any use of drugs in children is always a goal in asthma management, so for that reason alone it may be worth considering chiropractic care for children with this chronic condition.

Headaches

Headaches in children are common. Like adults, children can develop different types of headaches, including migraine or stress-related (tension) headaches. Children can also have chronic daily headaches.

Causes of headaches can range from lack of sleep to skipping meals, poor food choices (high sugar, high caffeine), or not drinking enough water and becoming dehydrated. Too many hours listening to loud music through earphones, watching TV or playing video games, using cell phones and computers, and needing to wear corrective glasses can all be potential triggers for headaches. Musculoskeletal reasons ranging from tight neck muscles due to poor posture to strains and sprains from athletic activities can all contribute to headaches. And in some cases, headaches in children are caused by a common cold, an ear or sinus infection, hormonal changes of puberty, high levels of stress or anxiety at home or at school, or minor head trauma. All of these are important triggers that can be uncovered with a little detective work during an office visit with the chiropractor. Sometimes just identifying the trigger and changing it resolves the problem. Sometimes the problem will require a referral to another type of physician. If it's a musculoskeletal issue, manual therapy may relieve the symptoms of a headache.

Although few studies have been done on the effect of manual therapies on headaches in children, a 2013 systematic review indicated that it may be useful in the treatment of these common forms of headache in adults.[21]

Back Pain

Back pain is not limited to the adult population but can be found, too frequently, in our youth. Whether linked to heavy backpacks, poor choices in or how they wear their shoes, increased sports activity, or poor posture while playing video games or sitting with their laptops and cell phones, more and more young people are presenting with complaints of low back pain. Although most low back complaints are associated with joint dysfunction and muscle weakness or imbalance and will respond well to a reasonable period of chiropractic treatment along with corrected posture or strengthening exercises and raised awareness of the body, a thorough exam (sometimes including diagnostic imaging like X-ray) should be performed to differentially diagnose any more serious underlying pathology and refer the patient to the appropriate health care providers.[10]

Sports Injuries

As youngsters begin to participate in organized sports at an ever-earlier age, injuries ranging from overuse and simple sprains and strains to dislocations and fractures may occur. Whether on the field or in the office setting, the chiropractor will evaluate the child's injury and make a differential diagnosis, sometimes needing to refer for X-rays or other appropriate tests and to another health care provider like an orthopedist or physical therapist to comanage and help the child return to normal activities (and "the game") as quickly as possible.

Adjusting the Older Child

The maturing anatomy of the older child allows the chiropractor to use more techniques than those used on infants and very small children, but the chiropractor will still be very careful to modify those techniques based on the individual child's size and developmental stage. The adjustments or manipulations will also be performed by hand or with an instrument, and there will more likely be cavitation of joints; the noise sometimes produced when a joint is mobilized, often referred to as a "crack" by laypeople, is simply the release of gas that has built up in a nonmoving joint as a result of cellular respiration. The mobilization of the joint not only restores the ability to move the joint but sends information to the brain from the mechanical receptors in the joint that help the body know where it is in space, improving balance and coordination and, at times, reducing the sensation of pain that can be associated with changes in a child's behavior.

After a careful evaluation and discussion with parents and patient to inform them of the clinical findings and treatment recommendation (and any possible side effects), the adjustments can be performed with the patient lying or kneeling on a chiropractic bench or seated on a chiropractic stool. Chiropractors will use their hands or a chiropractic instrument to mobilize the joint, taking patient preference into consideration. There may be brief discomfort or some muscle soreness after treatment, which is usually allayed by gentle movement or the application of a cool cloth or an ice pack for a few moments.

Ethics and Responsibility as Practitioners

The "best practices" recommendations cited throughout this section were the result of the deliberations of a multidisciplinary panel of chiropractors and other health care providers, who were able to reach consensus regarding the chiropractic approach to the pediatric chiropractic patient "based on both scientific evidence and clinical experience."[12,13] This demonstrated an effort on the part of the profession to establish standards to guide practicing clinicians. Research into the effectiveness of chiropractic care for pediatric patients has lagged behind that of adult care, but this is being addressed through educational programs where research is now being incorporated into academic tracks to attain advanced chiropractic degrees. The responsibility of ethical and safe practice lies within the profession. This begins with an acknowledgement that mastery of both an academic foundation and clinical expertise in the art, science, and philosophy of chiropractic are necessary. Chiropractic is a profession, not a technique, and chiropractors are responsible for diagnosis and appropriate management of any case they accept. However, the usual measures of necessity of care, such as disability and pain, may not be applicable to pediatric patients. The pediatric patient may be evaluated using these traditional criteria but may also have other objective findings that support the necessity for chiropractic care, like the presence or absence of infant reflexes or relative attainment of developmental milestones secondary to neurologic or motor impairment (such as feeding, sitting, crawling).

Therefore, an understanding of child development is critical when treating pediatric patients.[15] Clinicians who are not appropriately trained in evaluating or treating children are strongly advised to become acquainted with colleagues who are competent. The chiropractor's responsibility goes beyond the application of chiropractic principles and practice and extends to the timely recognition of critical red flags and the need for referral for collaborative treatment to other appropriate health care professionals. Evidence for the effectiveness and safety of chiropractic care for children is gradually progressing, thanks to the dedication of academicians and clinicians around the world. It is important that the problems of infants and children, which cause suffering to children and families and use significant health care and community resources, be high on the list of conditions to investigate.

Summary

Studies in the United States show that over the last several decades, chiropractors have been the most common complementary and integrative medicine providers visited by children and adolescents. Chiropractors continue to seek integration with other health care providers to provide the most appropriate care for their pediatric patients. In the interest of what is best for the pediatric population, collaborative efforts for research into the effectiveness and safety of chiropractic care as an alternative health care approach for children should be negotiated and are welcomed.

Older Adults

By the year 2050, one in five Americans will be over age 65. Seniors are the fastest-growing segment of the population in many countries; this age wave is a global phenomenon. This section will explore the role chiropractic may play in contributing to the health of older adults.

Chiropractic Education on Aging

All accredited chiropractic colleges are three- to four-year educational programs with busy schedules of 30 or more classroom hours per week. Most of the courses in the chiropractic curriculum are in the basic (such as anatomy, physiology, and biochemistry) or clinical sciences (such as physical diagnosis and radiology). Of course, they also include specialized coursework in manipulation/adjusting techniques, soft tissues techniques, and physical modalities, such as ultrasound or inferential current (*see Chapters 4 and 5 for detailed descriptions*). Chiropractic colleges all include at least one course dedicated to issues of caring for "special populations," including older adult patients. The typical course in "special populations" at a chiropractic college includes about 30 total hours of classroom time. In 2001, the U.S. Health Resources and Services Administration Bureau of Health Professions funded a series of projects to develop and disseminate a model course in geriatric education for chiropractic students. This course was then shared with all North American chiropractic colleges. Some colleges use part or all of the model course to prepare chiropractic students to care for older adult patients.[22]

What Health Issues Cause Older Adults to Seek Chiropractic Care?

The most common reason older adults seek the care of a chiropractor is musculoskeletal pain, most often lower back pain.[23] Spine pain is a significant problem among older patients, with a 2011 report showing that about one-fourth of people over age 75 experience back pain.[24] According to a recent Gallup survey, about 28 percent of people aged 50 to 64 and 18 percent of those aged 65 and older have visited a chiropractor in the past 12 months.[25] Chiropractors are well suited to care for patients with spinal complaints since chiropractic or spinal manipulative therapy is one of several evidence-based treatments for patients with back pain.[3] In the interview found in Box 13.1, an older chiropractic patient describes his experience with and views on chiropractic.

Box 13.1

Interview with "Henry," Age 69, a Retired Counselor

What has been your experience with chiropractic?

"I never thought chiropractors did much, through most of my life. But, about 30 years ago, I hurt my back and the doctor wanted to do back surgery. I refused surgery and tried physical therapy and over-the-counter medications, but I really suffered for about five years. My wife dragged me to the chiropractor, and I tried flexion-distraction technique. I came off the table with *no pain!* The pain never came back like it was before. Then a few years ago, I hurt my back. After many weeks of putting up with it, I had given up many of my activities and gained about 20 pounds. I finally went to see my medical doctor, and all he wanted to do was prescribe painkillers and muscle relaxants. I didn't like that approach, so I went to see the chiropractor. Within two weeks I was much better and was able to start riding my bike and getting back in shape. I continued under chiropractic care and lost 35 pounds and felt stronger and healthier than I had in a long while. I think you guys (chiropractors) have the right approach; helping people help themselves get well and take some responsibility for their own health.

"I think chiropractic does great benefit to society because it uses natural methods (not drugs) and it allows the body to heal itself. Chiropractors really get to know their patients. Also, chiropractors look at whole health, and care about the mental health as well as physical health as all being important."

What Is Included in a Typical Chiropractic Office Visit for an Older Adult?

Chapters 2 and 3 provide details of a typical chiropractic office visit. For older adults, a more detailed health history is likely to be taken, especially if the patient has several chronic conditions, which increases in likelihood with age. Also, the examination may include vision, hearing, and mental status, if these seem appropriate. History of falls and assessment of balance and gait are particularly important in the older age group, and chiropractors are trained in these issues.

Comanagement

Because older adults often have chronic conditions, chiropractors usually comanage these patients with, or refer them to, other types of providers to ensure that all the patients' needs are addressed. The chiropractor will therefore focus primarily on various nondrug, nonsurgical methods to manage pain, increase mobility, and help the patient either regain or maintain his or her ability to live independently and enjoy being active.

Chiropractic Adjustive/Manipulative Techniques

Chapter 4 explains chiropractic adjustments, or manipulation, in detail. Patients in general, and frail older adults in particular, often seek out a chiropractor whose method of care matches their personal preferences as well as their health care needs. Many older adults, especially those in poor health or with some degree of frailty, may choose a chiropractor who has a gentler touch and uses a lower-force method of chiropractic adjusting. Most chiropractic offices use more than one chiropractic technique, tailoring care to the different states of health and ages of patients they see.[23]

Lower-Force Chiropractic Techniques

Most chiropractors use several different chiropractic adjusting techniques, enabling them to choose a technique to suit different patients' needs. While traditionally, chiropractic may be associated with the "popping" or "cracking" of the spinal joints, numerous low-force techniques have been developed within chiropractic as gentler, yet effective, alternatives.

Table 13.1 lists several commonly used chiropractic adjustive techniques, along with a brief explanation of the method by which the biomechanical force is applied. Patients may want to ask chiropractors which of

Table 13.1   Chiropractic Techniques Commonly Used in Care of Older Patients

Technique	Description	Procedure and Goal	Potential Advantages	Potential Limitations
Diversified	Traditional and most commonly used	A manual thrust to a joint to increase motion and restore alignment	• Amount of force used can be modified • Increases joint mobility	• May need to be modified for patient comfort and safety
Instrument-Assisted	Instrument (usually hand-held) used to deliver controlled amount of force to joint	Doctor applies instrument to joint or soft tissue	• Higher speed and lower force than traditional methods • Instrument can be used on lower-force settings for frailer patients • Very specific application of force • Adjustments done without rotating the neck or back	• Use of instrument eliminates much of the "hands-on" element of the care • May put less motion into joints than traditional manual techniques

Table 13.1 (Continued)

Technique	Description	Procedure and Goal	Potential Advantages	Potential Limitations
Thompson Terminal Point	Uses special table with pieces that drop away as the adjustment is given	Lower force to the patient, as the table pieces drop away during the adjustment	• Lower force depending on settings of the table's drop pieces • Adjustments done without rotating the neck or back	• Dropping away of table sections may be unpleasant to some patients
Sacro-Occipital	Patient placed on padded wedges to adjust pelvis	Uses minimal force, weight of patient and gravity, over longer amount of time to reduce misalignment of pelvic bones	• Minimal force • Addresses pelvis and postural distortions • No rotation or extension vectors used	•Imparts less motion into joints than traditional manual techniques
Flexion-Distraction	Uses specialized table that gently tractions the spine	Introduces motion into lumbar spine, to reduce joint stiffness and fixation	• May increase joint mobility and pliability of soft tissues • May promote the influx of fluid into disc	• Motorized version of table may not be tolerated by some patients • Eliminates some of the "hands-on" element of care • Not a full spine technique

(*Continued*)

Table 13.1 (Continued)

Technique	Description	Procedure and Goal	Potential Advantages	Potential Limitations
Logan Basic	Uses low-force thrust or pressure on sacrotuberous ligament (near tailbone) to balance the pelvis	Uses very low force over longer time to correct misalignment in pelvis, particularly of sacrum	• Minimal force • Addresses pelvis and postural distortions in depth • No rotation or extension vectors used	•Imparts less motion into joints than traditional manual techniques
Upper Cervical	Techniques focusing on the neck	Theoretically affects central and autonomic nervous system to correct problems distant from location of adjustment	• May range from exceedingly gentle to moderate force • Some upper cervical techniques avoid turning the neck to the side	• Specific to the neck • May put less motion into the neck than some other techniques

these techniques they use, in order to find the chiropractor who will best meet their needs and preferences. There are many adjusting techniques that do not rotate the spinal joints and do not entail the popping sound characteristic of the most commonly used chiropractic technique, which is called "diversified" or "high-velocity, low-amplitude manipulation." The alternate techniques may include the use of specialized tables, adjusting instruments, or padded blocks, which, when properly positioned, allow the patient's body weight to gently ease the spinal joints back into a normal position. Such lower-force techniques are designed to improve patient safety and comfort with chiropractic care, but additional research on whether these techniques are equally, or more or less, effective is necessary. Two studies have compared the results of use of a lower-force versus more traditional manual chiropractic technique. Both of these studies showed that patients improved with either type of chiropractic approach.[26,27] The second study, however, found some temporary advantage for using traditional manual adjustments (diversified) of the spine compared with an instrument-assisted technique. However, the differences between these two approaches was negligible within a few months of initiating care.[27]

Chiropractic Care for Balance and Fall Prevention

Older adults struggle with some specific health issues that chiropractors can help with as a part of the health care team. Falls are a leading cause of injuries in older adults. Some studies have investigated the role of chiropractic adjustments for the prevention of falls.[28] This is an important area for continued research, given the aging of the world's population.

However, it is already known that lowering the risk of falls in older adults is best achieved using a multifactorial approach that addresses mobility and gait, risk factors in the environment, and vitamin D supplementation.[29] Some appropriate fall prevention strategies include the following:

- completing a home safety assessment and eliminating fall hazards in the home
- strengthening leg muscles to improve steadiness of gait and ability to avoid falls
- improving balance through training or practice
- improving posture, to keep patients' center of balance over their hips

Virtually all of these strategies can be done or instructed by DCs, as allowed by their scope of practice.

Cervicogenic Vertigo

Vertigo is a health issue that can be very disorienting and frightening, and it becomes more common as we age. Beyond just dizziness, vertigo is a condition wherein the patient feels like the room is spinning. It may result in nausea, vomiting, visual disturbance, and an inability to get around. Cervicogenic vertigo (CV) is vertigo related to the cervical spine or neck. There are few, if any, effective treatments in the medical field, and patients may be quite disabled from vertigo as a result. Patients experiencing vertigo may not be able to drive a car, walk for long distances, participate in athletics, and so on. Chiropractic care for CV has been studied, and there is moderate-quality evidence that spinal manipulation may be an effective treatment.[3]

The Safety of Chiropractic Care for Older Adults

Chapter 6 discusses the issue of safety in detail. A few recent studies have looked specifically at the safety of spinal manipulation and/or chiropractic care for older adults. No serious adverse events have been reported in any clinical studies involving spinal manipulation among older adults.[30] Two recent studies analyzing data from Medicare patients found no evidence of injuries caused by chiropractic care and demonstrated no risk of stroke related to chiropractic manipulation.[31,32]

"Best Practices" for Chiropractic Care for Older Adults

A set of recommendations detailing the safest and most effective approach to chiropractic care of older adults was developed by a multidisciplinary group for the chiropractic profession.[33] This ensures that DCs follow a standardized approach to provide the best care for this population. This "best practice" set of recommendations covers examination, manipulative and other types of treatment, and advice on lifestyle for older adults.[33]

A Very Special Population: Hospice Care

Barry Wiese, DC, shares his unique experience practicing chiropractic in hospice care. Dr. Wiese is currently director of Integrated Health Centers at Logan University in Chesterfield, Missouri.

Hospice care is quite an unusual practice setting for chiropractors. How did you get into this type of practice?

"New York Chiropractic College, my employer at the time, had an opportunity to develop a working relationship with a local home care/hospice agency. This relationship entailed having an 'on-site' chiropractor who would be available to see employees, including admin staff and home care based therapists, nurses, and others. This person was also to be involved with treating hospice patients on a referral basis. I was working in two additional teaching clinics for NYCC (long-term care and geriatric hospital and private college health center) so my experience and availability played a role in my assignment to this clinic, which was limited to two half-days per week and occasional weekend work."

What type of preparation did you have?

"I didn't have the benefit of any specific preparation leading up to opening this admittedly unique clinical setting. I did have some experience within integrated environments, but other than some intermittent personal experience I was not well prepared for what I was about to be involved in.

"I initially believed my educational background would give me some advantages as I grappled with this relatively unheard of application of chiropractic care. At the time (2005) I had over 10 years of clinical experience, a diplomate in chiropractic neurology, and a couple of certifications related to sports medicine. While my clinical judgment may have been sharpened, it did very little in allowing me to avoid initial mistakes."

What type of preparation did you wish you had but had to catch up on later?

"Two specific areas I was lacking, and both were immediately apparent. First, I found that there is much to learn on the subject of death and dying. I knew almost nothing when I started (save for personal experience) but was fortunate to have been surrounded by "mentors" in the form of hospice nurses (angels on Earth if you ask me), hospice doctors, and most importantly, leaders in the hospice field who worked as administrators in the same hallway I occupied. All I needed to do was listen. Second, I did not have an appropriate mind-set when treating my first few hospice patients. My approach with musculoskeletal conditions—to that point—had always involved working steadily toward a resolution of symptoms. Sometimes this meant a bit of soreness or other type of discomfort as a result of treatment, but in the long view this was acceptable when positive clinical results were achieved. In hospice (i.e., palliative) care, this is an absolute no-no when it can be prevented. While it's possibly true that with a little 'extra' work these patients may experience longer-lasting or perhaps permanent resolution to their problems, this cannot come at the expense of transient soreness so often accepted with more traditional care settings.

"Here's an anecdote from my experience that drives home this point: George (not his real name) was my second hospice patient. He was referred to me for lower back and associated leg pain, a condition he had reportedly experienced for many years. When I visited him for the first time, portable table in hand (all hospice visits were performed in the patient's home or a specialized hospice facility) I was pretty confident in my ability to eliminate his sciatica pain, or at least minimize it. I (mistakenly) saw him as a condition, and not as a hospice patient. Following examination, I decided that the best course of action was side posture mobilization/manipulation on this 80-year-old man with terminal cancer. My plan included a gentle approach, although at my core I believed that if I restored some reasonable amount of motion to his lower lumbar spine I would be able to positively impact his life, and quickly. And I believe this notion got the better of me. My treatment was not comfortable for George, although such discomfort is a common reaction to chiropractic care and easily tolerated by most patients, even older adults. I arrived for a scheduled follow-up and George met me at the door. He informed me he didn't want me to see him again as a patient because of the amount of pain he endured during and after his initial visit, even though it was now resolved. I was floored; I've had some adverse reactions to treatment procedures before, but I knew immediately how much of a mistake I had made. Although I had not done him any actual harm, I had caused him significant discomfort. I failed to balance my treatment plan against his other conditions; more importantly, I failed to consider how my treatment choices might negatively impact his life. Hospice patients have a very limited amount of time left to them, so even a transient reaction, easily tolerated by other patients, may not be acceptable to them.

"George passed away less than a month later. I have never forgotten him and the lesson he taught me about how to consider patients' entire circumstances when formulating treatment plans. I only wish I had another chance to make it right.

"Remember: these patients often have only months, weeks, or sometimes days remaining in their lives. Your role is to make them as comfortable as possible during this time. If it's possible to remedy a condition without any adverse reaction, that's a plus. If some discomfort results from care, even if there's a belief that ultimately a positive benefit will be seen at the other end, you have 'stolen' some precious, comfortable time from them. I find that unacceptable and very quickly I learned to avoid this possibility."

What did you find most interesting, fulfilling, inspiring?

"Hands down: hospice nurses. Several became patients of mine, and I attribute this to the rapid growth of this clinic. These individuals involve themselves in the lives of their patients like nobody I've seen before or since. They are there to care for, listen to, and support patients and their families in likely the most difficult form of health care imaginable. Then after a patient passes, they mourn in their own way and get back to doing the same with another patient. In my opinion, this is the purest practice of health care."

Do you have an experience that sums up or somehow captures the essence of this practice?

"There were many, many 'successes' and smiling moments. It's always good for the soul when you realize how much you've helped another person, especially when you've managed to reduce or remove pain.

"One example of how I was able to help can be illustrated with a patient I will call Sam (not his real name). Sam had been diagnosed with a degenerative spinal cord disease for nearly a year when I first saw him, and the effects of the disease were quite obvious. He had difficulty with movement, of course, and he spent nearly the entire day, each day, in a bed on the lower level of his home. When I arrived his wife told me that the biggest favor I could do for him was to help with the pain and limited motion of his right arm. This was especially important for Sam because he used his right arm to reach for things—and the most valuable object in Sam's world was the TV remote control. He needed to reach it and raise his arm toward the TV to change channels. In spite of wasting muscles and an ever-increasing difficulty to speak, having the ability to use the TV remote represented one last 'normal' function he struggled to maintain control over.

"Working with Sam I was able to improve shoulder and elbow active range of motion at each visit, a benefit that would last two to three days. He was enormously grateful for this, as was his wife and his caregivers, who had put up with his remote control woes for quite a while!

"The simple things add up to a lot with hospice patients, and I feel chiropractors have much to offer when it comes to restoring some elements of a normal life to these patients—even if only for a short time. Although at this time chiropractic is not one of the reimbursed forms of hospice care, I can speak from firsthand experience when I say: the patients provided me with gratitude on a level a chiropractor may never experience anywhere else. And that just might be payment enough."

Conclusion

This chapter gave the reader a view of chiropractic across the life-span, from the very beginning, in pregnancy, through to the very end, in hospice. We hope that this chapter will inform those who have not yet explored the benefits of chiropractic care so that they may consider it as a safe, valuable health care option for people of all ages.

Note: Portions of this chapter are adapted from Vallone SA, Miller J, Larsdotter A, and Barham-Floreani J. Chiropractic approach to the management of children.
Chiropr Osteopat. 2010;18:16.

References

1. Stuber KJ, Wynd S, Weis CA. Adverse events from spinal manipulation in the pregnant and postpartum periods: a critical review of the literature. *Chiropr Man Therap.* 2012;20:8.

2. Borggren CL. Pregnancy and chiropractic: a narrative review of the literature. *J Chiropr Med.* 2007;6(2):70–74.

3. Clar C, Tsertsvadze A, Court R, Hundt GL, Clarke A, Sutcliffe P. Clinical effectiveness of manual therapy for the management of musculoskeletal and non-musculoskeletal conditions: systematic review and update of UK evidence report. *Chiropr Man Therap.* 2014;22(1):12.

4. Diakow PR, Gadsby TA, Gadsby JB, Gleddie JG, Leprich DJ, Scales AM. Back pain during pregnancy and labor. *J Manipulative Physiol Ther.* 1991;14(2): 116–118.

5. Pistolese RA. The Webster Technique: a chiropractic technique with obstetric implications. *J Manipulative Physiol Ther.* 2002;25(6):E1–9.

6. Black LI, Clarke TC, Barnes PM, Stussman BJ, Nahin RL. Use of complementary health approaches among children aged 4–17 years in the United States: National Health Interview Survey, 2007–2012. *Natl Health Stat Report.* 2015(78):1–19.

7. Miller J. Demographic survey of pediatric patients presenting to a chiropractic teaching clinic. *Chiropr Osteopat.* 2010;18:33.

8. Hestbaek L, Jørgensen A, Hartvigsen J. A description of children and adolescents in Danish chiropractic practice: results from a nationwide survey. *J Manipulative Physiol Ther.* 2009;32(8):607–615.

9. Ndetan H, Evans MW, Jr., Hawk C, Walker C. Chiropractic or osteopathic manipulation for children in the United States: an analysis of data from the 2007 National Health Interview Survey. *J Altern Complement Med.* 2012;18(4): 347–353.

10. Gleberzon BJ, Arts J, Mei A, McManus EL. The use of spinal manipulative therapy for pediatric health conditions: a systematic review of the literature. *J Can Chiropr Assoc.* 2012;56(2):128–141.

11. Todd AJ, Carroll MT, Robinson A, Mitchell EK. Adverse events due to chiropractic and other manual therapies for infants and children: a review of the literature. *J Manipulative Physiol Ther.* 2015;38:699–712.

12. Hawk C, Schneider M, Ferrance RJ, Hewitt E, Van Loon M, Tanis L. Best practices recommendations for chiropractic care for infants, children, and adolescents: results of a consensus process. *J Manipulative Physiol Ther.* 2009;32(8): 639–647.

13. Hawk C, Schneider MJ, Vallone S, Hewitt EG. Best practices for chiropractic care of children: a consensus update. *J Manipulative Physiol Ther.* 2016;39(3): 158–168.

14. Miller J. Cry babies: a framework for chiropractic care. *Clin Chiropr.* 2007;10:139–146.

15. Hewitt E, Hestbaek L, Pohlman KA. Core competencies of the certified pediatric doctor of chiropractic: results of a Delphi consensus process. *J Evid Based Complementary Altern Med.* 2016;21(2):110–114.

16. Dobson D, Lucassen P, Miller J, et al. Manipulative therapies for infantile colic. *Cochrane Database Syst Rev.* 2012 Dec 12;12:CD004796.

17. Fry LM. Chiropractic and breastfeeding dysfunction: a literature review. *J Clin Chiropr Pediatr.* 2014;14(2):1151–1155.

18. Hash J. Deformational plagiocephaly and chiropractic care: a narrative review and case. *J Clin Chiropr Pediatr.* 2014;14(2):1131–1138.

19. Davies, NJ. Chiropractic management of deformational plagiocephaly in infants: an alternative to device-dependent therapy. *Chiropr J Australia.* 2002; 32(2):5255.

20. Bronfort G, Evans RL, Kubic P, Filkin P. Chronic pediatric asthma and chiropractic spinal manipulation: a prospective clinical series and randomized clinical pilot study. *J Manipulative Physiol Ther.* 2001;24(6):369–377.

21. Schetzek S, Heinen F, Kruse S, et al. Headache in children: update on complementary treatments. *Neuropediatrics.* 2013;44(1):25–33.

22. Borggren CL, Osterbauer PJ, Wiles MR. A survey of geriatrics courses in North American chiropractic programs. *J Chiropr Educ.* 2009;23(1):28–35.

23. Examiners NBoC. *Practice Analysis of Chiropractic 2015.* Greeley, CO: National Board of Chiropractic Examiners; 2015.

24. Docking RE, Fleming J, Brayne C, Zhao J, Macfarlane GJ, Jones GT. Epidemiology of back pain in older adults: prevalence and risk factors for back pain onset. *Rheumatology (Oxford).* 2011;50(9):1645–1653.

25. Weeks WB, Goertz CM, Meeker WC, Marchiori DM. Public perceptions of doctors of chiropractic: results of a national survey and examination of variation according to respondents' likelihood to use chiropractic, experience with chiropractic, and chiropractic supply in local health care markets. *J Manipulative Physiol Ther.* 2015;38(8):533–544.

26. Hondras MA, Long CR, Cao Y, Rowell RM, Meeker WC. A randomized controlled trial comparing 2 types of spinal manipulation and minimal conservative medical care for adults 55 years and older with subacute or chronic low back pain. *J Manipulative Physiol Ther.* 2009;32(5):330–343.

27. Schneider M, Haas M, Glick R, Stevans J, Landsittel D. Comparison of spinal manipulation methods and usual medical care for acute and subacute low back pain: a randomized clinical trial. *Spine (Phila Pa 1976).* 2015;40(4):209–217.

28. Holt KR, Haavik H, Elley CR. The effects of manual therapy on balance and falls: a systematic review. *J Manipulative Physiol Ther.* 2012;35(3):227–234.

29. USPSTF. *Guide to Clinical Preventive Services.* Washington, DC: Agency for Healthcare Research and Quality; 2014.

30. Dougherty PE, Hawk C, Weiner DK, Gleberzon B, Andrew K, Killinger L. The role of chiropractic care in older adults. *Chiropr Man Therap.* 2012;20(1):3.

31. Whedon JM, Mackenzie TA, Phillips RB, Lurie JD. Risk of traumatic injury associated with chiropractic spinal manipulation in Medicare Part B beneficiaries aged 66 to 99 years. *Spine (Phila Pa 1976).* 2015;40(4):264–270.

32. Whedon JM, Song Y, Mackenzie TA, Phillips RB, Lukovits TG, Lurie JD. Risk of stroke after chiropractic spinal manipulation in Medicare B beneficiaries aged 66 to 99 years with neck pain. *J Manipulative Physiol Ther.* 2015.

33. Hawk C, Schneider M, Dougherty P, Gleberzon BJ, Killinger LZ. Best practices recommendations for chiropractic care for older adults: results of a consensus process. *J Manipulative Physiol Ther.* 2010;33(6):464–473.

CHAPTER FOURTEEN

Sports Chiropractic

Russ Ebbets, DC

The Evolving Role of Sports Chiropractic

Over the last decade, the settings in which chiropractic care is offered have expanded significantly. Chiropractic care is now found in hospitals, Veterans' Administration centers, and other types of multidisciplinary practices.

One of the great obstacles these pioneering efforts have faced is the question, "What exactly does the chiropractor do?" While evolving efforts in research and application of evidence-based practices have helped bridge this knowledge gap, questions remain. In spite of the rapidly changing health care environment, research results come slowly with competing political and economic interests diluting the promise of validating efforts and confusing both the innovative gatekeepers and the general public.

A possible exception is the athletic arena. In a time of multimillion-dollar contracts and longevity of careers measured in dog years, the vetting process of the effectiveness of chiropractic care has been fast-tracked to days and weeks versus months or years.

A successful team requires cooperation, which sets a model for the health care staff. Multiple disciplines must be on the same page in an effort to minimize injury downtime, accelerate recovery, and enhance performance.

Complicating this scenario are the rigorous drug policies professional and Olympic sports have adopted. No longer are the traditional pharmaceutical "go-to" therapies of steroids, amphetamines, and narcotic painkillers allowed. Violation of league or organization drug policies can result in stiff penalties that are likely to negatively impact an individual's career and may prove crippling to a team's seasonal aspirations.

This reality offers a unique opportunity for the non-drug-based health care practitioners (chiropractic, physical therapy, massage, nutrition), especially the chiropractor. Proactive efforts with respect to planning and preventive care may lessen injury downtime while also enhancing performance.

The problem that arises, once again, is evidence. In this time of evidence-based care, anecdotal reports may tweak curiosity, but the lack of hard data dilutes the message to the scientific community. The science of one is the science of none.

A second complicating issue is the chiropractor's understanding of his or her role on the athletic health care team. Traditionally, most sports chiropractors have graduated from the athletic training ranks. Even chiropractic's certified chiropractic sports physician program (designed by a former athletic trainer) is based on the athletic training model, which is reactive care—that is, care after the injury has occurred.

With this preparation, the role and function of the sports chiropractor often defaults to that of the athletic trainer. With minimal variation comes a duplication of services, creating a win-lose situation. An increasing role for the chiropractor represents a loss of role for the athletic trainer. The current reality is that the athletic trainer is already well vested politically and culturally, and it could be argued that he or she represents the standard of care for on-field recognition, management, and care of sports-related injuries, at least in the United States.

When viewed in this light, the reality is that the chiropractor's contribution may be seen as duplicative rather than complementary. While this reality may seem troubling, it also presents an opportunity in terms of ownership of the proactive efforts: recovery therapies and performance enhancement.

Recovery is a concern in modern-day athletics because of a combination of training and time. With most professional careers lasting fewer than five years, refining the training process has become paramount. Too much training produces illness and injuries, which may limit potential development and shorten the athlete's career. Diligent recovery efforts help to normalize body function (another term for this is "return to homeostasis"). This allows the athlete a longer period of rest before the next competition or workout.

Performance is enhanced by aiding the expression of the athlete's biomotor skills. There are five biomotor skills that make an athlete athletic: these are *strength, endurance, speed, flexibility,* and *coordination.* The ability of athletes to more efficiently express these skills in their running, jumping, or throwing ultimately translates to enhanced performance. Part of the job of a coach is to manage the stress of training in order to enhance the development of bio-motor skills.

Modern sports training is an outgrowth of Hans Selye's general adaptation syndrome (GAS).[1] In the 1950s, Soviet physiologists experimented with progressive overloads and measured athletes' ability to adapt.[2] Over the last 60 years, the concepts of periodization and training theory have been employed worldwide for the perfection of human effort.[3,4] Improvements in athletic performance are the result of stress management. The pattern of stress, recovery, and adaptation is a simplified version of Selye's GAS.

Training theory is by its very nature proactive. One is introducing a stress to the body in the hope of producing a desired future result. Critical to this training process are accelerated recovery times so that more work can be done in less time. This, in theory, raises the adaptive levels of the athlete and subsequently improves his or her performance outcomes.

The Role of Chiropractic Care in Performance Enhancement

Chiropractic care is used to enhance performance by optimizing the expression of the five biomotor skills, although evidence of this effect is mostly anecdotal, with only a few controlled studies having been done at this time.[5,6] Additionally, it is thought that spinal manipulation may play a role in normalizing body functions, which suggests the possibility of accelerating recovery times. The only comprehensive literature review on the enhancement of sports performance by chiropractic care found that the evidence was insufficient to make a definitive conclusion and that more research is needed.[6]

Traditional sports medicine might be graphically represented by a two-circle model consisting of (1) first response/life support or emergency care and (2) treatment of non-life-threatening injuries or conditions. The chiropractor's chief role can then be represented by the addition of a third circle that represents proactive care, or preventive care. This is the *athletic triage model.*

Promotion of the athletic triage model offers a clear distinction as to the role and function of the chiropractor in the current athletic health care setting. Through the application of Hans Selye's GAS and Yakolev's model, the chiropractor fills a position that is complementary rather than duplicative.

Additionally, the athletic triage model applies joint manipulation and soft tissue work, which are thought to contribute to accelerated recovery and performance enhancement.

This chapter will explain the sports chiropractic approach to treating athletes, an approach that emphasizes prevention of injuries and enhancement of performance rather than focusing primarily on treating injuries.

The Power of Language

In communication science, there are a number of theories to explain how humans communicate with each other. Our ability to communicate on various levels is critical for expressing needs and wants, hopes and desires, and joys and fears. As time marches on, language continues to evolve, adding new concepts and words that 20, 10, or even 5 years ago did not exist (such as "selfies," "megabytes," "iPad," and "cell phone").

There is an old teaching adage that "words cue action," but, if that is true, words can also cue inaction. This may happen when personal or group interests clash with needs and desires. Exactly who gets to decide what a word means?

In modern societies, the arbiter of new words and the lexicon is the dominant social group. At the most basic level, the dominant social group, by dictating language, can dominate reality by defining it. This is a minor point in homogenous societies where the group interests are all the same—that is, they are "homogenized." But in the multicultural, diverse world of the 21st century, the old model begins to break down.

Kramerae's "muted group theory of cultural communication" neatly summarizes this problem.[7] It states that in any social situation, the dominant social group determines the lexicon. In a homogenous society, it serves the needs of the homogenous group. In a culturally diverse society, it serves the needs of the dominant social group, possibly to the exclusion of all others.

Traditional sports medicine follows a reactive care model. An athlete receives care when something is "wrong." The "wrong" could be an acute, non-life-threatening injury, like a sprained ankle, or a contact collision or unguarded fall that may present with a life-threatening consequence. Sports medicine delivers care "after the fact."

Care "after the fact" is consistent with the conventional biomedical model of care. It is the presence of symptoms, pain, or injury that spurs a patient to seek help. No sane person would go to an emergency room for a wellness visit.

This presents a problem for the sports chiropractor. "Sports chiropractic" will be defined here as manual spine and extremity adjusting, soft tissue work, and stretching. For most athletes, chiropractic care is used proactively, when nothing is "wrong."

But why would an athlete seek chiropractic care when nothing is "wrong"? For many, the simple answer is that it makes them feel better. Some believe it helps them perform better, and others who get treated feel it aids their recovery. Well-being, performance enhancement, and accelerated recovery lead many athletes to seek chiropractic care. These are all aspirations to proactive states heavily supported by anecdote, minimally supported by data.[6] But this proactive care presents a problem for traditional sports medicine, which operates on a model of reactive care. In the U.S. health care arena, the mainstream medical approach is that of treating symptoms.

To complicate this point, within the lexicon of traditional medicine's Stedman's, Dorland's, Mosby's, or Taber's medical dictionaries, the concepts of athletic performance enhancement, accelerated recovery, and restoration and regeneration are not mentioned. Whoever controls the definitions, controls the reality.

Sport in Context

Is it accurate to refer to both a person who runs a five-hour marathon and another who participates in the NBA Championship and averages 20 points a game as "athletes"? Are those involved in aesthetic sports, such as figure skating, gymnastics, and synchronized swimming, also considered "athletes"? And who is the athlete in horse racing or the equestrian sport or dressage—the human or the horse?

One might be dismissive of these questions, noting that what is being compared is "apples and oranges." That is, these are activities whose demands are so unrelated they almost defy comparison. But regardless of any differences among these diverse sports, all could agree that each endeavor requires *athleticism*.

There are actually four levels of sport. When viewed in this context, a more meaningful comparison can be made, despite the individual demands of each sport. These levels are the fundamental level, fitness level, and performance level, which is divided into two parts—pre-hab and rehab.

Fundamental Level of Sport

The basic level of sport is the fundamental level. This represents the entry level and includes youth programs. The structure of practices is a combination of self-discovery and guided discovery as the developing child learns the fundamentals of movement. Additionally, cooperation, sharing, team work, and putting forth effort in a competition are encouraged so that this early socialization leads to a more enlightened integration as an adolescent or adult team member. Ideally, emphasis on winning takes a back seat to the development of values that can be built upon as the child matures.

Fitness Level of Sport

The second level is that of fitness. This stage enjoys the highest level of participation. It is not competitive, per se, but rather its goals are health maintenance, cardiovascular fitness, and strength development, combined with weight management and social opportunities. The time commitment may range from daily practice to at least three to four days per week. Winning is not so much the goal of this level, rather the focus is on improving one's own level of fitness.

Two Levels of Performance: Pre-hab and Rehab

Performance is the top level. This is where competitive performance is the preeminent goal. As was taught at the Institute of Sport and Physical Culture in the former Soviet Union, training at this elite level is not a natural or healthy thing to do to the body. Personal bests, won-lost records, individual and team rankings, statistics, and daily practices characterize this stage.

The fourth level actually has two parts. Athletic involvement brings with it an inherent risk of injury. To that end "pre-hab" efforts, actions, and movements done to prevent injury (balance work, core stability, anatomical adaptation, focused bodybuilding) would necessarily be done to ensure a more healthful participation. This pre-hab is *neuromuscular education* of the body to meet the demands of one's chosen activity.

One of the realities of sports participation is that injuries happen. The return to a pre-injury state is accomplished through specifically designed exercises to strengthen the body's broken links and restore movement patterns that will allow for safe return to play. Rehabilitation work is *neuromuscular reeducation*, teaching the body how to do things in a biomechanically sound way.

Pre-hab efforts should play a significant role in the three other stages of athletic participation. From the fundamental stage, the pre-hab efforts of a dynamic warm-up can develop and refine movement skills that last a lifetime. For the fitness participant, pre-hab efforts can counter the linear nature of most fitness activities (e.g., exercising on treadmills or ellipticals; jogging, cycling,), toning the dynamic stabilizers that suffer disuse atrophy as one moves through life. Pre-hab efforts for the performance-based athlete may lengthen the career, improve competitive effectiveness, and lessen the severity of repetitive microtrauma or the damage of contact macrotraumas by strengthening weak areas of the body by preemptively bolstering them.

When sport is viewed in this context, the demands of the competitive effort can be recognized by all. And while the nuances of each level could be argued, the importance of pre-hab preventive efforts must be emphasized.

Training Theory

Once upon a time, the concept of stress as it is used today did not exist. Canadian endocrinologist Hans Selye dedicated his life to the study and justification of this series of alarm reactions by the body. His landmark book, *The Stress of Life*, was published in 1954 and introduced the concept of stress into the common vernacular.[1]

Selye came to understand that the body reacts similarly to various threatening situations and that there is a subtle connection via the sympathetic and parasympathetic nervous systems that includes the adrenal cortex of the kidneys, the pituitary gland, and the hypothalamus. The collective response of these tissues and the release of their individual hormones effects the body's systems (circulation, assimilation, recovery, and elimination). Selye called this multisystem whole-body reaction the "general adaptation stress" (GAS) syndrome.[1]

By 1956, Russian physiologists had adapted Selye's work on the body's ability to adapt to stress, experimenting with how the body adapts to incremental bouts of work stress. The cycle of stress-recovery-adaptation came to be represented by a sine-wave pattern called "Yakolev's model." With this representation, the concept of modern training theory and periodization as used for athletic development was born.[2]

In Yakolev's model, the X-axis represents homeostasis, the normal basic metabolic rate (BMR) of an athlete. Traveling in a +X direction represents a period of time. This time could be an individual training component (e.g., a set of the bench press, a running interval, the execution of a series of technical elements), the work of a day, one week, one season, or a career.

The Y-axis represents fatigue. At the lowest point, the training session ends and the body begins the recovery process. Coe and Martin have named this lowest point the "Valley of Fatigue."[8] It represents a programmed state that triggers Selye's alarm reaction. Traveling too far down the Y-axis is represented in the fatigue syndromes of overtraining, illness, and injury (both mental and physical).[9] Of special note is that overly motivated individuals and those with an obsessive-compulsive personality (good enough is never enough) eventually become injured as their focus is imbalanced, ignoring or denying the importance of recovery.

From the Valley of Fatigue, the curve begins to travel up the Y-axis and eventually peaks before gradually returning to the BMR over time. This high point is the body's adaptation to the stress of the workout. When done with methodical intention, this stress-recovery-adaptation curve can be repeated daily, and the gradual adaptation of the body to the demands placed upon it results in measurable performance improvements.

This stress-recovery-adaptation model is critical to the performance-based athlete whose goal is improving performance. For the fitness athlete, improved performance is of minimal concern. For the child athlete, application of Yakolev's model presents a dilemma. Is the focus of the fundamental stage growth and development or training and competition?[9] Philosophies differ widely on this issue.

Understanding Yakolev's model makes application of the concepts of periodization, progressive overload, specificity of training, individualization of training, and multilateral development all the more powerful. Over the last 60 years, scientifically validated studies have developed any number of "best practices" that allow the skillful coach and dedicated athlete to capitalize on training efforts that maximize practice time, allowing one to maximize individual potential. But at its most basic level, the discussion necessarily must begin by asking the question, "What quality or qualities get trained?" The simple answer to this question is "the five biomotor skills." The focal design of daily, weekly, monthly, seasonal, or career training sessions is to enhance the expression of the five biomotor skills, the skills that make an athlete athletic.

It is through the periodic and systematic application of the stress-recovery-adaptation pattern that the expression of the biomotor skills and their various combinations are improved and performance is enhanced.

The Biomotor Skills

What makes an athlete an athlete? While people may debate what constitutes a sport and which sport is more difficult, the argument is really moot as the various sports have few common factors with which to make a fair comparison. The exception is the biomotor skills necessary to successfully compete and excel at these sports.

Speed, strength, endurance, flexibility, and coordination are the five components of all sports and athletic activities. Musicians, dancers, weekend warriors, professional athletes, even chiropractors use the five biomotor skills to a greater or lesser degree to ply their trade.

What differentiates the various activities is the degree of expression of the individual skills. Applied sports (that is, individual events of track and field) highly prize the individual biomotor skills of speed, strength, and endurance.

Ball sports may prize these same individual biomotor skills but due to the nature of the game repackage the skill to suit the demands of that sport. Speed and strength would generally be necessary for a successful four-second football play from scrimmage, but the quality of endurance would not be evident until the fourth quarter, at the end of a long drive, or deep into a 12-, 14-, or 16-week season. To that end, it becomes useful to analyze individual sports, even positions within the sports, to see which qualities are necessary to excel.

Sports coaches ought to create an environment that allows for the fullest expression of the desired qualities. To a certain extent, exercise science and strength and conditioning coaches have begun to address these individual demands.

A synopsis of each biomotor skill is useful to illustrate each biomotor skill's greater or lesser contribution to athletic participation.

Speed

"Speed" is defined as the ability to move the body or a body part quickly. Sprinting is the most common expression of speed. Speed is actually a vector-dependent quality (from point A to point B) that is by definition essentially a linear movement.

With speed thus defined, it is important to note that none of the biomotor skills can be expressed by themselves. To express speed, one must have strength, body symmetry, coordination, and balance. Additionally, a stable core musculature is necessary for the rapid concentric, isometric, and eccentric contractions of the hip musculature of top-end sprinters who are able to take up to five strides per second.

Strength

"Strength" is defined as the "ability of a muscle or muscle group to generate muscular force under specific conditions."[3]

Once again, the quality of strength is actually determined by a combination of the biomechanics of the joints, functional movement patterns, and physiologic processes and is often combined with the speed with which these actions can be executed to produce power.

Strength at the basic motor unit level is enhanced by clarity and development of one's nervous system, and this quality can be trained with progressive overload[4] and enhanced with therapeutic interventions.[5]

Of particular note is Siff's belief that "strength and skill are the foundation of all fitness."[10] This is fitness from the view of the speed-strength paradigm. This thought can be contrasted with Kenneth Cooper's aerobic paradigm, which emphasizes cardiovascular fitness and is credited with starting the running boom in the United States in the 1980s.

This dichotomy underscores the importance of defining which level of athletic participation one is referencing from the four levels of sport. While the aerobic paradigm may allow one to enjoy the benefits of participation in the fitness level, success at the performance level in all sports and individual disciplines hinges on one's ability to exhibit the qualities of the speed-strength or power paradigm.

Endurance

"Endurance" is defined as the ability to resist fatigue.[4] Fatigue is actually a defense mechanism of the body. While most would see endurance as the ability to do the same activity repeatedly, it is the depletion of one's energy stores (ATP, oxygen) that signals the end of one's efforts and is therefore the measure of endurance.

Psychological factors can override the body's warning signals and defense mechanisms, driving one to compete for excessively long periods. This type of mental effort creates a temporary imbalance of the mind-body-biochemical system that will warrant special recovery measures upon completion.

To continually ignore these signals creates a state of "overtraining," a situation where the training regimen has continually exceeded the capacity of the body to recover. This, in turn, creates a situation where the body is highly susceptible to illness, physical injury, psychological imbalance, and most likely a combination of all of these. The "female athletic triad" (anorexia, amenorrhea, and osteoporosis) is a classic example.

Cardiovascular efficiency enhances the quality of one's endurance, but other factors, such as efficient biomechanical movements, speed of execution of the movements, and body weight can also play a significant role in one's endurance. There is an old coaching maxim that the loss of

10 pounds equates with a 60-second faster 10k time. But there comes a point of diminishing returns, at which the weight one loses is no longer a loss of nonproductive fat but is composed of the driving force of muscle tissue. When this occurs, performance suffers.

Flexibility

"Flexibility" is defined as the ability to move the body parts through a wide range of motion.[4] Flexibility should be optimized, not maximized. That is, it is possible to have too much flexibility. Flexibility is also the only noncompetitive biomotor skill. Flexibility has different requirements for different sports. While a dynamic, unencumbered range of motion is desirable, the amount of flexibility that would be considered a "dynamic and unencumbered range of motion" can vary widely in different sports.

Related to the issue of flexibility is overstretching, which is an effort to maximize the excursion possibilities of a joint. Overstretching may dampen the stretch reflex. This will, in turn, dampen the responsiveness of a muscle. A dampened strength reflex or stretch-shortening cycle can decrease force production and increase ground contact times. This may have a negative effect on speed, strength, and power production.

A dampened stretch reflex can also negatively impact the summation of forces that the performance of technical elements (e.g., martial art katas, gymnastic moves, figure skating jumps) or techniques (e.g., overhand pitching, shot putting) require. It is this coordinated series of stretch reflexes that capitalizes on the elastic qualities of the body's soft tissues.

Flexibility of the holding elements of the joints (tendons, ligaments, and fascia) is also an important consideration. The primary job of these tissues is to stabilize the joints. With too much rigidity, the stress of movements is transferred to the musculoskeletal junctions, requiring these tissues to contract and stabilize at the same time. If these holding elements allow too much movement, the joint capsules can become unstable. The stress resulting from routine shearing and torqueing forces can produce injuries that range from the microtears of a common tendonitis to catastrophic tissue failure, such as a torn anterior cruciate ligament (ACL).

Isometric positions combined with slow, rhythmic movements at these tissues' end range can increase collagen deposition at the stress points. This creates a more stable joint complex. The functional integrity of these tissues should be one of the primary foci of the above-mentioned pre-hab efforts.

Coordination ABCs

The ABCs (agility, balance, coordination, and skill) are collectively defined as the ability to move body parts with specific objectives. In many respects, the ABCs are a final catch-all of the five biomotor skills. It is the refinement of these abilities that often makes the difference between the gradations of success one achieves in performance-based sport.

Agility is the ability to move the body in a lateral or evasive manner. Agility will play a greater or lesser role, depending on the particular demands of a sport. Interestingly, the Russian sport coaches also saw agility in a broader context, including the mind in their definition. This "agility of the mind" is what is commonly called "cleverness." Agility of the mind is the thought process behind agile or evasive patterns.

Balance is undoubtedly the most important biomotor skill, but, unfortunately, it is also the one most taken for granted. Surprisingly, even people with no symptoms of a balance problem can experience dramatic improvements with specific training.

Balance is critically important because one cannot express any other biomotor skill without it. Any improvements in balance can play a significant role in force production, technical execution of movement, decreased ground contact times, and efficiency of movement, which are of critical importance in short-duration efforts and a critical concern for energy-efficient movements in endurance efforts. This refined movement decreases the wear and tear of career-long training, thereby playing a significant role in short-term injury prevention and long-term health.

Coordination deals with the symmetry of body movements, especially in sports and activities that repeat the same movements (e.g., running, swimming, crew). But coordination also comes into play in the sequencing of the body's stretch reflexes for an efficient summation of forces and a non-energy expenditure of enhanced force application.

The final component of the ABCs is *skill*. The ability to hit a golf ball or sink a foul shot are pertinent skills of golf and basketball respectively. The acquiring of skills is closely tied to learning. "Learning" is the refined expression of a sport's particular skills with acquisition following Maslow's whole-phase-whole-method of learning. In this regard, skill refinement is a career-long process of self-discovery combined with a coach's guided discovery. To that end, skill identification, acquisition, refinement, and expression are both a daily and career-long concern.

Because of this, skill acquisition is dependent on multiple factors, including coaching, facilities, motivation, learning environment, and the ability of the athlete to manage change, as improvement necessitates expressing the biomotor skills in new ways.

In summary, an understanding and appreciation for the biomotor skills is necessary in any discussion of sport at whatever level (fundamental, fitness, performance, rehab/pre-hab). Leading training theorists have made numerous attempts to illustrate the interconnectedness of the biomotor skills, yet these attempts have proven to be cumbersome and incomplete. The difficulty lies in the dynamic nature of individual sports, which defies simple comparisons.

The ability of the athlete to express the five biomotor skills is at the core of what makes an athlete athletic. The identification, development, and career management of these five biomotor skills is a daily, weekly, season-, and career-long training concern.

Meticulous time management is one of the components of preparing an athlete for competition. With the career of an athlete spanning just 10 to 12 years, any downtime spent on rehabilitation efforts or misguided training is lost time, never to be regained. Careful attention to and systematic development of these five biomotor skills is the core factor in giving the athlete more time to train, recover, develop, and excel.

Rehabilitation and Sport

Injuries and sports participation seem to go hand in hand. Football, with its collisions and high level of contact, is reported to have a 100 percent seasonal injury rate among its players. Other sports, although less violent in nature, present with their own characteristic injury patterns of bone, joint, and tissue damage due to misuse and overuse syndromes.

While the susceptibility to injury can be lessened with a skillful preparation of the athlete in the pre-hab phase of training, the reality is that for most, long-term involvement in athletic activities creates a breakdown in the body due to a sport's repetitive nature or asymmetrical demands.

Injuries are the result of the classic triune of force, frequency, and duration (e.g., an episode of too much force that happens too fast for the body to accommodate or a force that lasts too long). In fact, injuries are usually a combination of these factors.

"Rehabilitation" is commonly defined as efforts to restore the ill or injured to a pre-injury state. The factors that are acted upon in rehabilitation are actually the biomotor skills. This has long been a focus of sports medicine efforts in a reactive care model. It warrants restating that although rehabilitation efforts are critical for the athlete to return to play, in the grand scheme of a career, rehabilitation efforts represent "lost" time for the acquisition, perfection, and expression of a skill.

While it is possible for an athlete to return to play "new and improved," it begs the question, why weren't these efforts made prior to the injury?

Box 14.1

Skill Classifications Continua

Cyclic, Acyclic, and Acyclic Combined
- Cyclic: same action repeated (running, cycling, swimming)
- Acyclic: action has beginning and end (pitching, foul shot, shot put)
- Acyclic combined: combination (dribble and shoot, long jump, pole vault)

Gross and Fine
- Gross: large groups of muscles (running, lifting)
- Fine: small groups of muscles (playing the piano, violin, golf shot)

Open and Closed
- Open: environment constantly changing (tennis game, soccer match)
- Closed: predictable environment, what to do and when to do it (foul shot, tennis serve)

Internal and External
- Internal: performer controls the rate of play (marathon)
- External: environment controls rate (ball games)

Discrete, Serial, and Continuous
- Discrete: clear beginning and end (foul shot, tennis serve)
- Serial: discrete skills strung together (hop, step, and jump)
- Continuous: has no beginning or end, end of one cycle is beginning of next (running, swimming, cycling)

Individual, Coactive, and Interactive
- Individual: performed in isolation (high jump, figure skating)
- Coactive: with others, without direct confrontation
- Interactive: with other performers directly involved (ball sports)

Simple and Complex
- Simple: straight forward (100m sprint)
- Complex: complicated (chess, sailing, quarterback)

Low and High Organization
- Low: not much attention needed (riding a bike)
- High: large number of skills linked together (figure skating, quarterback, basketball)

Self-Paced and Externally Paced
- Self-paced: action started by performer (downhill skiing)
- Externally paced: clock timing not controlled by performer (100m sprint)

Variable and Fixed Practice
- Variable: tactical application of skill (boxing, martial arts)
- Fixed: drilled motor sequence (plays in ball sports)

Mass and Distributed Practice
- Mass: without breaks, high level of fitness required
- Distributed: rest breaks provided

This would constitute pre-hab efforts, which would pay particular attention to the prevention of overuse syndromes.

Therefore, rehabilitation should be clearly seen as a reactive-type care—care given after the fact. So, while this form of treatment makes an invaluable therapeutic contribution to the participation and career of an athlete, it must also be seen for what it is, time lost, never to be regained for athletic skill development.

Recovery

To a degree, the body adapts to the stresses placed upon it. The physical laws of Davis and Wolff have been used for over a century to describe the physical adaptations soft tissues (ligaments, tendons, muscles, and fascia) and bone undergo in response to lifestyle and environmental challenges.

Recovery is the upswing portion of the curve on Yakolev's model. It is the time after the state of fatigue has been reached, the exercise or work ceases, and the body is allowed to normalize and return to its homeostatic state.

One of the goals of a controlled training situation is to raise the adaptive levels of the body through progressive overloading that leads to a heightened level of performance.[4] From an intellectual standpoint, one may reason that this progressive overload is simply a straight-line progression that climbs steadily without break throughout life. In fact, the continued evolution of the athlete is actually a series of days, weeks, and months of intricately connected training cycles that allow for both taxing challenge and necessary recovery, alternating a series of hard-medium-easy work days into weekly, monthly, and seasonal training cycles.

Another essential factor is the development of a smooth transition from the stress-recovery-adaptation portions of Yakolev's model. These phases should not be seen as independent points but rather as smoothly blended transitions within a unified whole.

Injuries are most likely to occur when the stressors become too great or are repeated too often, creating an overtraining situation.[9] Another complicating factor would be minimal or incomplete recovery efforts that compromise or negate any adaptation.

While passive recovery efforts may be of passing concern to the fitness athlete, they are central to that of the performance athlete. Bompa has stated that 50 percent of athletic performance hinges on one's ability to recover.[11]

The process and importance of recovery is different for each level of sport. In the fundamental level, the admonition "don't fatigue the system" is applicable. This level emphasizes daily routine activities combined with healthy lifestyle habits, such as hydration, sleep, and proper nutrition.

For the fitness athlete, the periodic bouts of work allow for one to two days of nonwork and time for the body to rest and regenerate. Once again, proper nutrition, hydration, and rest complement this training state.

In the fundamental and fitness levels, recovery is essentially a passive process. Recovery happens naturally with routine, day-to-day activities. There is little effort to make recovery happen more quickly or more effectively.

One of the things that differentiate performance-based athletes from all other levels is the frequency and volume of their training. Top-level athletes, depending on the stage of the season, may have between 7 and 15 practice sessions per week. Additionally, they may spend three or more hours per day honing their skills. In fact, there is a training maxim that states one should "recover as hard as one trains." While this may be an unnecessary concern to the weekend warrior, within the scope of the performance-based sport this is a critical concern.

Inattention to one's recovery with passive efforts prolongs the time spent in the "Valley of Fatigue" and possibly presents a situation where the athlete attempts the next bout of training work while not fully recovered. While this situation should raise concern on a short-term basis, it can prove to be disastrous if the pattern proves to be a long-term habit that results in overtraining, illness, and injury.

Recovery for the elite performer becomes yet another opportunity to manage how time is spent. Directed efforts, such as active rest (e.g., complementary activities to remove metabolic wastes) and restorative modalities (e.g., hydrotherapies, sauna, massage, joint manipulation) need to be planned into the athlete's day. This planning may direct or dictate the athlete's lifestyle, exemplifying what Gambetta has called the "24-hour athlete."[3]

Recovery for the elite performer becomes a critical training component because of the concept of time. Planned recovery efforts can help accelerate the rate of recovery of the body's systems, helping the athlete return to a homeostatic BMR so the next bout of exercise can be more safely attempted.

The limiting factor in athletic development is lack of time. The career of a top performer is counted in dog years and may last only 10 to 12 years. Because of this fact, all time must be judiciously accounted for.

The implications of a quicker recovery are that the athlete may be "fresher" or better rested, allowing the next bout of exercise to be more challenging or to happen sooner in the weekly training cycle, which will cumulatively result in more training days over the course of a week, month, or season, thereby increasing the athlete's work capacity.

A quicker recovery also has important implications during the championship portion of a season. Successive days of competitions with multiple rounds or a quick succession of games (as in the Olympics or the NBA play-offs) illustrates the competitive advantage a well-rested, well-recovered athlete or team may have. Note that at the fundamental or fitness levels, this is not a concern.

It has been established that the increase in work capacity is one of the critical factors necessary for performance-based efforts. For the elite athlete, programmed attention to hydration, supplementation, various therapeutic interventions, and *recovery* plays a central role in both the ascension to elite status and the longevity of one's athletic life as an elite performer.

Performance Enhancement

In the early 1900s, the word "training" came into the lexicon of athletic preparation. "Training" was defined as specific efforts to enhance or sharpen the expression of the skills necessary to compete and excel in sport. One did speed work to enhance speed, strength work to enhance strength, stretching to optimize flexibility, skill work to coordinate actions (e.g., a basketball foul shot) or to create synchronous actions within a team (e.g., a basketball fast break), and lengthened the time of workouts to create endurance.

Even with a minimal understanding, one would recognize the qualities being trained as the five biomotor skills. The level of sophistication in this area has risen to the point that most colleges and professional teams have a coach whose sole responsibility is the development and enhancement of these qualities—the strength and conditioning coach.

While application of these qualities may have been formalized in the early 1980s, this position existed in part and to varying degrees within the various sports well before then. Thoughts such as "lifting will make you tight" and "swimming is bad for a field-based athlete" may be seen as ridiculous statements today, but barely 30 years ago they were dominant thoughts, especially in America. It wasn't until the advent of sport science—the application of science to sport for performance enhancement or accelerated recovery—that common locker-room myths were superseded by the scientific method. The Soviet physiologists of the 1950s are credited with being the driving force behind this change.

The Soviet physiologists modified Selye's general adaptation syndrome to sport. Yakolev's model of stress recovery and adaptation was a way to safely and systematically overload the body, generating a stress reaction that led to an adaptation on the part of the body. So, while "stress" per se generally has a negative connotation in society, this managed stress leads to a desired adaptation within the body—what Selye termed "eustress," or positive stress.

Repeated consistently, this eustress produces a training effect that includes an increased work capacity and, theoretically, improved performance, but only up to a point. The Soviet physiologists found out that the repeated, relentless dipping into the "Valley of Fatigue" potentially accelerated or exceeded the body's ability to recover from stress. Therapeutic interventions were necessary to lessen or delay this damage.

One simple intervention was the use of drugs. While ergogenic aids (e.g., steroids, amphetamines, barbiturates) skirted the bounds of fair play, they were initially undetectable (c. 1960). Over the following decades, drug cheats and regulators have played a cat-and-mouse game that has continually challenged the investigative skills of regulators. To complicate this issue, different sports organizations have significantly different approaches to the problem, from minimal attention (NHL) to strict enforcement (Olympic sports).

As the penalties for drug use have escalated, coaches and athletes have sought other restorative measures to enhance performance and accelerate recovery. The use of sports chiropractic (joint and spinal manipulation/adjusting, stretching, and soft tissue work) has come to the fore. But does sports chiropractic care enhance performance? And more to the point—what constitutes performance enhancement?

Claims of chiropractic care and its role in enhancing performance have been many and enthusiastic over the last few decades. But the unfortunate reality is that most of the claims have been anecdotal in nature. Confounding this reality is that there is no clear agreement as to what exactly was enhanced. Some authors note speed, others note strength, but efforts to translate these findings into team accomplishments produce fuzzy interpretations of any data produced. The only literature search on the topic concluded, "at this time there is insufficient evidence to support the notion that treatment by a chiropractor can directly improve performance."[6] This narrative review of peer and non-peer-reviewed literature clearly illustrates the often-repeated "enthusiastic and anecdotal" claims of sports chiropractors that lack the evidence to support conclusions. It is interesting to note that the review did not evaluate the effect chiropractic care has on the expression of the five biomotor skills.

It stands to reason that if what makes an athlete an athlete is the expression of the five biomotor skills, then any intervention that improves these skills, be it training focus, illicit drug use, or treatment, would qualify as performance enhancement.

Before going any further, it warrants mention that performance enhancement here is on an individual basis. Efforts to make sweeping generalizations to team sports are problematic and blur the focus of the discussion. Team sports by their nature involve tactics, strategies, and team skills that necessarily must be presented collectively. Although individual efforts make up a team, it is the synchronous actions of the team, where the whole is greater than the sum of its parts, that leads to success.

Traditional Sports Medicine

Traditional sports medicine is, for the most part, reactive care, although taping and bracing might be considered preventive.

The main players in traditional sports medicine are the athletic trainer and the emergency medical services (EMS) provider. Both professionals treat conditions after symptoms have presented—that is, after something has gone wrong. It is absurd to consider going to the EMS provider for an external arterial defibrillator treatment or the athletic trainer to get a knee taped as preventive care.

Within the social milieu of an athletic contest, the defined role of the athletic trainer is well established as the "first responder" for athletic injuries (again, something has gone "wrong"). The athletic trainer then must recognize what the problem is, determine the severity of the injury, and initiate the appropriate action, whether that be further off-field evaluation, activation of an emergency plan, or release of the athlete for return to play.

The EMS personnel are present for life support. These professionals possess the equipment, experience, and expertise to maintain life in situations where transport to a hospital emergency room is deemed necessary. EMS personnel have the experience to handle life-threatening situations. Motor vehicle crashes, acts of violence, cardiac arrests, and other potentially dire situations are part and parcel of their daily routine, not random occurrences.

The training of most sports chiropractors comes after chiropractic college in the 120-hour certified chiropractic sports physician (CCSP) program or 300-hour diplomate program. Both programs are weekend seminars with no practical component or on-field experience required. While both life-saving techniques and taping and bracing are studied, this knowledge is "textbook knowledge" with no practical application opportunities outside of one's private practice.

Both programs follow a curriculum based on the athletic trainer model—reactive care. One of the significant differences is the lack of any on-field, practical experience for the chiropractor. Furthermore, although the chiropractors who undertake this training are able to apply newfound knowledge in their private practice, there has as yet been no systematic effort to integrate the chiropractor into current sports medicine teams.

The CCSP and diplomate programs are based on the traditional sports medicine model of reactive care. Any contribution the sports chiropractor makes to this paradigm is that of duplication of services. And this duplication of services, no matter how well intentioned, can threaten the current power structure.

For some sports chiropractors, this presents the obvious choice to "go it alone." With the proliferation of sports leagues and the reality of limited budgets, underserved sports will willingly accept a "sports chiropractor," especially one who advertises the ability to "do it all," including athletic training services, EMS/first aid/CPR, and chiropractic services. In this setting, the sports chiropractor works in isolation and may have an untested level of expertise in critical areas.

Much of the political thrust of the last two decades within the American Chiropractic Association has been to integrate chiropractic care into the mainstream medical model. This has been achieved to an extent with Veterans Administration appointments and hospital rotations. In the sports world, there has been an expanding acceptance of chiropractic, driven in large part by the demands of athletes.

But, if pressed, athletes may not be able to explain why they choose chiropractic care, beyond feelings of general well-being. In an informal study conducted over three successive years in New York, the study team conducted patient satisfaction surveys on three significantly different athletic populations: middle-aged women runners, college-aged crew athletes, and college-aged track-and-field athletes (total of 135 respondents). In all three groups, the results were similar. Of particular note were the respondents' reports of improved mood (23%) and more energy (22%).

A third obstacle to true integration is the answer to the question, "What exactly does the chiropractor do?" The educational training of the athletic trainer and EMS personnel does not include any descriptions regarding the training of the chiropractor, the skill set and abilities, or the potential contribution the chiropractic professional can make to athletes' welfare. Concepts such as performance enhancement, accelerated recovery, restoration, and regeneration, all critical steps in the daily, weekly, and monthly training cycles of an athlete, are similarly left out.

Prior to 2011, in over 9,000 pages of evidence-based textbooks from the previous 20 years, there is not one chapter, one page, one indexed reference to any of these concepts. In texts published since 2011, there is a total of two references to chiropractic with one of the texts categorizing chiropractic as part of the "peripheral team" with the student assistants and equipment manager and the other stating that chiropractors "restore normal function by manipulating bones, specifically at the spinal column" but that they are not physicians.[12]

A Paradigm Shift: The Athletic Triage Model

Inductive reasoning is when one takes a limited number of facts and makes a sweeping generalization. The thought process moves from the specific to the general. It relies on the use of anecdotes instead of data. The problem is that within the scientific method, inductive reasoning may or may not lead to a valid conclusion. To infer that something is therapeutic for all because it helped one person is to make a sweeping generalization from a single fact.

Rehabilitation efforts repair and restore the five biomotor skills. In spite of the fact that there are only five biomotor skills, this therapeutic intervention is the evidence-based standard of care for the systematic repair treatments of the ill and injured. There are literally thousands of scientific studies that validate this claim.

Rehabilitative care plays a significant role in the life of an athlete. The athlete's constant striving to exceed previous efforts or meet the challenges of the competition place the her or him in a state of perpetual risk. The stresses and strains of elite performance present planned or unplanned circumstances that are not natural or healthy for the body.

Because of the short span of athletic life, it becomes incumbent on athletes and their supporting cast of trainers, coaches, and health care support staff to use strategies that capitalize on the time that is available. Current league and international rules of competition ban the use of drug therapies to enhance performance or accelerate recovery. By necessity, other nondrug therapies are being evaluated in an effort that may attain elusive goals in the near future.

And while the chiropractic profession has a long history of peripheral involvement in sport, often making significant contributions to the welfare and performance of athletes, attempts to alter the old sports medicine model of reactive care has presented its challenges, not the least of which is duplication of services.

The athletic triage model proposes the development of a new model of sports health care that services the established components of acute, non-life-threatening care, life support with the emergency medical services, and the proactive components of performance enhancement and accelerated recovery.

The athletic triage model presents a model of sports health care that is complementary to the current sports medicine model, not conflicting, and represents integration of the unique services a chiropractor provides for the benefit of the athlete, not a duplication of the services already provided.

In the reactive care model of traditional sports medicine, the concept of performance enhancement is not on the radar screen. Performance enhancement is not studied in undergraduate or graduate courses on athletic training or EMS as evidenced by its total absence from the textbooks used to teach these disciplines. And why would they be? Performance enhancement as a concept is proactive in nature and not within the constructs of the job description of an athletic trainer (first response to acute, non-life-threatening care) or EMS personnel (life support) whose most important jobs come after something has happened.

Sports chiropractic heightens the expression of the five biomotor skills. While the evidence of this fact is not to the same magnitude as the research on the effect of rehabilitative efforts on the biomotor skills, it is nonetheless there.

The athletic triage model adds a third circle to traditional sports medicine and creates a unique place for services that are minimally offered and poorly understood yet within the construct of modern training theory and critical to the overall development of athletes.

The athletic triage model represents a paradigm shift that recognizes the fact that the limiting factor in athletic development is time and that efforts directed at performance enhancement effectively speed recovery, giving the coach and athlete more time to train.

Accelerating recovery helps minimize the damaging effect of the continual stress of high-performance efforts on the body. Remember that time spent in rehabilitation efforts is downtime, never to be recovered, which negatively affects the possibility of achieving one's potential.

To this end, it is incumbent on the sports chiropractors of the future to promote their services of performance enhancement and accelerated recovery. The athletic triage model offers a clear definition of the therapeutic services rendered by these professionals and highlights the unique contribution sports chiropractic can make.

Additionally, the athletic triage model integrates the services of each provider on the team, promoting the unique contribution of each without the loss of status or duplication of efforts.

Athletes are the ultimate beneficiaries of this new paradigm. In their daily pursuit of excellence, athletes leave no stone unturned in their quest to achieve their goals. Yet this quest for excellence is not without its physical and emotional challenges. The various support staff play a critical role in athletes' attempts to reach their absolute potential.

Conclusion

In coaching, training theory and periodization are part of the landscape, as are the immediate and long-term goals of performance enhancement and accelerated recovery. The reactive care model is a dated health care paradigm that only partially addresses the needs of the modern-day athlete. The athletic triage model offers the sports chiropractor the opportunity to showcase a unique skill set that makes a significant contribution that is safe, effective, and complementary and beneficial to athletes at whatever level they reside.

Below is an interview with a sports chiropractor, including how she became one and what her practice is like.

Interview with a Sports Chiropractor

Emma Minx, DC, CCSP, MS, is a sports chiropractor with a DC from Logan University as well as a master's degree in sports science and rehabilitation. She is also a certified chiropractic sports physician. She now practices sports chiropractic at Bannockburn Chiropractic and Sports Injury Center in Bannockburn, Illinois.

How did you get into this practice?

"When I was in high school, I was a patient at the office I now practice in! I was being treated by Dr. Stuart Yoss, the head chiropractor and owner, for elbow and shoulder tendinitis. Dr. Yoss saved my career as a softball player because my injuries were severely affecting my performance and jeopardizing my chance to play collegiate softball. However, not only did his treatment resolve my elbow and shoulder pain, but I started playing better than I did before I was injured. At the time, I had plans to become an ER doctor. As I got into college, I considered doing orthopedics, but due to my own chiropractic experience, I decided to pursue a career in chiropractic. Throughout chiropractic school, I would return home to shadow Dr. Yoss. He became my mentor. Because of his success and reputation as a chiropractor, I sought his advice on what techniques and seminars to take. With aspirations to join his practice, I knew I had to become full-body certified in Active Release Technique (ART), because that was a requirement of all the doctors in his practice. Finally, I asked to do my preceptorship with him, and out of that opportunity, he decided to hire me. He wanted to start another office in my hometown and brought me on to build that office, using my connections."

What type of preparation did you have to become a sports chiropractor?

"There were two main things that most prepared me for this type of practice. First was becoming full-body certified in ART. The other was being selected to be in the Biofreeze Human Performance Clinic while I was in my last year in chiropractic school. At this clinic, I saw many patients with sports injuries, and we used soft tissue treatment and corrective exercises, which was the perfect preparation for my current practice."

What type of preparation did you wish you had but had to catch up on later?

"Being in a sports practice requires a lot of comanagement with other health professionals—PTs, orthopedists, strength coaches, personal trainers, nutritionists, functional medicine practitioners, podiatrists, athletic trainers—and others! I wish that there was preparation in chiropractic college in how to comanage and communicate with other health professionals. Luckily, I had to do an internship to complete my master's in sports science and rehab. I chose to do mine with my alma mater, which was also the local high school in the town I was going to practice in. I worked with the athletic trainers in the training room. This was where I learned about working with other health professionals.

"You have to change your mind-set and realize you are on a team. The goal of the team is to take care of each athlete. On a team, you have to put your ego to the side and also realize each person is valuable to the team.

We each have our strengths, so I had to learn when to step in and when to just take a back seat. I think that helped me a lot in practice when comanaging patient cases with other health professionals—especially PTs (physical therapists)."

What do you find most interesting, fulfilling, inspiring?

"There is a smile people get when they feel better—I see it especially with kids and adolescents. When I am done treating, I ask them to stand up and see how they feel. If I see that smile, I know how they are feeling before they even say anything. It is gratifying to see because you know they walked in with pain and now they are leaving smiling.

The other most fulfilling feeling is when an athlete can finally return to their sport. I always said that what Stuart did for me as a patient, I wanted to do for my patients. So when an athlete comes into the office in pain, thinking they can't play, but then they leave with little to no pain and actually can go play—it is an incredible feeling. You know you made them happy."

Do you have an experience that you feel sums up or somehow captures the essence of this practice?

"One athlete who stands out in my mind is a competitive cheerleader. She had lots of low back pain from all the tumbling and stunts she had to do in cheerleading and she also had headaches and tension in her neck and upper back. When they came in, her dad said she didn't want to come because she was afraid I was going to tell her she was going to have to take a break from cheerleading. She cheers for a competitive program and sitting out isn't an option. Her dad promised I would do everything I could to keep her active in cheerleading.

"I began the exam and I considered a stress fracture because she had pain with extension. However, stork test and spinal percussion (orthopedic tests) were negative in the lumbar spine (lower back). I noticed while testing the lumbar flexion and extension (leaning forward and backward) that there was an imbalance and she was stressing the right side more.

"After I treated her with adjustments and ART (Active Release Techniques), her biomechanics greatly improved. The imbalance was 95 percent resolved, and she only had slight pain on extension. She was pretty quiet throughout the treatment, but when she got up, she had a smile on her face, and I knew she felt much better—she didn't have to say anything! I told her she could keep cheering but would need a few follow-up visits. Her team went on to win a state championship in cheerleading, and she never had to take time away from her sport. She now comes in every few weeks for maintenance adjustments because she knows how good she feels afterward. That's one of my favorite cases so far."

What is your advice for other DCs who would like to become involved in this type of practice?

"I think having a soft tissue technique in your tool belt is key to being able to work with athletes. It allows you to treat a lot more issues than a traditional chiropractor; for example, rotator cuff, plantar fasciitis, elbow tendinitis, iliotibial band syndrome, trochanteric bursitis, ankle sprains, etc. Yes, you can argue that plantar fasciitis can be because of a rotated pelvis so only spinal adjustments may be needed, but having a soft tissue technique can help accelerate the healing of the injured tissue in the foot.

"Also, a lot of times, the stereotype with chiropractors is that after an adjustment, you feel good for a few hours but the pain returns. I believe the problem is that the muscles haven't been addressed, so if they are tight or imbalanced, it is going to pull the joint back to where it was prior to the adjustment. Adjusting, then doing soft tissue will help make the adjustment hold longer.

"Learning the joint-by-joint approach by Gray Cook is important because it gets you to look above and below the injured tissue. For example, problems in the foot can be traced to the hip, or knee pain could be a lack of ankle mobility. It is necessary to have an advanced understanding of anatomy and biomechanics.

"The techniques I find important are ART, kinesiology taping, instrument-assisted soft tissue manipulation (IASTM), and corrective exercises."

What type of athletes do you usually treat? That is, which sports?

"I treat all different types of athletes—young and old. I have treated a child as young as eight, who played basketball and baseball, and a 93-year-old woman who took a spin class five days a week—she had neck pain and was concerned about missing her workouts! The type of injuries coming into the office also depends on the time of the year: tennis and golf (elbows) in the summer, paddle tennis (calves and Achilles tendon) in the winter, and triathletes year round.

"If you claim to be a sports practitioner, you need to have a good understanding of any and all sports. I'm terrible at golf, but I understand the golf swing so that I can help and understand my patients. For example, if they have medial elbow pain, they likely are gripping the club too hard or hitting too many divots."

Do you only see athletes in your practice, or do you see people who just do sports and exercise as leisure activities?

"I see both. However, I would argue that those doing sports just as leisure activities are athletes too. 'Leisure' athletes have similar injuries to those playing organized sports at the club, high school, collegiate, or professional levels. Although my office is a sports practice, we still see a lot of general population patients. Even though they may not have a game to play, it is just as gratifying when a patient can barely walk into the office and leaves standing up straight."

What are some of the most notable types of patients you've seen?

"Due to doctor-patient confidentiality, I can't reveal the specifics of who I have treated. However, I have worked on Olympians, professional athletes, CrossFit athletes, Iron Man triathletes, high school and collegiate athletes. As an office, we are the team chiropractors for the Chicago Bulls (NBA), Blackhawks (NHL), and Sky (WNBA).

"Although it is a pretty impressive part of my job treating professionals, I have realized that the average person who walks into my office is just as important. At the end of the day, they want to feel better and get back to the activities they want to do."

References

1. Selye H. *The Stress of Life.* New York: McGraw Hill; 1956.

2. Viru A. Early contributions of Russian stress and exercise physiologists. *J Applied Physiol.* 2002;92:1378–1382.

3. Gambetta V. *Athletic Development.* Champaign, IL: Human Kinetics; 2007:261–275.

4. Bompa T. *Periodization: Theory and Methodology of Training.* Champaign, IL: Human Kinetics; 1999:95–146.

5. Hedlund S, Nilsson H, Lenz M, Sundberg T. Effects of chiropractic manipulation on vertical jump height in young female athletes with talo-crural joint dysfunction. *J Manipulative Physiol Ther.* 2014;37:116–123.

6. Miners A. Chiropractic treatment and the enhancement of sports performance. *J Canadian Chiropr Assoc.* 2010;54:4.

7. Griffin E, Ledbetter A, Sparks G. *A First Look at Communication Theory.* 9th ed. New York: McGraw-Hill; 2014.

8. Martin D and Coe P. *Better Training for Distance Runners.* Champaign, IL: Human Kinetics; 1997.

9. Ebbets R. Children and sport. *J Clin Chiropr Pediatrics.* 2010; 11(1):707–712.

10. Siff M. *Supertraining.* Denver, CO: Supertraining Institute; 2004: 442–465.

11. Bompa TO, Haff GG. *Periodization: Theory and Methodology of Training.* Champaign, IL: Human Kinetics; 2009.

12. Cartwright L, Pitney W. *Fundamentals of Athletic Training.* Champaign, IL: Human Kinetics; 2011.

Index

About the Editor and Contributors

Editor

Cheryl Hawk, DC, PhD, CHES, is an author on over 100 publications in peer-reviewed scientific journals and is the lead author of the 2013 book *Health Promotion and Wellness: An Evidence-Based Guide to Clinical Preventive Services.* She received her doctor of chiropractic degree in 1976 from the National University of Health Sciences and practiced full time for 12 years. In 1991, she earned a PhD in preventive medicine from the University of Iowa and became a certified health education specialist. She is former cochair of the Research Working Group of the Academic Collaborative for Integrative Health. She has been named Researcher of the Year by the American Chiropractic Association and the Foundation for Chiropractic Education and Research.

Contributors

Lyndon Amorin-Woods, BAppSci(Chiropractic), MPH, has practiced for over 30 years and was named Chiropractor of the Year by the Chiropractors Association of Australia in 2013. He has practiced in various multipractitioner settings and at present maintains a private practice alongside his role as senior clinical supervisor at Murdoch University. He is a member of the steering committee of ACORN, Australia's chiropractic practice-based research network, and is actively involved in chiropractic research and advocacy.

Emily Canfield, DC, MS, ATC, is an instructor at New York Chiropractic College. She is the director of the sports chiropractic program, where she teaches lower extremity technique. She is a 2010 graduate of Northwestern Health Sciences and holds an MS in sports studies from High Point

University. She is also a certified athletic trainer. Dr. Canfield is an adjunct professor at Corning Community College and has maintained a private practice in Elmira, New York, since 2014.

Clinton Daniels, DC, MS, DAAPM, is a staff chiropractor for the Veterans Affairs Puget Sound Health Care System in Tacoma, Washington. He was a member of the inaugural class of the Veterans Affairs chiropractic residency program. He is a diplomate of the American Academy of Pain Management and a member of the Scientific Commission of the Council on Chiropractic Guidelines and Practice Parameters, and he holds faculty appointments with Logan University and the University of Western States.

Russ Ebbets, DC, is a level-three coach in U.S.A. Track and Field (USATF) coaching education. He has spoken at the High-Performance Summits on improving distance running in America. Since 1999, he has edited *Track Coach*, the technical journal for USATF. He has presented at the International Federation of Sports Chiropractic World Conference on sport and training theory. He has directed complementary chiropractic care at 250+ events.

Marion W. Evans Jr., DC, PhD, MCHES, is professor and department head of Food Science, Nutrition, and Health Promotion at Mississippi State University. He holds a PhD from the University of Alabama in health promotion. He is a master certified health education specialist and a certified wellness practitioner with the National Wellness Institute. He is the author, with Cheryl Hawk, DC, PhD, CHES, of a 2013 text entitled *Health Promotion and Wellness: An Evidence-Based Guide to Clinical Preventive Services*.

Brian J. Gleberzon, MHSc, DC, is a professor at the Canadian Memorial Chiropractic College. He teaches courses on healthy aging, jurisprudence, and chiropractic technique systems. He has authored two textbooks, *Chiropractic Care of the Older Patient* and *Technique Systems in Chiropractic*, and 60 articles in peer-reviewed journals. In 2007, he was elected to the licensing body that oversees chiropractors in Ontario, and in 2001, he was named Researcher of the Year by the Ontario Chiropractic Association.

Bart Green, DC, MSEd, PhD, is a full-time corporate health chiropractor and a part-time faculty member at National University of Health Sciences. He is the editor-in-chief for the *Journal of Chiropractic Education*. He has extensive experience working in interdisciplinary pain management teams for patients with chronic noncancer pain.

Shawn Hatch, DC, is a 2006 graduate of Western States Chiropractic College. He has practiced in a variety of settings, including multidisciplinary clinics and private practice in Peru. Since 2011, he has been working as an attending chiropractic physician in the Campus Health Center at the University of Western States. Having a lifelong interest in sports and exercise, he achieved certification as diplomate of the American Chiropractic Board of Sports Physicians in 2011.

Dennis M. J. Homack, DC, MS, CCSP, is an associate professor at New York Chiropractic College. He also teaches postgraduate courses in ergonomics and a certification program in advanced lower extremity movement analysis. He is a 1997 graduate of New York Chiropractic College and holds an MS degree in ergonomics from Cornell University. He is also a certified chiropractic sports physician. Dr. Homack has maintained a private chiropractic practice in Seneca Falls, New York, since 1998.

Claire Johnson, DC, MSEd, PhD, is a professor at National University of Health Sciences and the editor-in-chief for *Journal of Manipulative and Physiological Therapeutics, Journal of Chiropractic Medicine,* and *Journal of Chiropractic Humanities.*

Lisa Zaynab Killinger, DC, is a professor of diagnosis at Palmer College of Chiropractic, where she received her chiropractic degree in 1983. She directed several U.S. Health Resources and Services Administration grants on geriatric education, including 10 years as a site coordinator for the Iowa Geriatric Education Center. Dr. Killinger has served numerous elected positions in the Chiropractic Health Care Section of the American Public Health Association. She has authored/coauthored eight book chapters and over 75 publications, primarily on geriatrics.

Robert A. Leach, DC, MS, CHES, is in full-time practice and has authored professional journal articles and *The Chiropractic Theories,* in its fourth edition and used worldwide by more than 20,000 chiropractors. His research spans topics from cervical hypolordosis and attention deficit hyperactivity to public health and chiropractic health education. He is a member of the Mississippi Chiropractic Association, the Society of Health and Physical Educators, and the American Public Health Association, and is a delegate to the American Chiropractic Association.

William J. Lauretti, DC, spent over 15 years in private practice in Maryland before joining the clinical science faculty at New York Chiropractic College in 2005. He is a spokesperson for the American Chiropractic Association who has been interviewed by major news outlets, including CNN, the *Washington Post*, the *Boston Globe*, and Reuters International News Service about the safety of chiropractic care.

Mark Pfefer, RN, MS, DC, graduated from Cleveland University in 1988 and practiced full time for 11 years. He is currently working as professor and director of research at Cleveland. In 2000, he earned an MS in exercise science from the University of Kansas. Dr. Pfefer has received research funding from the National Institute for Chiropractic Research and is certified by the American Chiropractic Association's Chiropractic Rehabilitation Council.

Robert M. Rowell, DC, MS, is a professor and researcher at Palmer College of Chiropractic. He teaches classes in diagnosis, rehabilitation, and therapeutic modalities. He is a 1992 graduate of Northwestern College of Chiropractic and holds a master's degree in clinical research. He is a two-time Association of Chiropractic Colleges award-winning researcher. He has published numerous papers in clinical and educational research.

Cami Stastny, DC, is a 2014 graduate of Texas Chiropractic College. She is an associate at NW Sports Rehab, in Federal Way, Washington. She practices chiropractic, functional rehabilitation, and nutrition. She coauthored the research study *Perspectives and Understanding of Pain Management Concepts among Chiropractic Students and Chiropractic Physicians*.

Sharon Vallone, DC, FICCP (Fellow in Clinical Chiropractic Pediatrics), celebrates 30 years of practice with a lifelong focus on maternal health, birth, and early childhood development. As an author, coeditor of the *Journal of Clinical Chiropractic Pediatrics*, and lecturer, she has had the great pleasure of meeting and working with fellow chiropractors and other health care providers around the world. Committed to collaborative excellence, Dr. Vallone practices in a multidisciplinary environment with a focus on the special needs child.

Robert Vining, DC, is a licensed doctor of chiropractic and the research clinic director at the Palmer Center for Chiropractic Research. His professional experience includes private practice, practice within the United States Department of Veterans Affairs, and chiropractic college academic faculty. Dr. Vining's professional focus includes implementing clinically oriented research studies, translating scientific evidence for practitioners, and developing integrated, team-based care models, including chiropractic.

John Weeks is an organizer, writer, speaker, consultant, and sometimes executive who for three decades has worked to transform the medical industry's reactive and reductive focus through advancing the movement for integrative health and medicine. Toward this end, he helped create and guide multiple interprofessional and multistakeholder initiatives. He is the publisher-editor of *The Integrator Blog News & Reports* and editor-in-chief of the *Journal of Alternative and Complementary Medicine*.

Francis J. H. Wilson, DC, MSc, PhD, is a chiropractor and senior lecturer at the Anglo-European College of Chiropractic in Bournemouth, England. He edited and contributed to the book *Chiropractic in Europe: An Illustrated History* (2007) and has written a variety of historical and sociological papers relating to the chiropractic profession. His academic interests include questions of identity and professionalism in contemporary chiropractic.

Jon Wilson, DC, is the assistant dean of chiropractic education at Cleveland University–Kansas City. He teaches chiropractic technique and is also actively involved with the university's research department. He has been a peer reviewer for the *Journal of Chiropractic Medicine*, the International Conference on Spinal Manipulation, and the Association of Chiropractic Colleges Research Agenda Conference.